Neurorehabilitation in Parkinson's Disease

AN EVIDENCE-BASED TREATMENT MODEL

Neurorehabilitation in Parkinson's Disease

AN EVIDENCE-BASED TREATMENT MODEL

Edited by

Marilyn Trail, MOT, OTR
Assistant Professor of Neurology
Baylor College of Medicine
Co-Associate Director of Education
Parkinson's Disease Research, Education and Clinical Center
Michael E. DeBakey VA Medical Center
Houston, TX

Elizabeth J. Protas, PT, PhD, FACSM
Interim Dean and Ruby Decker Endowed Professor
Senior Fellow, Sealy Center on Aging
School of Health Sciences
University of Texas Medical Branch
Galveston, TX

Eugene C. Lai, MD, PhD
Professor of Neurology
Baylor College of Medicine
Director, Parkinson's Disease Research, Education and Clinical Center
Michael E. DeBakey VA Medical Center
Houston, TX

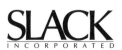

Delivering the best in health care information and education worldwide

www.slackbooks.com

ISBN: 978-1-55642-771-8

The procedures and practices described in this book should be implemented in a manner consistent with the professional standards set for the circumstances that apply in each specific situation. Every effort has been made to confirm the accuracy of the information presented and to correctly relate generally accepted practices. The authors, editor, and publisher cannot accept responsibility for errors or exclusions or for the outcome of the material presented herein. There is no expressed or implied warranty of this book or information imparted by it. Care has been taken to ensure that drug selection and dosages are in accordance with currently accepted/recommended practice. Due to continuing research, changes in government policy and regulations, and various effects of drug reactions and interactions, it is recommended that the reader carefully review all materials and literature provided for each drug, especially those that are new or not frequently used. Any review or mention of specific companies or products is not intended as an endorsement by the author or publisher.

SLACK Incorporated uses a review process to evaluate submitted material. Prior to publication, educators or clinicians provide important feedback on the content that we publish. We welcome feedback on this work.

Published by: SLACK Incorporated
                     6900 Grove Road
                     Thorofare, NJ 08086 USA
                     Telephone: 856-848-1000
                     Fax: 856-853-5991
                     www.slackbooks.com

Contact SLACK Incorporated for more information about other books in this field or about the availability of our books from distributors outside the United States.

Library of Congress Cataloging-in-Publication Data

Neurorehabilitation in Parkinson's disease : an evidence-based treatment model / [edited by] Marilyn Trail, Elizabeth Protas, Eugene C. Lai.
    p. ; cm.
  Includes bibliographical references and index.
  ISBN 978-1-55642-771-8 (alk. paper)
  1. Parkinson's disease--Patients--Rehabilitation. 2. Evidence-based medicine. I. Trail, Marilyn. II. Protas, Elizabeth. III. Lai, Eugene C.
  [DNLM: 1. Parkinson Disease--rehabilitation. 2. Evidence-Based Medicine. WL 359 N49488 2008]

RC523.N49 2008
616.8'3306--dc22

                         200704622

Printed in the United States of America.

Last digit is print number: 10 9 8 7 6 5 4 3 2 1

DEDICATION

To Adrian and Dolores and in memory of my parents, Nicholas and Dorothy Trail.
MT

I dedicate this book to my husband and son for their support and interest in what I do.
EJP

I dedicate this book to my loving wife and family for their understanding and support.
ECL

CONTENTS

Acknowledgments

The editors wish to thank our contributors for sharing their expertise, our patients and their families for their hope and courage, and the institutional support of The Michael E. DeBakey Veterans Affairs Medical Center in Houston, Texas; Baylor College of Medicine, Department of Neurology, Houston, Texas; and the University of Texas Medical Branch, School of Allied Health Sciences, Galveston, TX.

About the Editors

Marilyn Trail, MOT, OTR is the Co-Associate Director of Education for the Parkinson's Disease Research, Education and Clinical Center (PADRECC) at the Michael E. DeBakey Veterans Affairs Medical Center and an Assistant Professor of Neurology at Baylor College of Medicine in Houston, Texas. She received her Bachelor of Arts degree in Anthropology from the University of Oklahoma and her Master of Occupational Therapy degree from Texas Woman's University.

Ms. Trail has years of experience mentoring graduate students in treatment of patients with Parkinson's disease and amyotrophic lateral sclerosis in the clinical setting. She is Chair of the Houston PADRECC Education Committee which sponsors yearly regionally recognized continuing educational conferences on Parkinson's disease and related movement disorders for allied health professionals and VA/community health fairs for patients with Parkinson's disease, editor of the National VA Parkinson's Disease Consortium/National PADRECC newsletter for movement disorder specialists, editor of the Houston PADRECC newsletter for Parkinson's disease patients and their families, a reviewer for peer-reviewed scientific journals, and a consultant and contributor to Practical Pointers for Patients wit Parkinson's Disease, a patient/family resource guide published by the National Parkinson Foundation.

Ms. Trail's research interests concern quality of life and activity in Parkinson's disease patients, and she is the principle investigator on several projects related to these issues. She has published numerous papers and abstracts in professional journals such as the Journal of Neurological Sciences, Journal of Palliative Medicine, Archives of Physical Medicine and Rehabilitation, Movement Disorders, and Annuals of Neurology. She was the recipient of the Lita Wallace Readers Digest Foundation Grant and the principal investigator for The Methodist Hospital Foundation Grant. For many years she worked as a clinical specialist in occupational therapy at The Methodist Hospital in Houston, where she focused upon the treatment and education of patients with Parkinson's disease and amyotrophic lateral sclerosis. She lectures widely on these topics.

Dr. Elizabeth J. Protas is the Interim Dean, School of Allied Health Sciences, University of Texas Medical Branch, Galveston, the Ruby Decker Endowed Professor, and a Senior Fellow of the Sealy Center on Aging. Her research and clinical interests focus on exercise, aging and physiological responses to exercise of individuals with chronic disabilities, particularly individuals who have had a stroke or Parkinson's disease. She has published over 50 manuscripts and book chapters. She has received grant funding from the National Institute of Health, the National Institute on Disability and Rehabilitation Research, the Department of Veteran's Affairs and the Foundation for Physical Therapy to support her research.

She was an investigator with the Veteran's Affairs Rehabilitation Research and Development Center of Excellence on Healthy Living with Disabilities and the Parkinson's Disease Research, Education and Clinical Center. Dr. Protas has been on the American College of Sports Medicine's Board of Trustees and is a Fellow of the College. She has also served as the past president and former executive director of the Texas Regional Chapter of the American College of Sports Medicine.

In 2007, the Council on Aging and Adult Development of the American Association for Active Lifestyes and Fitness awarded Dr. Protas the Herbert H. deVries Award for Distinguished Research in the Field of Aging. The University of Texas Health Science Center at Houston College of Nursing awarded the Joseph C. Valley Gerontological Professional of the Year to Dr. Protas in 2000. At Texas Woman's University, she implemented the 3rd doctoral program in physical therapy in the country, and the only postdoc-toral fellowship program in physical therapy in the nation. She has been on the Committee for Post-doctoral and Doctoral Awards of the American Physical Therapy Association. For the Foundation for Physical Therapy, Dr. Protas has chaired the Doctoral Research Awards Committee, and has been a member of the Foundation's Advisory Committee and the Research Awards Committee. She serves as an accreditation site visit team leader for the Commission on Physical Therapy Education Accreditation and has been a member of the Cardiopulmonary Specialty Council and the American Board of Physical Therapy Specialties. Dr. Protas is a Founding Fellow of the American Association of Cardiovascular and Pulmonary Rehabilitation. She received her BS in Physical Therapy in 1968 and her PhD in Education in 1981 from the State University of New York at Buffalo.

Eugene C. Lai, MD, PhD is a Professor of Neurology at Baylor College of Medicine and the Director of the Parkinson's Disease Research, Education and Clinical Center at the Veterans Affairs Medical Center in Houston, Texas. Dr. Lai received his bachelor of science degree in Biochemistry from the University of Wisconsin and his doctorate degree, also in Biochemistry, from the University of Washington. He then studied Medicine at Baylor College of Medicine and completed his Neurology residency training at Baylor Affiliated Hospitals in Houston.

Dr. Lai is a clinician-scientist who has special interests in the causes and treatments of neurodegenerative diseases, such as Parkinson's disease, Alzheimer's disease, and amyotrophic lateral sclerosis. He also has expertise in the assessment of motor function and quality of life. He is the principal investigator or co-investigator of many clinical research studies. He has more than one hundred scientific publications and abstracts, and has lectured widely on topics in neurodegenerative diseases. He also enjoys teaching residents and fellows in his clinical practice.

He is board certified in Neurology and is also a member of the American Medical Association, American Academy of Neurology, Texas Medical Association, Harris County Medical Society, and Society for Neuroscience. He is on the Medical Advisory Board of the Parkinson Foundation of Harris County and on the Executive Board of the Houston Area Parkinson Society. He is the past President of the Houston Neurological Society and has also served as the Vice-President of the Texas Neurological Society. He has been recognized as one of American's Top Physicians, Texas Super Doctors and Houston Super Doc.

About the Contributors

Julie A. Alvarez, PhD
Department of Psychology
Tulane University
New Orleans, LA

Mary Frances Baxter, PhD, LOT
Associate Professor
School of Occupational Therapy
Texas Woman's University
Houston, TX

Mark Bishop, PhD, PT
Assistant Professor
University of Florida
Department of Physical Therapy
Gainesville, FL

Denis Brunt, EdD, PT
Professor and Chair
Department of Physical Therapy
School of Allied Health Sciences
East Carolina University
Greenville, NC

Jill Cable, MS, CCC-SLP
Speech-Language Pathologist
Banner Good Samaritan Rehabilitation
Institute
Phoenix, AZ

Michelle R. Ciucci, PhD, CCC-SLP
Post-Doctoral Fellow
Department of Psychology
University of Texas
Research Associate, Post-Doctoral Fellow
Department of Otolaryngology
University of Wisconsin
Madison, WI

Fiona Dobson, BScPT, PhD
School of Physiotherapy
The University of Melbourne
Australia

Becky G. Farley, PhD, PT
Assistant Research Professor
Department of Physiology
University of Arizona
Tucson, AZ

Pamela Fok, BScPT
School of Physiotherapy
The University of Melbourne
Melbourne, Australia

Cynthia M. Fox, PhD, CCC-SLP
Research Associate
National Center for Voice and Speech
Denver, CO
Research Lecturer
Department of Neurology
University of Arizona
Tucson, AZ

Angela Halpern, MS, CCC-SLP
Research Associate/Speech-Language
Pathologist
National Center for Voice and Speech
The Denver Center for Performing Arts
Denver, CO

Jyh-Gong Gabriel Hou, MD, PhD
Assistant Professor of Neurology
Baylor College of Medicine
Associate Director of Research
Parkinson's Disease Research, Education
and Clinical Center
Michael E. DeBakey VA Medical Center
Houston, TX

Frances Huxham, PhD
Geriatric Research Unit
Kingston Centre
Cheltenham
Australia

Robert Iansek, PhD
Geriatric Research Unit
Kingston Centre
Cheltenham
Australia

Nancy Lowenstein, MS, OTR, BCPR
Clinical Assistant Professor
Department of Occupational Therapy &
Rehabilitation Counseling
Sargent College of Health & Rehabilitation
Sciences

Boston University
Boston, MA

Leslie A. Mahler, PhD, CCC-SLP
Assistant Professor
Department of Communicative Disorders
University of Rhode Island
Kingston, RI

Hylton B. Menz, PhD
Musculoskeletal Research Centre
La Trobe University
Australia

Kimberly J. Miller, BScPT, MSc
School of Physiotherapy
The University of Melbourne
Melbourne, Australia

Meg E. Morris, BScPT, Grad Dip (Geron),
MAppSc, PhD
School of Physiotherapy
The University of Melbourne
Melbourne, Australia

Sheila Mun-Bryce, OTR, PhD
Department of Neurology
University of New Mexico Health Science
Center
Albuquerque, NM

Naomi D. Nelson, PhD
Associate Professor of Neurology
Baylor College of Medicine
Co-Associate Director of Education
Parkinson's Disease Research, Education
and Clinical Center
Michael E. DeBakey VA Medical Center
Houston, TX

Pagamas Piriyaprasarth, BScPT
School of Physiotherapy
The University of Melbourne
Melbourne, Australia

Lorraine Olson Ramig, PhD, CCC-SLP
Professor, Department of Speech, Language,
Hearing Sciences
University of Colorado
Boulder, CO

Senior Scientist, National Center for Voice
and Speech
Denver Center for the Performing Arts
Denver, CO
Adjunct Professor, Columbia University
New York, NY

Shimon Sapir, PhD, CCC-SLP
Associate Professor, Department of
Communication Sciences and Disorders
Faculty of Social Welfare and Health Studies
University of Haifa
Haifa, Israel

Aliya I. Sarwar, MD
Assistant Professor of Neurology
Baylor College of Medicine
Associate Director of Patient Care
Parkinson's Disease Research, Education
and Clinical Center
Michael E. DeBakey VA Medical Center
Houston, TX

Rhonda K. Stanley, PT, PhD
Associate Professor, Physical Therapy
Arizona School of Health Sciences
AT Still University
Mesa, AZ

Linda Tickle-Degnen, PhD, OTR/L,
FAOTA
Professor, Occupational Therapy
Director, Health Quality of Life Lab
Tufts University
Medford, MA

Michele K. York, PhD
Assistant Professor of Neurology
Baylor College of Medicine
Neuropsychologist
Parkinson's Disease Research, Education
and Clinical Center
Michael E. DeBakey VA Medical Center
Houston, TX

PREFACE

Patients with Parkinson's disease present a challenge for rehabilitation specialists due to the distinct nature of their cardinal symptoms: postural instability, bradykinesia, impaired gait, tremor, and rigidity and to the degenerative process itself. Health care professionals who work with this group of patients require special knowledge of the disease process, its assessment, and its treatment.

The purpose of this text is to provide a much needed comprehensive theoretical, clinical, and evidence-based resource for physical therapists, occupational therapists, speech-language pathologists, psychologists, physiatrists, and other health care providers working with this group of patients. We brought together contributors, selected for their expertise in the subject matter, to write the book for advanced students, clinicians, and educators to use as both a primary text and a resource.

Parkinson's disease is a progressive central nervous system disorder that affects over one million Americans, with the highest frequency in the over 60 age group. With enhanced life expectancy throughout the industrialized world, the World Health Organization expects a large increase in the number of persons with Parkinson's disease who will require health care. While pharmacologic treatment provides benefit, the disorder slowly progresses, resulting in significant disability and functional limitations. Alternative therapies, specifically those provided by physical therapists, occupational therapists, speech-language pathologists, psychologists, and physiatrists, play an important role in the treatment of this patient population.

Few could argue that as health care professionals we have a responsibility to provide our patients with the best possible care and the most effectual treatment methods available. Evidence-based practice arose from a concern that patients were receiving interventions unsupported by the scientific data. We must be accountable not only to our patients and their families but to third party reimbursers, the community at large, and our colleagues in health care. There is a growing recognition that if we are to deliver effective services, we must expand the research base of our respective disciplines. Practicing evidence-based therapy means we deliver treatment that has been recognized as most successful. Throughout this text, our intent is to supply the evidence, and apply it to actual practice while providing clinicians with tools for treatment.

We chose to present the information through an interdisciplinary approach, believing that knowledge shared among health care providers enhances collaboration, facilitates learning, combines resources, and promotes mutual respect between professions. We hope the case studies and vignettes written by physical therapists, occupational therapists, speech-language pathologists, neurologists, and psychologists help readers clarify and incorporate both the theoretical and the empirical information provided herein. Comprehensive bibliographies at the end of each chapter provide access to the evidence presented and further reading for those interested in the topics.

The text contains chapters on physical therapy, occupational therapy, and speech-language pathology evidenced-based treatment interventions for patients with Parkinson's disease as well as separate chapters on home programming for each discipline. Other topics include an overview of the disease, neuroplasticity and Parkinson's disease, and cognitive and psychosocial issues associated with the disease. We've allowed an entire chapter on assessment and outcome measures for Parkinson's disease commonly used by clinicians and researchers and included facsimiles of the actual instruments, plus a chapter on assistive and adaptive technology recommended for patients with this diagnosis. We hope this book fills the gap in the present literature and that it benefits your needs.

FOREWORD

The authors and editors of *Neurorehabilitation in Parkinson's Disease* have presented a thorough configuration of the problems that both a client and a professional will face once the medical diagnosis of Parkinson's disease is made. The book bases the information and the integration of that information on current research evidence within the literature.

The complexity of management of the medical and the movement dysfunctions created by this progressive pathology frustrates not only the individual, family, and friends, but also individuals within the health care delivery system. This text helps to inform and direct those professionals toward clinical decision making based on today's clinical evidence. Although few professionals will have the expertise or the credentials to practice within all the professional settings presented within this text, each reader will gain a more integrated understanding of the interaction of all professions when providing service to an individual with Parkinson's disease. When dealing with movement dysfunction that changes with medication, with therapeutic intervention, and with progressive and active ongoing disease, therapists need to differentiate clinical signs in order to accurately communicate why clinical symptoms exist and change. Placing realistic expectations and encouraging clients to set functional goals that match the complexity of this central nervous system problem is an integral part of the practice of occupational, physical, and speech therapies. This text helps guide colleagues through the process of evaluation and identification of specific movement dysfunctions, and potential treatment selections made by therapists and patients as an individual progresses through various stages of the disease process. The authors and editors of this new text have taken a very complex clinical problem and presented recommendations that will help many health care professionals in the future as our population ages and more medical diagnoses are made.

Darcy Umphred, PT, PhD, FAPTA

Overview of Parkinson's Disease: Clinical Features, Diagnosis, and Management

Jyh-Gong Gabriel Hou, MD, PhD; Eugene C. Lai, MD, PhD

Introduction

Parkinsonism is a syndrome manifested by part or all of the symptoms of rest tremor, rigidity, bradykinesia, and postural instability.[1] Parkinson's disease (PD) is a specific chronic, progressive neurodegenerative disease that affects about 1 million people in the United States.[2] The etiology of PD is still largely unknown, and it is also referred to as idiopathic or primary PD. Associated symptoms include smaller handwriting (micrographia), shuffling gait, speech disturbance, and dysphagia. Non-motor complications, including sleep disturbance, depression, autonomic dysfunctions, and cognitive impairment, can significantly impair quality of life. The progressive and disabling features are the major burden to the patients themselves, their families, and society as a whole.

Although the etiology is unknown, it is generally believed that a combination of genetic and environmental factors play a role in the pathogenesis of PD.[3] The primary pathology involves the basal ganglia, especially the substantia nigra. Several subcortical nuclei compose the basal ganglia and play a role in the initiation and control of movements. Dopaminergic neuronal loss in the substantia nigra leads to a decrease in the level of dopamine and results in parkinsonian symptoms.[1,3]

HISTORICAL ASPECTS

PD was first described by Dr. James Parkinson in 1817. In his "Essay in Shaking Palsy," he wrote, "Involuntary tremulous motion, with lessened muscular power, in parts not in action and even when supported with a propensity to bend the trunk forwards and to pass from a walking to a running pace: the senses and intellects being uninjured."[4] However, this essay did not receive much attention at the time. It was not until the 1860s to 1870s, as Jean-Martin Charcot tried to differentiate tremors of multiple sclerosis from other disorders, that the condition was more recognized and thoroughly studied. Charcot virtually identified all four cardinal symptoms of PD: rest tremor, bradykinesia, rigidity, and balance impairment.[5] Brissaud drew attention to midbrain lesions as the cause for PD.[6] However, the pathological hallmark—degeneration of the substantia nigra—was not described until the early 20th century by Tretiakoff.[7] The delineation of the selective cell loss, depigmentation, and degeneration of the substantia nigra became clearer only in the 1960s.[7] More recently, a new concept of the pathology of PD at different disease stages was further described by Braak et al.[8]

Surgery involving the basal ganglia circuitry to ameliorate symptoms of PD was first performed by R. Meyers in 1939, and pallidotomy and thalamotomy became popular in the 1950s.[9] Surgeries were less commonly performed after levodopa was introduced in the late 1960s. Levodopa, the precursor to dopamine, effectively improved PD symptoms in several early studies,[10,11] and several other medications for PD have been introduced in recent decades. However, when the limitations of medical therapy became apparent in the late 1980s, functional stereotactic surgeries regained attention. Deep Brain Stimulation (DBS) was first introduced in the mid-1990s and has now become a helpful surgical treatment for PD when the best medical treatment is unable to control the symptoms or causes unacceptable side effects.[12]

EPIDEMIOLOGY

The reported prevalence of PD varies widely among different studies, mainly because there is no biomarker to confirm the diagnosis. Some epidemiologic studies had higher prevalence rates because parkinsonism syndromes rather than expert-confirmed idiopathic PD were included. One such study in Boston, MA found a high prevalence of parkinsonian symptoms, with 29.5% in individuals between ages 75 to 84; more than half were older than 85 years.[13]

In a Minnesota study, the average annual incidence rate of PD in the age group 50 to 99 years was 114.7; incidence increased steeply with age from 0.8 in the age group 0 to 29 years to 304.8 in the age group 80 to 99 years. The cumulative incidence of parkinsonism (assuming no competing causes of death) was 7.5% to age 90 years.[14] Overall, it is generally estimated that at least 1 million Americans are affected.[2] European studies revealed about a 1.6% prevalence rate, although studies varied.[15,16] Another European study demonstrated that crude prevalence rate estimates ranged from 65.6 to 12,500 per 100,000 people, and incidence estimates ranged from 5 to 346 per 100,000 people per year.[17] Overall, the prevalence in America and Europe seems to be higher than that of the Far East.[18-20] However, whether Caucasians have higher prevalence rates of PD than Asians or Africans is not yet clear.[21] Several studies were conflicted in results regarding prevalence in people of different races. In an Upper Manhattan study, blacks had a one-third lower prevalence rate than Hispanics or non-Hispanic whites.[22] However, Schoenberg et al reported similar prevalence rates for blacks and whites in a biracial county in Mississippi.[23] Thus far, no firm evidence of racial difference in PD has been established.

Age is an important risk factor for PD. An estimated 2% of the population older than age 65 is affected, and PD is rare in people prior to age 40.[24] The previously mentioned Boston study also indicated more parkinsonian symptoms among the older groups.[13] In terms of gender prevalence, men are more affected than women by about 1.5 to 2-fold.[25,26] Whether this is a result of biological, environmental, or lifestyle differences between the genders requires further investigation. A recent study found a sex gene present in men that may play a role in their higher incidence of PD.[27]

The personal and socioeconomic burdens of PD are huge. Direct expenses related to PD include medical services, medications, and medical therapies. Indirect costs have even broader ranges. Patients may suffer loss of productivity, income, and quality of life. Furthermore, patients' families will need to spend extra time, money, and effort to care for them. In a recent study, the total estimated annual direct costs were $23,101 per patient with PD versus $11,247 for controls. The regression-adjusted incremental direct cost of PD versus controls was about $10,349. Adding $25,326 in indirect costs, and multiplying by 645,000 cases of PD in the United States, the total cost is projected to be $23 billion annually.[28] The socioeconomic impact is similar in other countries.[29,30]

ETIOLOGY

No definite single etiology is confirmed for primary PD. Most of the cases are idiopathic, whereas some have been linked to genetic mutations. Pathology is characterized by dopaminergic neuronal degeneration in the substantia nigra. Lewy bodies are found mainly in the basal ganglia. How this neurodegeneration occurs is still uncertain. It is generally believed that environmental factors, possibly infectious agents, toxins, drugs, or endocrine disorders, could potentially affect and induce the manifestation of the underlying defects in genetic expression in these patients. Many cellular mechanisms have been proposed, including oxidative stress, premature apoptosis, loss of neurotrophic factors, glutamate toxicity, inflammatory processes, mitochondrial dysfunction, neuromelanin degeneration, and so on.[31-34] The studies on familial forms of PD found several gene abnormalities in the ubiquitin-proteosomal system and the mitochondrial cytochrome C chain.[33,35] Therefore, no one single etiology is able to satisfactorily explain the entire pathogenesis of primary PD.

A study of the World War II Veteran Twins Registry demonstrated an overall similarity in concordance for monozygotic and dizygotic twins.[36] In this study, 71 monozygotic and 90 dizygotic twin pairs were identified. The concordance was 13%—above background level but not significantly higher. When the inquiry was restricted to patients over age 50, concordance was equal in monozygotic and dizygotic twins. The researchers concluded that genetic influences were not important to the etiology of typical PD. However, among the few pairs with early onset PD, these genetic influences might be stronger. A positive family history is more common for the patients with symptom onset under age 40. Lucking et al found a substantial number of young-onset PD patients with parkin gene mutations, even in the absence of an affected relative.[37] A mutation in the gene for α-synuclein on chromosome 4q has been associated with autosomal dominant PD in several families.[38] Currently, more and more gene mutation foci have been found to be related to familial PD. Patients with autosomal dominant and autosomal recessive gene mutations usually present with parkinsonian symptoms at a younger age and have strong family histories. Another group of patients who possess PD susceptible genes that carry higher risk of developing the disease may acquire symptoms without following Mendelian rules. Table 1-1 lists the current data on genes related to PD.

Environmental toxins that may be responsible for inducing PD have been widely investigated. Researchers found an association with rural living and agricultural work. There is evidence that exposure to pesticides and herbicides may increase risks.[39] Results from dietary studies are controversial, but there appears to be an increased risk of PD associated with dietary iron, manganese, and heavy metal intake.[36] Folic acid deficiency may also be related.[40,41]

Cigarette smoking has been a topic of interest. Several studies indicate that there is an inverse relationship between smoking and PD.[42-44] Smokers are 50% less likely to have PD, but the reason for this association is not known. Whether nicotine or other ingredients in cigarettes are neuroprotective is unclear.[45] Coffee consumption also seems to decrease the incidence of PD. Findings from the Honolulu-Asia study suggested that the risk of PD was five times higher in non-drinkers when compared with individuals who consumed more than seven cups of coffee a day.[46,47] Possible involvement of caffeine in blocking adenosine 2A receptors (A2A) has been proposed. A2A antagonist has been shown to be neuroprotective.[48,49] Further studies are needed.

Secondary parkinsonisms are a group of disorders with parkinsonian symptoms, but their causes are more defined. There is a long list of these conditions with different etiologies that render the brain susceptible (Table 1-2). They include etiologies caused by drugs (neuroleptics, antiemetics), infection (postencephalitic), tumors, basal ganglia calcification, atherosclerotic vascular disease, traumatic brain injuries, and various toxins such as MPTP (1-methyl-4-phenyl-1,2,3,6-tetrahydropyridine), carbon monoxide, cyanide, carbon disulfide, manganese, and so on.[45] These conditions likely cause damage to the substantia nigra and other parts of the basal ganglia. The clinical features are usually different from the typical presentations of primary PD. Their differential diagnoses will be discussed later in this chapter.

BASAL GANGLIA PATHOPHYSIOLOGY

Neuropathological examination of brains from patients with PD reveals a loss of pigmented neurons from the pars compacta of the substantia nigra. These neurons contain neuromelanin and produce the neurotransmitter dopamine (DA). Loss of 50% to 60% of these cells from the substantia nigra results in critical DA deficiency in the striatum.[50,51] Involvement is usually bilateral, but typically uneven in severity, which explains the asymmetric nature of PD symptoms. Other subcortical nuclei, including locus ceruleus and dorsal vagal nucleus, may also be affected.[51] DA cell losses in the pigmented brain stem nuclei, the intermediolateral column of the spinal cord, and the sympathetic ganglia are reported, suggesting associated autonomic dysfunction in PD patients.[52,53] Lesioning in the nucleus basalis and the ventral tegmental area may account for cognitive deficits.[54,55] Microscopically, concentric hyaline intracytoplasmic inclusions, termed *Lewy bodies*, can be found in several subcortical nuclei of the surrounding basal ganglia. Lewy bodies contain accumulations of α-synuclein ubiquitin and protein.[56,57] Involvement of the cortical areas may explain hallucination, psychotic symptoms, and cognitive decline in PD.[55,58]

Voluntary movement is initiated from cerebral cortex and regulated by complex feedback loops that involve the cortex, thalamus, basal ganglia, and cerebellum. The basal ganglia consists of the caudate, putamen, globus pallidus (interna and externa), subthalamic nucleus, and substantia nigra. The cerebral cortex is the command center of the brain and it sends signals to the striatum (putamen and globus pallidus) by two pathways: direct and indirect. The direct pathway exits from the putamen to the globus pallidus interna (GPi).[59,60] The indirect pathway exits from the putamen to the globus pallidus externa (GPe), to the subthalamus nucleus (STN) and then reaches GPi. These

TABLE 1-1

Single Gene Mutations Related to Parkinson's Disease

Locus	Mutated Genes	Mode of Inheritance	Gene Locus Location	Features	Regions Reported
PARK1	α-Synuclein	AD	4q21	Early onset, rapid progression, response to levodopa, Lewy body+	Italy, Greece
PARK2	Parkin	AR	6q25.2-27	Juvenile onset, susceptible to leprosy, no Lewy body	Japan
PARK3	Unknown	AD	2p13	Juvenile to late onset, Lewy body+	Germany
PARK4	α-Synuclein, gene triplication	AD	4p15, 4q21	Cortical involvement, Lewy body+	Iowa
PARK5	Ubiquitin C-terminal hydrolase; UCHL-1	AD	4p14	Affect α-synuclein degradation and Parkinson's disease susceptibility	Germany
PARK6	PINK1	AR	1p36	Early onset (28 to 35 years old), all cardinal features of PD	Italy, various Asia regions
PARK7	DJ1	AR	1p36	Early onset (before age 40), with typical parkinsonian symptoms and psychotic episodes	Netherlands
PARK8	Unknown, may be LRRK2	AD	12q12	Unilateral onset. Mean age 50. Response to levodopa. Pure nigral degeneration without Lewy bodies or neurofibrillary tangles.	Japan, Spain, Nebraska
PARK9	Unknown	Susceptible	1p36	Pallidopyramidal degeneration, juvenile onset. Responded to levodopa.	Jordan
PARK10	Unknown	Susceptible	1p32	A susceptibility gene for age at onset (AAO) PD.	Various
PARK11	Unknown	Susceptible or AD	2q36-q37	Increase susceptibility of PD without parkin mutations	North America

continued

TABLE 1-1, CONTINUED

Single Gene Mutations Related to Parkinson's Disease

Locus	Mutated Genes	Mode of Inheritance	Gene Locus Location	Features	Regions Reported
PARK12	Unknown	Susceptible or X-linked	Xq21-q25	Consistent evidence of linkage to chromosomes 2 and X. It supports the hypothesis that gene-by-gene interactions are important in PD susceptibility.	North America
PARK13	HTRA2	Unknown or susceptible	2p12	Typical PD symptoms, responded to levodopa. Possible mitochondrial involvement.	Germany

TABLE 1-2

Causes of Secondary Parkinsonism

Toxins

      MPTP (methyl-4-phenyl-tetrahydropyridine)
      Manganese
      Carbon monoxide

Vascular Disease

      Basal ganglia lacunae
      Binswanger's disease

Brain Structural Damage

      Tumor
      Trauma
      Chronic hepatocerebral degeneration
      Hydrocephalus
      Wilson's disease

Drugs

      Neuroleptic drugs
      Metoclopramide, prochlorperazine
      Dopamine depleting agents (reserpine, tetrabenazine)

Infections

      Postencephalitic parkinsonism
      Creutzfeldt-Jakob disease
      Acquired immunodeficiency disease

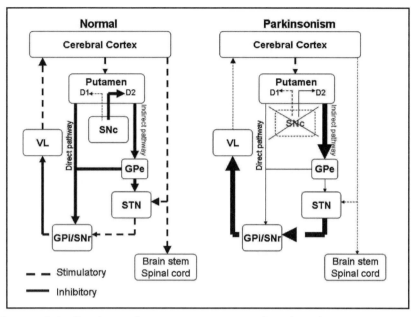

Figure 1-1. Basal ganglia circuitry in normal and parkinsonism patients (Modified from Wichmann T, Delong MR. Functional anatomy of basal ganglia and motor systems. In: Watts RL, Koller WC, eds. *Movement Disorders: Neurologic Principles and Practice.* New York: McGraw-Hill Company; 1997:87-97.).

nuclei in putamen, GPi and GPe use gamma-aminobutyric acid (GABA) as the primary neurotransmitter, which functions as an inhibitory function to the postsynaptic neurons. DA in the substantia nigra regulates the putamen by using different DA receptors to enhance the GABA inhibitory effect on the direct pathway and attenuate the GABA effect on the indirect pathway. Thus, a decreased DA level will cause disinhibition of STN and GPi and subsequently inhibit output from the thalamus to the cerebral cortex, leading to various motor manifestations of parkinsonism, including resting tremor, bradykinesia, and rigidity. This basal ganglia circuit theory also becomes the pathophysiological basis for the surgical treatment of PD[59-63] (Figure 1-1).

CLINICAL MANIFESTATIONS

Parkinson's disease is a complex neurodegenerative disorder. Although the main symptoms are caused by the disrupted control of body movement, there are many concomitant non-motor symptoms, including cognitive decline and psychiatric manifestations.

The four main motor symptoms of PD are resting tremor, bradykinesia, cogwheel rigidity, and postural instability. Generally, the presence of resting tremor in addition to one of the other symptoms, or the presence of the other three symptoms in the absence of resting tremor, will indicate the clinical diagnosis of PD. Other supportive diagnostic features are good response to levodopa treatment and the presence of dyskinesia after long-term usage of levodopa. The typical parkinsonian symptoms are asymmetric, and the pattern of asymmetry persists throughout the disease, even as late as 15 years after symptom onset.[64,65]

Figure 1-2a. Finger tapping is one of the examination methods to test hand dexterity in PD patients.

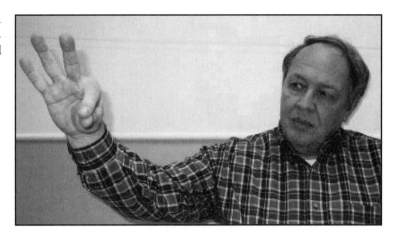

Motor Systems

Resting Tremor

Tremor is usually the first symptom noticed by patients or their family members. It occurs in the resting position and disappears or diminishes on hand motions, especially in the early stages of the disease. The frequency is typically slow, about 4 to 6 Hz.[66] Hands are the most common anatomical sites with tremor. In addition, legs, chin, mouth, and tongue may also be affected. It often starts on one side of the body and gradually involves the other side as the disease progresses. However, the side with the initial symptoms is usually more severely affected and the tremor remains asymmetric throughout the course of the disease. Flexion of the fingers and rotation of the wrist joint during tremor are characteristic. Amplitude will vary, and will become more pronounced when the patient is under stress.[67,68] In some patients, after a short disappearance of their tremor when their hands are held in front of the body, a postural tremor with the same frequency as their resting tremor may appear. This is called *re-emerging tremor* and is characteristic of PD.[69] As the disease progresses, patients often have both resting and action tremors. This may sometimes present diagnostic challenges to differentiate the diagnosis from essential tremor.

Bradykinesia

At the beginning stage of PD, many patients may not perceive the subtle symptoms, which present insidiously. One symptom that may be present before noticeable tremor is *bradykinesia,* meaning slowness of movement. Patients may experience slowness or difficulty in performing some simultaneous or repetitive motor acts, such as writing or playing a musical instrument. Gradually, every motor act becomes less fluid and more labored. On examination, the limb movements have decreased motion amplitude and loss of dexterity. Finger taps with index finger and thumb, hand movements with hands opened and closed in rapid succession, rapid alternating movements with pronation-supination movements of hands, and leg agility with heels tapping on the ground in rapid session are the four most common tests of the patient's dexterity (Figure 1-2a). Handwriting becomes smaller (*micrographia*), walking is slower (with shuffling), and the patient has more difficulty rising from a low chair. The patient's voice also becomes softer with reduced volume (*hypophonia*). In addition to hypophonia, the speech is fast, prosody is not normal, and there is sometimes stammering, stuttering, or *pallilalia* (perseverative repetition of syllables). There is also difficulty and slowness in handling utensils, chew-

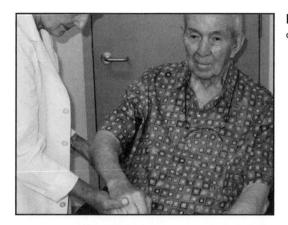

Figure 1-2b. A patient is being tested for upper extremity rigidity.

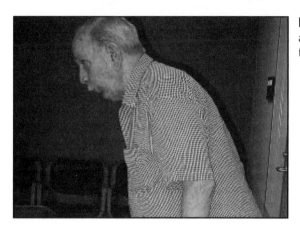

Figure 1-3. A patient with PD demonstrates a moderately stooped posture when bending forward.

ing food, and buttoning. It can affect the trunk, causing difficulty turning in bed or getting in and out of a car, and reduced facial expression (*hypomimia* or masked facies).

Rigidity

PD patients experience an increase in muscle tone, which results in rigidity. *Cogwheel rigidity* is a ratchet-like quality felt when patients' joints are passively moved (Figure 1-2b). It is sustained and resistant to passive movement not related to movement velocity, as opposed to other types of rigidity such as lead-pipe phenomenon. The resistance to externally imposed joint movement is present at very low speeds of movement and does not exhibit a speed or angle threshold. Simultaneous co-contraction of agonist and antagonist muscles may occur, and this is reflected in an immediate resistance to a reversal of the direction of movement around a joint. The limb does not tend to return toward a particular fixed posture or extreme joint angle. Both limbs and trunk (including the neck) can be affected. While a patient is actively performing a voluntary movement with one limb, increased tone in the contralateral limb may result. This maneuver may help an examiner sense the rigidity if it is not detected initially. In addition, many PD patients suffer *dystonia*, especially in their feet, such as toe curling or foot twisting. The typical features of early morning dystonia involve both lower extremities that cause cramping pain and difficulty in gait when patients first awake in the morning. Rigidity also causes stooped posture and forward shift of the center of gravity (*propulsion*), resulting in postural instability. Patients also manifest flexed limbs and decreased arm swing when walking (Figure 1-3).

Figure 1-4. The clinician examines the patient's postural stability by pulling his shoulders from behind.

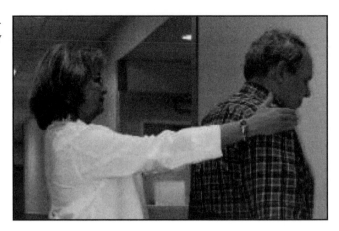

Postural Instability

Postural instability is likely to be the combined effect of rigidity and bradykinesia and generally occurs in patients with more advanced PD. It is mainly due to the loss of postural reflexes, which causes difficulties in positional adjustments. The patient's trunk is flexed to the stooped posture, and he or she presents with shuffling gait. The patient with PD tends to walk more quickly due to involuntary propulsion, and he or she may take smaller and faster steps (*festination*) and fall forward as a result. In addition, PD patients frequently have *freezing gait*, or sudden inability and hesitancy in moving their legs. Freezing is most often seen in gait initiation and on turns. Once gait is initiated, the patient can walk more naturally, as if "thawed." Patients with freezing gait have particular difficulty walking through narrow passages or reaching a destination (such as a chair) before sitting down. Falls can easily occur during these freezing episodes. The clinician may examine a patient's ability to balance by performing the "pull test" from behind. This test examines the patient's response to a sudden, strong posterior displacement produced by a pull on the shoulders while the patient is erect with eyes open and feet slightly apart. The patient is prepared and can practice prior to the test (Figure 1-4); however, patients with more severe PD may fall if not caught by the examiner.

These symptoms resulting from postural instability are unfortunately relatively resistant to pharmacological treatment. Patients may require physical therapy or rely on walking aids.

Non-Motor Symptoms

Motor difficulties are not the only problems for PD patients. A variety of non-motor symptoms that lessen the patient's quality of life include psychiatric symptoms (depression, anxiety), autonomic dysfunctions, sleep disturbances, sensory disturbances (especially pain), and dementia.

Cognitive Impairment

Dementia in PD may not be evident until the later stages. Although the cognitive decline reported in early stage PD is subtle and does not often interfere with daily functioning, PD patients have been shown to demonstrate cognitive slowing and executive functioning problems at early stages.[70] Furthermore, longitudinal research has described PD-related cognitive deficits in language, visuospatial functioning, long-term memory, and executive functioning that are greater than what would be expected to occur as a result of normal aging. The percentage of PD patients with cognitive deficits is estimated to be approximately 20%.[71,72] Generally, the cognitive impairment in PD is different from cortical dementia, which is found with Alzheimer's disease. The subcortical dementia found in PD patients encompasses the clinical symptoms of cognitive slowing, impaired memory recall and retrieval, and executive deficits, which arise from dysfunction between subcortical areas (eg, thalamus, striatum) and cortical areas. However, about 15% to 30% of demented patients with PD may also have coexisting Alzheimer's disease, and reveal symptoms of affected language, memory, and visuospatial functioning early in the course of the disease, including the presence of aphasia, agnosia, and apraxia.[73-76] Cognitive dysfunction in PD may be a consequence of disruption not only in the primary motor circuit, but also in a number of interconnected pathways from the basal ganglia to the cortex. Dopamine depletion in the lateral orbitofrontal and the dorsolateral prefrontal circuits has been suggested as a possible mechanism of cognitive impairment in PD.[77]

Those PD patients at higher risk of developing dementia include:[78-80]

- Over 70 years of age
- Unified Parkinson Disease Rating Scale (UPDRS) score above 25 (moderate to advanced impairment)
- Depression
- Development of mania, agitation, disorientation, or psychosis when treated with levodopa
- Facial masking at presentation
- Exposure to psychological stress
- Presence of cardiovascular abnormalities
- Low socioeconomic status
- Low educational level
- Patients presenting with bradykinesia and postural and gait disturbances. Tremor or other parkinsonian signs are less associated with dementia

Psychosis

Hallucinations may occur during later stages of PD. Psychosis and visual hallucinations are commonly related to dose-dependent adverse effects of the anti-PD medications in combination with disease progression and medical illnesses. Risk factors include advancing age, presence of dementia, and poly-pharmacy. Patients who experience hallucinations generally have some degree of cognitive decline. Hallucinations are usually visual in nature rather than auditory. Patients may report seeing small animals, insects, children, or their deceased relatives or friends. In the early stages, patients are aware that the hallucinations are not real. Symptoms are commonly more severe toward the evening, when lighting is reduced (*sun-downing*).[81] Patients may experience frightening dreams or night terrors that can lead to acting or lashing out during the dream state, and these can be aggravated by dopaminergic and other psychoactive medications. Any medical illness, even an upper respiratory tract infection or diarrhea, may trigger or worsen the dementia or psychotic symptoms. They are best managed by either reducing the evening or daily total dose of levodopa or discontinuing dopamine agonists. Quetiapine or clozapine may be used at bedtime to relieve such symptoms.[82]

Depression

Depression is a very common feature in patients with PD; studies report prevalence between 16% to 70%.[83-85] Norepinephrine and serotonin play important roles in depression by linking with DA deficiency. The characteristics of depression in PD are decreased energy and motivation; losing interest; feelings of sadness, helplessness, and hopelessness; changes in weight, sleep, and appetite; irritability; and thoughts of suicide. Approximately 7% to 32% of PD patients are diagnosed with major depression according to *Diagnostic and Statistical Manual of Mental Disorders, Fourth Edition* (DSM-IV) criteria.[86] The patient may fluctuate between a normal affect and a depressive state, with more frequent episodes of depression during the "off" medication stage and improvement when the motor symptoms are better treated. The relationship between depression and cognitive functioning in PD has not been established definitively.[87]

PD patients may also experience periodic anxiety and panic attacks, which contribute substantially to morbidity and caregiver burden. Anxiety disorders are more prevalent in patients with PD than age-matched controls, although they are often underdiagnosed.[88] Panic attacks easily occur in patients who develop erratic motor fluctuations during "off" periods.[89-91] *Reactive* depression is another form of depression experienced by newly diagnosed patients and others with more advanced disease who are losing independence and control because of changes in motor functioning and feelings of helplessness.[92] Other social factors, including job loss with subsequent changes in income or loss of identity, may also contribute to depression. Concurrent memory difficulty, communication problems, and sleep interruptions all add to the severity of depression and anxiety.

Sleep Disturbance

Sleep disturbance is a common problem in PD patients. Because of depression and/or hallucinations, patients may become restless at night and have difficulty falling asleep. Excessive daytime sleepiness occurs from lack of sleep during the night and sets up a vicious cycle for poor sleep hygiene. This sleepiness is common and very real, often approaching levels observed in narcolepsy.[93] A significant portion of patients may suffer restless legs syndrome, which can cause insomnia.[94-96] Even after falling asleep, patients may wake up frequently due to stiffness or urinary urgency.

Those at higher risk for pathological sleep are male patients with advanced disease, cognitive impairment, drug-induced psychosis, and orthostatic hypotension.[93] REM behavior sleep disorder (RBD) is very likely to occur. It is characterized by loss of atonia during REM sleep, resulting in excess motor activity during dreams. It is highly related to neurodegenerative disorders, including PD.[97,98] Recent studies suggested RBD may occur well before the emergence of PD symptoms. Approximately half of the patients with RBD will eventually develop PD, and so RBD may be an indicator of presymptomatic PD.[99]

Autonomic Dysfunctions

Autonomic dysfunctions include orthostatic hypotension, excessive drooling (partly due to decreased dexterity of oral muscles), constipation, regurgitation, decreased gastrointestinal functionality, urinary frequency or incontinence, sexual dysfunction, and excessive sweating or intolerance of heat or cold.[100,101] Orthostatic hypotension is a particular concern. It may be a subtle sign in the early stage of PD, but may not manifest as a major problem until the later stages.[102] Treatment is symptomatic. Patients are encouraged to drink appropriate amounts of water. They should also get up slowly from sitting and stand for a while before initiating gait to prevent a sudden drop of blood pressure. Dopaminergic medications usually do not significantly help, and they may even worsen the symptoms. Those who are also taking anti-hypertensive medications may need to lower their dosages. In more severe cases, additional medication may be necessary to improve their blood pressure responses.

Gastrointestinal symptoms are common, and constipation is the most frequently encountered problem. Slower bowel movement and decreased mobility exacerbate the severity of constipation. Patients are advised to consume plenty of high-fiber food and fluids and get regular exercise. Artificial fibers and laxatives may also help relieve symptoms.[103]

Another common symptom is urinary urgency or incontinence due to spastic bladder. Roughly 27% to 39% of PD patients experience these problems.[104] Nocturnal urinary urgency is also very common, and can often be relieved by the appropriate dosage of anticholinergics or alpha-blockers. Sexual dysfunction, such as erectile difficulty, loss of libido, and anorgasmia, is common in male PD patients.[105] Despite the impact of sexual dysfunction on quality of life, patients rarely offer this information. Sildenafil has been reported to be effective for patients without obvious cardiovascular risk factors.[105]

NATURAL PROGRESSION

The progression of PD varies among patients. It affects the upper and/or lower limb asymmetrically, and eventually, most patients will be affected on both sides. There are several well-established instruments that are helpful to track the symptoms and progression of PD. One common measure is the UPDRS, which is composed of four main parts: 1) mentation, behavior, and mood; 2) activities of daily living (ADL); 3) motor examination; and 4) complications of therapy.[106] There are five scores in each single item to rate the severity of symptoms and signs of PD. Other well-recognized rating scales include the Modified Hoehn and Yahr Staging, which grades clinical severity,[107] and the Schwab & England Activities of Daily Living Scale, which evaluates the functional abilities of PD patients to manage their daily activities. These evaluation instruments will be discussed in Chapter 3.[108]

The initial symptoms of PD are usually mild. In early PD, parkinsonian signs may be particularly subtle and patients may only experience slowness, stiffness, and difficulty with handwriting. Physicians may initially diagnose arthritis, depression, or normal aging. By paying particular attention to the history of tremor (even if not visible during examination), to slowness of fine motor control, to a slightly flexed posture and gait changes, and to micrographia, the clinician can diagnose PD in its early stages.[109] Eventually, patients will experience asymmetry of parkinsonian signs, obvious resting tremor, a clinically significant response to levodopa, and little or no balance problems in the first months and years of the disease.[1] The speed of progression varies, but may be related to different subtypes. Clinical subgroups are often classified into tremor-predominant versus postural instability gait disorder (PIGD) variants. Another group is young-onset (usually between age 21 and 40 years) versus later onset PD.[110] When PD begins in an elderly patient, decline is more rapid than in middle-aged onset patients, and bradykinesia, rigidity, and balance problems predominate over tremor.[111] The tremor-predominant patients generally have a slower decline in motor function than the akinetic/rigid patients. Young-onset patients have more preserved cognitive function and fewer falls than those with late disease onset.[112,113] The responses to medical treatment vary individually. However, most of the PD patients will benefit from dopaminergic medications, especially in the beginning stages of the disease. Symptom presentation and progression may differ substantially among affected individuals, therefore, management also needs to be individualized.

During the moderate stages of PD, although patients are still having good responses to dopaminergic medications, they may gradually need more doses or a combination of medications to maintain their motor functioning. The major problems that patients experience after several years of treatment for PD are symptom fluctuations (both motor and non-motor), dyskinesias, and behavioral or cognitive changes.[114-116] The most common form of motor fluctuation is a predictable decline in motor performance occurring near the end of each medication dose ("wearing off"). This gradually occurs from "on" with a good medication response to an "off" period 30 minutes to 1 hour before the next medication dose is taken. Less commonly, sudden and severe cataclysms of motor fluctuation may occur, with ambulatory patients becoming immobilized over just a few seconds ("sudden on-off").[117] As time goes on, many patients experience involuntary choreiform movements, called "on-time dyskinesia," as a peak-dose complication after medications are taken, or sometimes at the end of a medication dose. This on-off fluctuation with on-time dyskinesia not only severely affects the patient's quality of life, but also becomes a challenge to the physician's management skills. It requires close cooperation from the patient, who can record the fluctuation of symptoms during the day to help the physician to adjust medication doses and dosing intervals. "On" without dyskinesia or "on" with non-troublesome dyskinesia are the management goals.[118] The mechanisms for motor fluctuation and dyskinesia are not well understood. Although the peak dose level of levodopa is probably related to this phenomenon, not all PD patients have such fluctuation. Some studies found that 22% of PD subjects might develop fluctuations.[119,120] The underlying pathophysiology of motor fluctuations and dyskinesias is not fully understood, and further studies are required to provide more information.

As the disease progresses, difficulties in motor, autonomic, and cognitive function may develop that eventually overshadow symptoms that arise from tremor, rigidity, or bradykinesia despite treatment with levodopa or other drugs. Several types of motor signs and symptoms may be recognized in patients with advanced disease. These problems include gait abnormalities, imbalance, dysarthria, and dysphagia. In other words, the involvement in limbs has progressed to the trunk. Generally, axial and lower-extremity symptoms tend to respond less well to medications.[121] Patients will experience more difficulties with ambulation and postural control, producing more freezing and festination, resulting in imbalance and falls. Freezing most commonly occurs when turning, initiating a step, or when navigating through doorways or other narrow spaces. In some patients, this occurs mainly as an "off" phenomenon,[122] but it may occur independent of bradykinesia and tremor or unrelated to drug treatment.[123] Imbalance also commonly does not respond well to levodopa treatment. In addition, non-motor symptoms, including cognitive impairment, depression, hallucination, sleep disturbance, and autonomic dysfunction, become more evident in advanced PD. As patients become less mobile, constipation, pneumonia, pressure skin ulcers, and opportunistic infections are more problematic, especially if they are wheelchair- or bed-bound. Their ADL are increasingly more dependent. Although the progression of PD itself is not fatal, the potential complications, including aspiration, infections, weight loss, and fall injuries, do increase the morbidity and mortality rates in these patients.[124]

In summary, PD symptoms are mild in the early stages and treatment is often not needed. When the symptoms progress and medications are still effective, this is called the "honeymoon stage." As the symptoms progress, patients often require increased medication doses, and the efficacy of the medications decreases and motor fluctuations occur, which may manifest as dyskinesias. Patients may experience postural imbalance that is not effectively treated by medications. Toward the later stages, patients will have decreased physical activities as they become wheelchair- or bed-bound. Many non-motor symptoms also become obvious and may overshadow the problems of motor symptoms.

Diagnostic Criteria and Differential Diagnosis

There is no single laboratory or imaging test to confirm the diagnosis of PD. Pathological diagnosis depends on finding Lewy bodies in the basal ganglia from an autopsied brain. Practically, the clinical diagnosis is made by experienced physicians through neurological examination. A commonly accepted diagnostic criteria is the finding of at least two out of the three cardinal symptoms of resting tremor, bradykinesia, or rigidity, in the absence of other apparent causes of parkinsonism.[125] Based on clinical characteristics, PD can be divided into two types: 1) tremor-predominant subtype and 2) PIGD subtype, depending on which symptoms are more predominant.[126] Patients should be thoroughly questioned on their clinical history of symptoms, medication history, coexisting medical illness, living environment, social history, and family history. Examination of eye movements, orthostatic blood pressure, sensory deficits, and distinction between pyramidal and cerebellar involvement will help differentiate PD from other movement disorders.

Response to levodopa can be used as a diagnostic indicator of likely primary PD. The absence of significant clinical improvement after 4 to 8 weeks of levodopa therapy should cast doubt on the diagnosis. If unexpected side effects occur to levodopa users early in treatment, specifically hallucinations, the diagnosis of PD should also be reconsidered.[127]

Conventional brain imaging, such as CT or MRI scans, is not useful for the diagnosis of PD. Positron emission tomography (PET) studies using 18F-fluorodopa demonstrates reduced uptake in the striatum, particularly marked in the putamen in PD patients.[128,129] Several ligands have been developed for the postsynaptic dopamine receptor and the dopamine transporter protein in the presynaptic terminals. Using single photon emission computerized tomography (SPECT) with dopamine transporter ligands, such as β-CIT or TRODAT, the level of dopamine in the basal ganglia can be quantitatively measured and a deficiency will indicate PD.[130-132]

The differential diagnosis of PD covers a broad range of disease categories. Any condition presenting with parkinsonian symptoms should be considered for primary PD, secondary parkinsonism, or parkinsonism plus syndromes. The causes of secondary parkinsonism include drugs or toxins, central nervous system infections, brain lesions including infarctions, metabolic disorders, or other neurological disorders affecting the basal ganglia. Several medications can be offending agents to induce tentative parkinsonian symptoms. Offending medications are usually dopamine antagonists, including neuroleptic agents (all typical and atypical except clozapine and quetiapine), dopamine depleting agents (tetrabenazine, reserpine), antiemetic drugs, calcium-channel antagonists (flunarizine and cinnarizine), amiodarone, valproic acid, and lithium.[133,134] The presenting symptoms are generally more symmetrical. Bradykinesia and rigidity usually manifest early, characterized by masked face, slowness of movement, and gait difficulty. Tremor is less frequent than primary PD, but does occur. It may take several months or longer to develop parkinsonian symptoms after the drugs are initiated. Once the drugs are discontinued, it may also take several months for the symptoms to be resolved, if at all. Treatment is by anticholinergics because dopaminergic agents may worsen the patients' underlying psychiatric conditions, although small amounts have been used with satisfactory results.[133,134]

Parkinsonism plus syndrome, different from secondary parkinsonism, is mostly idiopathic. This includes progressive supranuclear palsy (PSP), multiple system atrophy (MSA), corticobasal degeneration (CBD), and dementia with Lewy bodies (DLB). All have some similar clinical characteristics of PD and clinicians may initially confuse them with PD. Other hereditary neurodegenerative diseases, including Huntington's disease, Wilson's disease, and neurodegeneration with brain iron accumulation may also present with parkinsonian symptoms.[135-137] Differential diagnosis among various groups of parkinsonism are discussed in several review references.[135,138,139]

MANAGEMENT

Treatment of PD includes pharmacological, surgical, and non-pharmacological options. No known medication is able to cure PD, although the effort to arrest its progression has always been a major focus of its treatment. Development of pharmaceuticals for symptomatic relief is the main goal of PD therapies. Surgical treatment aims to help advanced PD patients whose symptoms have become intractable to medical treatment. Non-pharmacological treatments include physical, occupational, and speech therapies. Various exercise programs as well as education and psychosocial support can also contribute to relieving symptoms and improving quality of life. Table 1-3 lists a general consideration of treatment options based on disease stages.

PHARMACOLOGICAL TREATMENTS

Medications are used to compensate DA deficiency resulting from degeneration of the substantia nigra. These include the DA precursor levodopa, DA agonists, and DA stimulating agent amantadine. Anticholinergic agents such as trihexyphenidyl reduce tremor by restoring the imbalance between acetylcholine and DA levels in the brain. Monoamine oxidase B inhibitor (MAOB-I) may have symptomatic and neuroprotective effects. Catechol-O-methyltransferase (COMT) inhibitor acts to prolong and stabilize DA levels by reducing its metabolism.

Levodopa

Levodopa is the most efficacious medication for treatment of PD. It is the precursor of DA that will be converted by dopa-decarboxylase (DDC) to DA once it is transported through the blood brain barrier (BBB) into the brain. DA is synthesized in the DA melanin-containing neurons in the substantia nigra and is released into the striatum on physiological stimuli for movement. Because DDC is also present in peripheral tissues such as gastrointestinal and vascular walls, levodopa can also be converted to DA outside of the brain, resulting in side effects such as nausea, vomiting, or orthostatic hypotension. Thus, a DDC inhibitor is combined with levodopa (carbidopa + levodopa or Sinemet; benserazide + levodopa or Madopar) as drug preparations that are now much more tolerable to patients. The DDC inhibitors do not cross the BBB and will prevent levodopa from being converted to DA in peripheral tissues. This will not only reduce levodopa side effects but also increase the availability of levodopa in the brain.

Levodopa is administered orally in three or more divided doses throughout the waking period. Taking it with meals may reduce gastrointestinal side effects. However, too much protein in the food content will affect its absorption. Starting doses are usually 50 to 100 mg/day and titration will be carried out slowly. The usual maintenance dose is 300 to 600 mg/day, although it can be much higher (>1000 mg/day) in some patients. In randomized trials comparing levodopa and dopamine agonists, levodopa improved ADL and motor symptoms by 40% to 50% as opposed to 30% with dopamine agonists.[140-143] The symptomatic improvement of gait difficulty by levodopa is not as striking as relief of tremor or rigidity.[144]

Side effects of levodopa include gastrointestinal (anorexia, nausea, vomiting), cardiovascular (arrhythmia, orthostatic hypotension), and psychiatric (mood disorders, sleep

TABLE 1-3

Treatment Considerations in Different Stages of Parkinson's Disease

Early Stages

- Neuroprotective considerations
  - -No definitive neuroprotective agents
  - -Possible trials of selegiline or rasagiline[166]
  - -Possible trial of coenzyme Q10 (1200 to 2400 mg/day)[253]
- Non-pharmacological approaches
  - -Frequent regular exercises, emphasis on stretching
  - -Biofeedback techniques
- Symptomatic relief
  - -Younger patients: Goal is to minimize long-term motor fluctuations and dyskinesia. Consider dopamine agonists or amantadine.
  - -Older patients: Goal is to minimize side effects, especially on cognitive effects. Consider levodopa.

Advanced Stages

- Maximize symptomatic relief and reduce motor fluctuations (wearing off)
  - -Combinations of levodopa, dopamine agonists, COMT inhibitor, and anticholinergics[198]
  - -Adjusting medication dosing and timing to avoid wearing off, evenly distribute medications throughout the waking period
  - -Injectable apomorphine for sudden wearing off symptoms[179]
- Treatment of dyskinesias[198]
  - -Reduce levodopa dose
  - -Increase levodopa dosing frequency
  - -Add amantadine
- DBS evaluation on patients presenting with either motor fluctuations or troublesome dyskinesias, or both[198]
- Treatment of freezing and falls
  - -Physical therapy evaluations
  - -Appropriate usage of assistive devices, including canes, walkers, and wheelchairs
  - -Environmental modifications to eliminate obstructions
- Treatment of non-motor symptoms
  - -Ask patients about individual symptoms
  - -Most are treatable symptomatically
  - -Rule out possible PD medication side effects

disturbances, and psychosis, such as hallucination or delusion) symptoms. These side effects are often temporary and can be controlled by adjusting the medication dosage and timing. However, the long-term side effects may be more bothersome to patients. The half-life of levodopa is about 1.5 hours.[145] Its effect usually commences 20 to 30 minutes after the medication is taken. Initially, each dose of levodopa is able to last 8 hours or longer for therapeutic benefit because the DA nerve terminals have the potential to store more DA for later use. However, as PD progresses, the nerve terminals are reduced and the reserve of DA in these terminals also decreases, resulting in a shortening in the duration of drug benefit. This is the reason why levodopa effectiveness may decline over time and result in motor fluctuations. Initially, patients will experience a loss of the beneficial drug effect before the next dose is due, known as "wearing-off" effect or "end-of-dose" deterioration. In the morning, because there is a lack of medication overnight during sleep, patients may report morning dystonia or nocturnal akinesia. Patients gradually need higher doses of levodopa in order to relieve parkinsonian symptoms, and this will result in the delayed "on" or drug-resistant "off" phenomenon. Further, "off" periods may change from the predictable "wearing off" phenomenon to unpredictable sudden "off," which is not related to the timing of medication dosing. To manage the aforementioned problems, physicians may increase the levodopa dosage or dosing frequency, or add other medications, such as a dopamine agonist or COMT inhibitor to enhance the levodopa effectiveness.[146-148] Several formulations of carbidopa-levodopa, including oral disintegrating tablets, combined with the COMT inhibitor entacapone, chronic release tablets are available and may also be used.

After using levodopa for several years, dyskinesias may emerge. Approximately 50% of PD patients may develop dyskinesias after 5 years on levodopa treatment, especially younger-onset patients.[149,150] It is an abnormal involuntary movement most often occurring when the patient is in the "on" state, but it can also occur during the "off" state. Peak-dose dyskinesia appears at the time of maximal drug effect, usually with choreic and dystonic movements. Diphasic dyskinesia occurs during the ascending or descending plasma levels of levodopa, presenting mostly with lower extremity repetitive dystonic or ballistic disabling movements. Off-period dyskinesia is usually dystonic in nature, occurring upon awakening or during "off" states, particularly in the evening.[151]

The pathophysiology of dyskinesia is still not known. It is thought to be related to dopaminergic neuron hypersensitivity, because younger-onset PD patients seem to develop the symptoms more often.[152,153] Pulsatile exposures of levodopa levels to postsynaptic dopaminergic receptors have been hypothesized as the cause.[151,154] However, controlled-release preparations of levodopa failed to prevent or prolong the occurrence of dyskinesia in the long term.[155,156] A recent study on repetitive transcranial magnetic stimulation of supplementary motor area (SMA) was able to reduce the therapy-induced dyskinesias, suggesting possible involvement of SMA.[157] However, the exact mechanisms still require further investigation.

Whether levodopa is neurotoxic to DA neurons has been argued for many years. In cultured cell and animal experiments, DA neuron damages caused by exposure to levodopa have been shown.[158-161] However, there is no evidence in humans showing DA neuron injury due to levodopa intake.[162,163] A previous international consensus meeting also concluded that there was no evidence to support the levodopa toxicity hypothesis and, hence, to sustain the belief that levodopa accelerates disease progression.[164] In an early versus late levodopa study (ELLDOPA), there was no significant difference in the beta-CIT scan in different groups taking various doses of levodopa, whether treated earlier or later.[165] The higher dose group improved the most on motor scale, but also had significantly more motor fluctuations. These clinical data suggest that levodopa either slows the progression of PD or has a prolonged effect on the symptoms of the disease. In contrast, the neuroimaging data suggest either that levodopa accelerated the loss of nigrostriatal dopamine nerve terminals or that its pharmacologic effects modified the dopamine transporter. The authors postulated that potential long-term effects of levodopa on PD remain uncertain.[165] The most recent practice guidelines published by the American Academy of Neurology suggested that levodopa does not appear to accelerate disease progression.[166]

Dopamine Agonists

These drugs have high affinities to DA receptors and mimic DA action by binding onto them. They are used as a primary drug treatment for PD or as an adjunct to levodopa. They act on the D2 dopamine receptor with certain concomitant effects on D1 or D3 receptors as well. Earlier drugs are ergot derivatives including bromocriptine, pergolide, and lisuride. Newer medications are non-ergot derivatives, including pramipexole and ropinirole, which usually generate fewer side effects than their ergot derivative counterparts. Apomorphine is a fast-acting agonist, administered by injection, that probably acts on D1 and D2 receptors to rescue patients out of a severe "off" state.[167] Rotigotine is the new dopamine agonist, administered in the form of a patch, that is indicated for early-stage PD.[168]

The clinical efficacy of DA agonists is well established. Several studies, including the pergolide study,[158] pramipexole study,[142,143] rotigotine study,[168] and ropinirole study,[169] all confirmed the positive clinical benefits. A DA agonist can be used as an initial treatment in newly diagnosed patients with PD or used as a combination therapy with levodopa. Its potential side effects, including sleep attacks, edema, weight gain, nausea, vomiting, hypotension, and hallucinations, may be more prominent than those of levodopa, especially when it is added to levodopa. A slow titration is necessary to avoid excessive side effects. Ergot derivative agonists tend to have more side effects than non-ergot derivatives. In a pharmacologic comparison between pramipexole and pergolide, the two had comparable effects on tremor reduction.[170,171] Pergolide has been withdrawn from the market due to its link to the development of cardiac valvular fibrosis.[172,173]

Despite potential side effects, many physicians consider using a DA agonist as the initial treatment for PD and reserving levodopa for supplemental therapy. One of the major reasons is that DA agonists seem to delay or decrease the risk of developing dyskinesia and motor fluctuation.[151,174] Early exposure of DA agonists before levodopa is given may also delay the onset of motor complications.[175] However, whether DA agonists are also neuroprotective and can delay disease progression is uncertain at this time, although there are reports regarding treatment with pramipexole or ropinirole that indicate a slower decline of striatal dopaminergic signals on neuroimaging studies compared to levodopa.[142,169]

In the practical clinical approach, it is reasonable to initiate a DA agonist on young-onset PD patients to help avoid possible early motor complications and gradually increase it to the maximally tolerated dosage. Usually after 1 to 3 years, levodopa will need to be added to better control the progressive parkinsonian symptoms. Levodopa is usually the first choice for elderly PD patients because of its more predictable benefits and lower side effects. In general, a combination of levodopa and a DA agonist is prescribed to adequately control the symptoms of PD.[176,177]

Apomorphine is a rapid-acting DA agonist. It has a potent D2 and a partial D1 activity. Its extensive first-pass hepatic metabolism has prevented its oral administration.[178] It is available as an subcutaneous formulation to treat PD. It is used in advanced PD patients who have "wearing off" phenomenon, troublesome or unpredictable "off" states or delayed "on" phenomenon. Once administered, this medication quickly produces symptomatic benefit within 10 minutes of dosing and maintains a duration of action for about 90 to 120 minutes.[179] Thus, it acts as a "rescue" therapy. Intermittent injections of apomorphine allow some decrease in the oral dopaminergic medications, and may reduce the risk of side effects. Apomorphine injection has its own substantial side effects, including yawning, dyskinesias, nausea and/or vomiting, somnolence, dizziness, rhinorrhea, hallucinations, edema, chest pain, increased sweating, flushing, hypotension, and pallor that need to be monitored closely. Patients need to take an anti-emetic medication before using apomorphine. Other routes of administration of apomorphine, including subcutaneous infusion, intravenous injection, intranasal spray application, and sublingual or rectal administrations, are still under investigation.[180]

Catecholamine-O-Methyltransferase (COMT) Inhibitors

COMT is widely distributed in glia cells in the human brain.[181] Most of the levodopa absorbed into the body is converted by COMT to the inactive metabolite 3-O-methyldopa before crossing the BBB into the brain. The accumulated 3-O-methyldopa then competes with levodopa absorption in the gut and the blood vessel wall, resulting in levodopa level fluctuations. The use of COMT inhibitor, such as entacapone or tolcapone, is to inhibit the action of this enzyme. Tolcapone may cause liver toxicity that needs to be monitored.[182,183]

COMT inhibitors are used as adjunctive therapy with levodopa and they are ineffective monotherapy for parkinsonian symptoms. They are indicated in PD patients with the signs and symptoms of end-of-dose wearing-off (so-called fluctuating patients). They serve to modestly improve motor function and reduce off time when added to levodopa.[184] Whether they will be beneficial for patients with early PD by stabilizing serum levodopa level and thus reducing the risk of developing subsequent motor fluctuations is still uncertain. Tolcapone has a longer half-life and is administered three times daily. Entacapone has to be taken with each dose of levodopa because its half-life is similar to that of levodopa. Entacapone is available as a single drug or as a combination drug with carbidopa/levodopa.[185] Major side effects include diarrhea, hyperkinesia, urine discoloration, fatigue, and hallucinations. In addition, it may worsen dopa-induced dyskinesia. It is recommended to reduce the levodopa dose slightly when entacapone is added.

Monoamine Oxidase-B (MAO-B) Inhibitors

Selegiline and rasagiline are the only available medications in this category. They are irreversible MAO-B inhibitors.[186-188] Initially, they were used as an adjunct to levodopa to inhibit the enzymatic degradation of DA by MAO-B in order to prolong its duration of action.[189,190] Later, they were used as neuroprotective agents in early PD patients to slow down the progression of the disease as well as delay the need for levodopa.[188,191-195] Recently, an evidence-based review indicated that selegiline has very mild symptomatic benefit with no evidence for neuroprotective benefit. Therefore, it is less commonly prescribed and is used in some early stage, younger PD patients only.

The newer rasagiline is a second generation irreversible MAO-B inhibitor. Clinical studies have revealed that rasagiline is associated with improved outcomes in patients with early PD and also reduces off time in patients with moderate to advanced PD with motor fluctuations.[196-198]

Anticholinergics and Amantadine

With decreased DA content in the substantia nigra, cholinergic neurotransmission in the striatum is then relatively more dominant. This DA/Acetylcholine imbalance is thought to be one of the causes for parkinsonian tremor. The anticholinergic agent, such as trihexyphenidyl, has some efficacy in controlling resting tremor but not effective for other symptoms such as rigidity, bradykinesia, or postural instability. It is mainly used in the early stages to delay the initiation of levodopa or as an adjunct therapy to treat symptomatic tremor.[199,200] Anticholinergics have substantial side effects, including dry mouth, blurred vision, urinary retention, constipation, confusion, memory impairment, or hallucinations, when used in higher doses and in elderly patients.

Amantadine is a drug used to treat influenza virus, but has been found to also improve PD symptoms. It is thought to stimulate DA release and inhibit glutamate neurotransmission. It has a mild effect to improve tremor, rigidity, and bradykinesia in early stage PD patients. It tends to lose its efficacy over time (approximately 1 to 2 years). However, for late stage PD patients, amantadine can again be used to reduce dyskinesias.[201,202] The mechanism is thought to be related to its glutamate inhibiting effect.[201] It is usually well tolerated by most patients, but edema, dizziness, confusion, and livedo reticularis of the skin can occur.[203]

SURGICAL TREATMENTS

As PD progresses, some patients develop worsening symptoms that are unresponsive to medication therapy with concomitant deterioration of their quality of life. The limitations of long-term medical treatment prompted development and revival of the surgical treatments for PD. Although surgeries on the brain to treat PD had been performed for more than eight decades, recent advancements in understanding of the functional organization of the basal ganglia and PD pathophysiology have prompted more intense interest in surgical therapies. The purposes of surgical treatment are to relieve the major symptoms of the disease and several medication-induced side effects, including motor fluctuations and dopa-induced dyskinesias. There are two main types of surgical options: electrical stimulation and brain transplantation. The target sites include the ventral intermediate nucleus of the thalamus (VIM), the internal segment of the globus pallidus (GPi), and the subthalamic nucleus (STN). Restorative therapy with surgical implantation of fetal cells, genetically engineered cells, or stem cells into the basal ganglia is still in an experimental stage at this time.[204-206]

As discussed earlier, DA deficiency in PD patients results in increased neuronal activities in GPi and STN. This overactivity subsequently inhibits thalamocortical motor circuits with resulting slowing and dampening of voluntary movements. Therefore, by pallidal or STN lesioning or electrical stimulation, the disinhibition of thalamocortical circuits may be reversed.

Ablative Surgeries

Ablative surgery results in a permanent lesion in the brain. Ablative surgery does not have the cumbersomeness of electronic devices embedded in the body and does not need frequent adjustment as required by electrode placements.

Thalamotomy

This procedure is performed to reduce parkisonian tremor as well as essential tremor. The lesion target is the ventral intermediate nucleus of the thalamus. Unilateral thalamotomy reduced contralateral limb tremor in 85% of patients.[207] Increased risks of speech and swallowing impairment have discouraged bilateral thalamotomy. As its benefit is only limited to improving tremor, this procedure is now less frequently performed than pallidotomy for treating PD.

Pallidotomy

This is one of the earliest ablative procedures performed, dating back about five decades ago. It became less popular due to advances in medical treatments. However, as the limitation of medical therapy became evident in advanced PD patients, especially for motor fluctuation and dyskinesias, pallidotomy has regained its popularity since the early 1990s.[208,209] This procedure is very effective in reducing or even abolishing contralateral tremor and dopa-induced dyskinesias.[210,211] Modest improvements on rigidity, freezing, and bradykinesia are also observed.[212,213] The total motor and ADL assessments are improved by 25% to 30% during the off state, but not significantly improved during the on state.[210,213] However, the benefits of pallidotomy may decline over time.

Pallidotomy can be performed with few neurological complications and its benefits are judged to overweigh the risks.[214,215] Currently, with increased deep brain stimulation (DBS) surgeries, pallidotomy is not performed as frequently as before. However, because DBS requires close monitoring and periodic adjustment of the stimulator that is also costly, pallidotomy is still appropriate for patients with unilateral disabling dopa-induced dyskinesias and resting tremor.

Subthalamotomy

The ablative surgery on the STN is much less commonly performed than pallidotomy. One of the major reasons is safety. STN is a small nucleus located just beside the midbrain. Focal neurological deficit may occur if part of the brain stem is damaged inadvertently during surgery. Nevertheless, several uncontrolled studies were reported.[216-219] A few complications such as cerebellar signs, increased dyskinesia, and chorea after the subthalamotomy have been observed. There were overall satisfactory results of decreased tremor, dyskinesias, and freezing gait. Further studies are needed to demonstrate the efficacy and risks of this surgical procedure.

Deep Brain Stimulation (DBS): Electrical Stimulation

DBS involves a surgically implanted, battery-operated medical device called a neurostimulator that delivers electrical stimulation to strategic areas of the brain to block abnormal signals in the circuitry of the basal ganglia and reduce PD symptoms (Figure 1-5). The DBS system consists of the lead, the extension, and the neurostimulator. The lead (or electrode) is a thin, insulated wire that is inserted through a small opening in the skull and implanted in the brain. The tip of the electrode is positioned within the targeted brain area. The extension is an insulated wire that is passed under the skin of the head, neck, and shoulder, connecting the lead to the neurostimulator. The neurostimulator (the "battery pack") is the third component and is usually implanted under the skin near the upper or lower chest or over the abdomen.[220,221]

The surgical procedure requires pre-surgery brain imaging and framing to conduct stereotaxic localization. Most surgeons use microelectrode recording to more specifically identify the precise brain target that will be stimulated. Once the system is in place, electrical impulses are sent from the neurostimulator along the extension wire and the lead to the brain. These impulses interfere with and block the electrical signals that cause PD symptoms. The common target areas are GPi and STN for PD.

Thalamic DBS

Similar to thalamotomy, thalamic DBS is mainly for uncontrolled tremor, especially essential tremor. It has the advantage of being safe even when implanted bilaterally. A

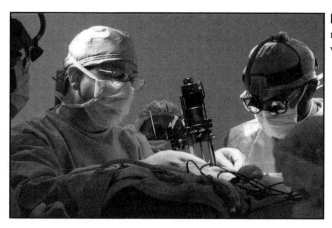

Figure 1-5. Surgeons implant a neurotransmitter into the brain of a patient with Parkinson's disease.

randomized trial showed that thalamic DBS had greater success in abolishing tremor than thalamotomy.[222] However, similar to thalamotomy, thalamic DBS is seldom used in treating PD as tremor reduction seems to be its only benefit.

Subthalamic DBS

This is the most commonly performed procedure in DBS surgery. This procedure reduces parkinsonian tremor, rigidity, and dyskinesia.[223] With appropriately selected PD patients, STN DBS improved off state motor scores by 60% to 65%.[224,225] Motor functions during the on state also improved.[225,226] Levodopa dosage could be reduced or even completely discontinued.[227] Thus, patients benefited from reduced dopa-induced dyskinesias. PD patients who do not respond to levodopa therapy usually do not benefit from DBS treatment.[228]

Complications from this procedure are usually minor and include sensory irritations, dysarthria, infection, cognitive or emotional changes, confusion and hallucinations. Major complications such as intracerebral hemorrhage or stroke are rare.

Pallidal DBS

This procedure places the leads at the GPi. If placed unilaterally, the benefits are similar to those of pallidotomy. However, GPi DBS can be placed bilaterally and still has much less risk for speech and other neurological complications. In several studies, motor functions in both "off" and "on" states improved after DBS placement.[226,229,230] Dyskinesias also decreased, especially with bilateral DBS.[231]

One of the major benefits of pallidal DBS is for treating generalized dystonia.[232,233] So far, there is no definitive conclusion on whether STN or GPi DBS has more potential benefits for patients with PD. In several open-label studies, STN DBS seemed to show improvement.[226,228,234] Both procedures are relatively safe.

Brain Transplantation

The underlying cellular biology lies in restoring degenerated DA cells. DA-producing neurons or growth factors for degenerating neurons, especially glial-derived neurotrophic factor (GDNF), are the main entities to be used. The first attempt was made by autologous adrenal medulla transplantation to the caudate nucleus.[235-237] Although the authors reported dramatic symptom improvement, similar results were not replicated by others. A double blinded, randomized trial of human embryonic DA neuron transplantation from fetal mesencephalon was reported in 2001.[237] Patients showed no improvement on the subjective global rating scale. However, 15% of the transplanted patients suffered persistent and severe dyskinesias.[238] Overall, the results were not dramatically encouraging. Currently, additional investigations include fetal porcine mesencephalic neuron and retinal pigment epithelial cell transplantation.[239,240] GDNF delivering system, GDNF-containing vector gene therapy, and stem cells are all possible choices under active investigation. Some of the advances will be discussed later in this chapter.

REHABILITATION THERAPIES

One of the most challenging goals in treatment is to correct the postural instability and gait difficulties of PD patients. Some patients respond to dopaminergic medications or DBS surgeries well by being turned "on" to improve their gait. However, many patients do not show good responses for postural balance, freezing gait, turning, initiation hesitation, and shuffling in spite of medical or surgical treatments. In addition, many higher level ADL skills such as driving, working, shopping, and cooking are affected even though the basic motor symptoms are improved by medications. Importantly, medications do not improve speech and swallowing problems. Rehabilitation services address all the aforementioned issues and allow patients to maximize their functioning and independence.

Physical Therapy

The physical therapist (PT) evaluates the PD patients' gait, balance, range of motion, coordination, and transfers (Figure 1-6). Therapists often initiate therapy with exercises for general conditioning, stretching, and strengthening. Individuals with PD are instructed to consciously process movement information, such as thinking about swinging the arms or taking large steps. The goal of therapy has been largely to help people maintain what motor capability they have for as long as possible and to help them adjust as their functional levels inevitably decline. It is now recognized that the brain has the ability to reorganize (ie, neuroplasticity) after disease and it can be facilitated through activity-dependent processes, including environmental enrichment, forced-use, complex skills training, and exercise[241-243] (see Chapter 2).

Occupational Therapy

The occupational therapist (OT) evaluates the patient's occupational performance, or ability to engage in self-care, work, and leisure. The OT looks at both the physical and psychosocial components of activity while assessing the patient's ability to perform ADL tasks. The OT will teach the patient and caregiver techniques and alternative strategies; recommend adaptive equipment such as elevated toilet seats, shower seats, adapted utensils, and button hooks; raise awareness of community resources such as books on tape and disabled parking; and instruct in energy conservation and motion economy techniques to maximize function. OTs will stress fall prevention and train the patient and family in home safety.[244] To increase productivity at home and at work is the ultimate goal so patients will enjoy activities and be able to better care for themselves.[245]

Speech and Swallow Therapy

PD frequently affects breathing, voice production, the richness of the voice, and clarity of speech. Coordination of speech and breath can be disrupted. Changes within the larynx can reduce speech volume, resulting in a softened or unsteady voice.[246] A patient may present symptoms that include soft voice, mumbled and fast speech, loss of facial

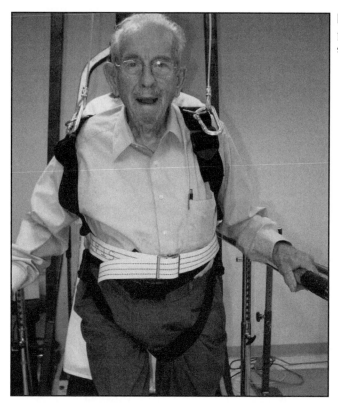

Figure 1-6. A patient is undergoing physical therapy for body weight supported treadmill training.

expression, and trouble swallowing. A speech language pathologist (SLP) evaluates and treats PD patients for such problems.[247] The Lee Silverman Voice Treatment (LSVT) is an intensive method that focuses on vocal loudness and has been effective for speech problems in PD.[248,249] For swallowing and aspiration, prevention is the most crucial aspect. Dysphagia therapy goals include improving the function of affected muscles through exercise, preventing the rate and degree of decline in swallowing function through exercise, and teaching compensatory strategies designed to make swallowing safer. In general, foods that are moist, slippery, and require less chewing are probably the best. However, for advanced PD patients with frequent choking, tube feeding may be the ultimate choice to prevent aspiration and to provide adequate nutrition.

Alternative Therapies

There are different terms for the treatment options other than conventional therapies. For many Europeans, these therapies are perceived as "supplementary" to conventional medicine, rather than as an "alternative," which is how they are typically considered in the United States. Many of these methods are culturally based. The use of these therapies is widespread, but their popularity differs among regions or countries. Because of the broad spectra of these therapies, it is often difficult to conduct randomized, controlled studies. As a result, their efficacy and safety issues are difficult to interpret or conclude. However, many patients do seek alternative therapies for PD, as there is currently no cure for this disorder. A study of the trends in alternative medicine in the United States showed an increase in the probability of visiting an alternative medicine practitioner from 36.3% to 46.3% from 1990 to 1997. The out-of-pocket expenses for alternative therapies in 1997 were around $27 billion, a sum almost identical to the out-of-pocket expenses for all physician services in that year.[250] The trend continues to grow.

Alternative therapies for PD can be roughly divided into two parts: oral supplements and physical activities. The oral supplements are either traditional herbs, or those agents that have been shown to be neuroprotective in the laboratories, but are not yet confirmed in humans. Known herbs include cowhage, which is commonly used in India and possibly contains levodopa, and Kampo kami-shoyo-san, a Japanese herb that is a mixture of different herbs and is reported to be effective in reducing the tremor associated with antipsychotic-induced parkinsonism.[251] The common "neuroprotective" supplements include:

1. Gamma-aminobutyric acid (GABA), an amino acid that acts as a neurotransmitter. It claims to help strengthen and relax the nervous system.

2. Alpha-lipoic acid, an antioxidant said to "recharge" other antioxidants in the body.

3. Coenzyme Q10, an oxygenating antioxidant that may help prevent free-radical damage and is important for cell renewal. Preliminary data in an open label trial revealed that high doses might benefit PD patients.[252]

4. Primrose oil and flaxseed oil that contain essential fatty acids (EFAs), which are reported to be deficient in people with PD.

5. Vitamin E, an antioxidant that possibly prevents free-radical damage. Recent clinical trials have raised questions about its safety and efficacy.[253]

6. Selenium, an antioxidant that may work with vitamin E. It may help increase circulation and tissue oxygenation, thereby limiting damage to nerve cells.

The aforementioned are just some examples of commonly used supplements for symptomatic treatment. However, no single supplement has been systemically studied to show significant benefits. At this time, there is not enough evidence for physicians to recommend any supplement to help combat the symptoms of PD.

FUTURE THERAPIES

Newer medications are continuously being developed to better benefit PD patients. Efforts have been geared toward smoother and steadier medicine levels in the system. There is a newer carbidopa/levodopa under preparation for smoother drug concentration in the body.[254] As of this writing, there is a new dopamine agonist administered as a skin patch that is also intended for smoother drug levels in the blood.[255] A new MAO-B inhibitor (rasagiline) has also been approved by the FDA for better symptom relief, decreasing dyskinesia, as well as possible neuroprotection.[256] Adenosine A2A antagonists are also under clinical trials for possible neuroprotection and anti-dyskinetic effects.[257]

More possibilities for breakthrough in treating PD lie in some highly advanced techniques. Among them, gene therapy and stem cell therapy are probably the two most promising approaches.

Gene Therapy

The insertion of foreign genes into cells produces new specific proteins that confer specific desired biological effects. The major challenge has been to deliver the selected genes to the appropriate target tissues. For this purpose, modified viruses have been adapted to carry the genes, as viruses are very effective at inserting their genetic material into cells. As a gene-transfer vector that lacks any disease associated with the original virus, the adeno-associated virus (AAV) can transfect non-dividing cells such as brain cells and produces stable, prolonged expression of the transgene.[258]

Because dopamine deficiency is the key feature in PD, introducing transgenes encoding enzymes involved in dopamine synthesis, or encoding neurotrophic factors will enhance dopamine production in the brain region that coordinates movement. Animal studies were conducted on transgenes encoding aromatic L-amino acid decarboxylase (AADC), which converted levodopa to dopamine, into the brains of rats and monkeys.[258] Other groups tried transgenes encoding GDNF and neurturin, and also reported favorable results from the rats and primates.[259,260] Probable human trials are on the horizon.

Stem Cell Therapy

Stem cell therapy is one of the most fascinating areas of biological research today, but like many expanding fields of scientific inquiry, research on stem cells raises scientific questions as rapidly as it generates new discoveries. Stem cells have two important characteristics that distinguish them from other types of cells. First, they are unspecialized cells that can renew themselves for long periods through cell division. Second, under certain physiologic or experimental conditions, they can be induced to become cells with special functions. There are two types of stem cells: 1) embryonic stem cells, which are derived from embryos that develop from fertilized eggs; and 2) adult stem cells, which are undifferentiated cell found among differentiated cells in an adult tissue or organ. These can renew themselves, and can differentiate to yield the major specialized cell types of the tissue or organ. Although they have different characteristics, both cell types have the potential to derive into specific neurons when the appropriate neuronal growth factors and environment are provided. Applying the techniques of stem cell therapy to PD has been a hot topic of research in recent years.[261]

In animal models, scientists have successfully introduced dopamine releasing cells from mouse embryonic stem cells and retained them in cell culture long term.[262] Other researchers have now shown a complete recovery from the methamphetamine-induced rotational response in mice that had unilateral 6-OHDA lesions in the nigrostriatal pathway about 60 days after transplantation of dopamine-rich cells from syngeneic or mouse embryos.[263] For human beings, the most useful three types of cells are human embryonic ventral mesencephalic tissue, embryonic and adult multipotent region-specific stem cells, and embryonic stem cells. Embryonic nigral cell implants were shown to improve reaction time and movement in patients with PD.[264] However, shortage of embryonic donor tissue limits large-scale clinical transplantation trials. Stem cell researchers also face many ethical issues. Nevertheless, trials of appropriate stem cell transplantation in PD patients will eventually reveal better understanding for the treatment of this degenerative neurological disease.

Case Study 1

Mr. X is a 62-year-old man who reports progressive difficulty in his right-hand dexterity for about 1 year. He has noticed right-hand tremor at rest in the last 4 months. The tremor disappears on hand motion, but causes him difficulty in performing fine motor tasks, such as playing the piano or handwriting. He also reports slight difficulty in getting out of a car or bed. It takes him twice as long to complete some daily tasks. Walking is normal with no falling, but his wife has noticed that he walks slower than before with occasional start hesitation. She also complains that his voice is becoming softer and she sometimes needs to ask him to repeat himself in order to catch his words. She also notices that his face is becoming less expressive. He has no previous exposure to neuroleptic medications or known hazardous exposures. There are no known family members with tremor or balance difficulty.

On examination, vital signs: normal. Mental status: normal. Cranial nerve: normal with symmetric facial expressions, although mild "poker" face is noted. His speech was clear although slightly soft in volume. Motor exam: no muscle wasting or fasciculations and is symmetrically normal strength. Mild cogwheel rigidity in the right elbow; left sided cogwheel rigidity is detected only on voluntary opening and closing of his right hand. Mild to moderate amplitude of resting tremor with pill-rolling motions at around 6 to 7 Hz is observed. In the rest position, his right hand reveals some metacarpal flexion as compared to the left. He has slower movements and occasional hesitancy with rapid hand movements. When asked to stand up without pushing, he needs multiple tries to finally get up from the chair. His posture is slightly stooped, but can be normal for an aged person. He walks with shorter steps. He has decreased arm swing in the right arm and its resting tremor is more obvious when he is walking. He takes one step back when he is pulled backwards but does not fall.

Discussion

This is a typical presentation of an early stage tremor predominant idiopathic PD. The patient presents with right-sided predominant symptoms of mild resting tremor, bradykinesia, and rigidity. His postural balance may be slightly affected, but overall well preserved. The presence of asymmetric resting tremor without signs of postural tremor distinguishes from essential tremor. There is no evidence to suggest possible secondary causes of his symptoms.

No known laboratory or imaging tests will confirm the diagnosis. An MRI of the brain does help rule out other possible intracranial lesions responsible for these symptoms. For treatment, there is a broad range of choices at this point. Levodopa is most commonly chosen because it usually has good immediate therapeutic effect with relatively fewer and milder side effects. Some may give a dopamine agonist, considering the possible long-term motor fluctuation complications of levodopa. Amantadine or anticholinergics may also be used to reduce resting tremor. MAO-B inhibitors such as selegiline or rasagiline may be considered for symptomatic improvement as well as possible (but not confirmed) neuroprotection. Each individual drug may improve these early PD symptoms. The more important issue will be patients' and caretakers' education. Education on dealing with PD in daily life, appropriate nutrition, adequate exercises, and psychological awareness is even more important than medications in preparing patients to live with PD for the long term.

Case Study 2

Mr. X is a 78-year-old man has a 12-year history of PD. His major symptoms are postural instability and gait difficulty, with some mild resting tremor. He takes a combination of medications, including carbidopa/levodopa CR 50/200, 1 tablet four times a day; entacapone 200 mg four times a day; pramipexole 1 mg three times a day; trihexyphenidyl 2 mg three times a day; and amantadine 100 mg twice a day. In the last 2 years, he has experienced more frequent end-dose wearing off while he took carbidopa/levodopa CR 50/200 1 tablet three times a day. He was panicky about being off because of freezing, rigidity, and difficulty walking. His medications were gradually increased to the current regimen over the past year. With these medications, he still experiences variable off states from 1 to 3 hours after his first morning dose of pills. He usually gradually "turns on" around 10:00 to 11:00 AM. However, he begins to have mild to moderate dyskinetic movements lasting through the rest of the day. The patient suffers vivid dreams at night. Over time, visual hallucinations have become more frequent. He reports that he sees animals, children, and deceased relatives in his room. They look so real that he is often confused about what he sees. He has difficulty getting a peaceful night's sleep. He wakes up frequently to urinate. On some occasions, he opens the door, trying to get out to "chase a kid running out of my house." As a result, he becomes sleepy and fatigued during the day. He often falls asleep on the sofa. His cognitive function is also declining. He has difficulty with short-term memory. His communication with people is often erratic because of forgetfulness and confusion. He requires more supervision and assistance with his basic ADL and frequently feels dizzy after standing. He has had several falls even during the on time, so that he has to rely on a walker for ambulation. His wife notices swelling in both of his feet. He also complains of constipation and may not have a bowel movement for 3 to 4 days.

Discussion

This is a common clinical scenario encountered in the more advanced and elderly PD patients. In terms of motor symptoms, a patient will experience more wearing-off and require more levodopa and other medications. However, this practice will also increase the risk of developing dyskinesia. Balance impairment may also become more obvious. In addition, non-motor symptoms, including cognitive decline, hallucination and psychosis, sleep disturbances, and autonomic dysfunctions may become more problematic than the motor symptoms. Addition of PD medications may even worsen the patient's non-motor symptoms.

Mr. X takes multiple medications for PD. He will require simplification of his medications because their benefits have been overwhelmed by their side effects. First, the absorption of carbidopa/levodopa 50/200 CR may be unreliable in the advanced PD patient. This is responsible for his delay to be turned "on" and the emergence of his "on"-time dyskinesia. It is better to change to regular carbidopa/levodopa 25/100 given at a shorter interval (eg, every 3 hours) to maintain his body levodopa concentration and reduce his motor fluctuations. Entacapone may cause more dyskinesia and should be discontinued. Trihexyphenidyl is an anti-cholinergic medication that may reduce resting tremor. However, it may cause confusion, cognitive decline, and dry mouth, especially for older patients. Thus, trihexyphenidyl should be discontinued. Amantadine may also have similar side effects, in addition to leg edema, but it may reduce his dyskinesia. Amantadine, in this case, should be reduced or stopped. Pramipexole, a DA agonist, may potentially cause hallucinations, daytime drowsiness, orthostatic hypotension, and leg edema. It also should be tapered off if the patient is still not doing well after discontinuation of amantadine and trihexyphenidyl.

Visual hallucination and cognitive decline suggest a possible dementing process in this patient. Mr. X should be referred for neuropsychological testing to determine his cognitive status and to rule out possible depression. Acetylcholine esterase inhibitor, such as rivastigmine or donepezil, has been shown to improve cognitive function in patients with PD. If the patient's hallucinations continue even after simplification of his medications, a low dose of quetiapine at bedtime can be tried for symptomatic treatment. A small dose of short-acting benzodiazepam may help his sleep. Autonomic dysfunctions such as urinary frequency, orthostatic hypotension, and constipation are common. They are probably caused by a combination of disease progression and medication side effects. More fluid intake is also important in improving orthostatic hypotension and constipation. As some of the patient's medications are adjusted, his undesirable symptoms may improve. Each patient's symptoms should be evaluated according to his unique situation and management needs to be individualized.

Freezing or gait starting initiation difficulty may be improved by levodopa. However, the patient's tendency to fall and worsening balance may not be easily treated. Rehabilitation with gait training is very important in this stage. Both physical therapy and occupational therapy will help increase mobility and daily activity skills. Mr. X should be encouraged to exercise as frequently as he can. The importance of daily stretching exercise cannot be overemphasized in patients entering the advanced PD stages. Assistive equipment such as a cane, walker, or push-cart may help prevent falls.

ACKNOWLEDGMENTS

The authors acknowledge Ellen Matthiesen and Marilyn Trail for their help and suggestions, and John Van for preparing the photographs in this chapter.

REFERENCES

1. Lang AE, Lozano AM. Parkinson's disease. First of two parts. *N Engl J Med*. 1998;339:1044-1053. Parkinson's disease. Second of two parts. *N Engl J Med*. 1998;339:1130-1143.
2. Tanner CM, Aston DA. Epidemiology of Parkinson's disease and akinetic syndromes. *Curr Opin Neurol*. 2000;13:427-430.
3. Siderowf A. Parkinson's disease: clinical features, epidemiology and genetics. *Neurol Clin*. 2001;19:565-578.
4. Parkinson J. An essay on the shaking palsy. 1817. *J Neuropsychiatry Clin Neurosci*. 2002;14:223-236. Discussion:222.
5. Goetz CG. Charcot on Parkinson's disease. *Mov Disord*. 1986;1:27-32.
6. Kapp W. The history of drugs for the treatment of Parkinson's disease. *J Neural Transm*. 1992;38(suppl):1-6.
7. Mettler FA. The substantia nigra and parkinsonism. *Trans Am Neurol Assoc*. 1964;89:68-73.
8. Braak H, Rub U, Jansen Steur EN, Del Tredici K, de Vos RA. Cognitive status correlates with neuropathologic stage in Parkinson disease. *Neurology*. 2005;64:1404-1410.
9. Speelman JD, Bosch DA. Resurgence of functional neurosurgery for Parkinson's disease: a historical perspective. *Mov Disord*. 1998;13:582-588.
10. Birkmayer W, Hornykiewicz O. The L-dihydroxyphenylalanine (L-DOPA) effect in Parkinson's syndrome in man: on the pathogenesis and treatment of Parkinson akinesis. *Arch Psychiatr Nervenkr Z Gesamte Neurol Psychiatr*. 1962;203:560-574. German.
11. Cotzias GC, Van Woert MH, Schiffer LM. Aromatic amino acids and modification of parkinsonism. *N Engl J Med*. 1967;276:374-379.
12. Benabid AL, Pollak P, Seigneuret E, Hoffmann D, Gay E, Perret J. Chronic VIM thalamic stimulation in Parkinson's disease, essential tremor and extra-pyramidal dyskinesias. *Acta Neurochir Suppl* (Wien).1993;58:39-44.
13. Bennett DA, Beckett LA, Murray AM, et al. Prevalence of parkinsonian signs and associated mortality in a community population of older people. *N Engl J Med*. 1996;334:71-76.
14. Bower JH, Maraganore DM, McDonnell SK, Rocca WA. Incidence and distribution of parkinsonism in Olmsted County, Minnesota, 1976-1990. *Neurology*. 1999;52:1214-1220.
15. de Rijk MC, Launer LJ, Berger K, et al. Prevalence of Parkinson's disease in Europe: a collaborative study of population-based cohorts. Neurologic Diseases in the Elderly Research Group. *Neurology*. 2000;54(suppl): S21-23.
16. de Rijk MC, Rocca WA, Anderson DW, Melcon MO, Breteler MM, Maraganore DM. A population perspective on diagnostic criteria for Parkinson's disease. *Neurology*. 1997;48:1277-1281.

17. von Campenhausen S, Bornschein B, Wick R, et al. Prevalence and incidence of Parkinson's disease in Europe. *Eur Neuropsychopharmacol.* 2005;15:473-490.

18. Li SC, Schoenberg BS, Wang CC, et al. A prevalence survey of Parkinson's disease and other movement disorders in the People's Republic of China. *Arch Neurol.* 1985;42:655-657.

19. Woo J, Lau E, Ziea E, Chan DK. Prevalence of Parkinson's disease in a Chinese population. *Acta Neurol Scand.* 2004;109:228-231.

20. Chan DK, Cordato D, Bui T, Mellick G, Woo J. Comparison of environmental and genetic factors for Parkinson's disease between Chinese and Caucasians. *Neuroepidemiology.* 2004;23:13-22.

21. Schoenberg BS, Osuntokun BO, Adeuja AO, et al. Comparison of the prevalence of Parkinson's disease in black populations in the rural United States and in rural Nigeria: door-to-door community studies. *Neurology.* 1988;38:645-646.

22. Mayeux R, Marder K, Cote LJ, et al. The frequency of idiopathic Parkinson's disease by age, ethnic group, and sex in northern Manhattan, 1988-1993. *Am J Epidemiol.* 1995;142:820-827. Erratum in: *Am J Epidemiol.* 1996;143:528.

23. Schoenberg BS, Anderson DW, Haerer AF. Prevalence of Parkinson's disease in the biracial population of Copiah County, Mississippi. *Neurology.* 1985;35:841-845.

24. de Rijk MC, Tzourio C, Breteler MM, et al. Prevalence of parkinsonism and Parkinson's disease in Europe: the EUROPARKINSON Collaborative Study. European Community Concerted Action on the Epidemiology of Parkinson's disease. *J Neurol Neurosurg Psychiatry.* 1997;62:10-15.

25. Kessler II. Parkinson's disease in epidemiologic perspective. *Adv Neurol.*1978;19:355-384.

26. Kuopio AM, Marttila RJ, Helenius H, Rinne UK. Environmental risk factors in Parkinson's disease. *Mov Disord.* 1999;14:928-939.

27. Shulman LM, Bhat V. Gender disparities in Parkinson's disease. *Expert Rev Neurother.* 2006;6:407-416.

28. Huse DM, Schulman K, Orsini L, Castelli-Haley J, Kennedy S, Lenhart G. Burden of illness in Parkinson's disease. *Mov Disord.* 2005;20:1449-1454.

29. Lindgren P, von Campenhausen S, Spottke E, Siebert U, Dodel R. Cost of Parkinson's disease in Europe. *Eur J Neurol.* 2005;12(Suppl):68-73.

30. Cubo E, Alvarez E, Morant C, et al. Burden of disease related to Parkinson's disease in Spain in the year 2000. *Mov Disord.* 2005;20:1481-1487.

31. Chun HS, Gibson GE, DeGiorgio LA, Zhang H, Kidd VJ, Son JH. Dopaminergic cell death induced by MPP(+), oxidant and specific neurotoxicants shares the common molecular mechanism. *J Neurochem.* 2001;76:1010-1021.

32. Fernandez-Espejo E. Pathogenesis of Parkinson's disease: prospects of neuroprotective and restorative therapies. *Mol Neurobiol.* 2004;29:15-30.

33. Mariani E, Polidori MC, Cherubini A, Mecocci P. Oxidative stress in brain aging, neurodegenerative and vascular diseases: an overview. *J Chromatogr B Analyt Technol Biomed Life Sci.* 2005;827:65-75.

34. Srinivasan V, Pandi-Perumal SR, Maestroni GJ, Esquifino AI, Hardeland R, Cardinali DP. Role of melatonin in neurodegenerative diseases. *Neurotox Res.* 2005;7:293-318.

35. Gandhi S, Wood NW. Molecular pathogenesis of Parkinson's disease. *Hum Mol Genet.* 2005;14:2749-2755.

36. Tanner CM, Ottman R, Goldman SM, et al. Parkinson disease in twins: an etiologic study. *JAMA.* 1999;281:341-346.

37. Lucking CB, Durr A, Bonifati V, et al. Association between early-onset Parkinson's disease and mutations in the parkin gene. French Parkinson's Disease Genetics Study Group. *N Engl J Med.* 2000;342:1560-1567.

38. Gwinn-Hardy K, Mehta ND, Farrer M, et al. Distinctive neuropathology revealed by alpha-synuclein antibodies in hereditary parkinsonism and dementia linked to chromosome 4p. *Acta Neuropathol* (Berl). 2000;99:663-672.

39. Giasson BI, Lee VMY. A new link between pesticides and Parkinson's disease. *Nature Neurosci.* 2000;3:1227-1228.

40. Muller T, Woitalla D, Kuhn W. Benefit of folic acid supplementation in parkinsonian patients treated with levodopa. *J Neurol Neurosurg Psychiatry.* 2003;74:549.

41. Chen H, Zhang SM, Schwarzschild MA, et al. Folate intake and risk of Parkinson's disease. *Am J Epidemiol.* 2004;160:368-375.

42. Benedetti MD, Bower JH, Maraganore DM, et al. Smoking, alcohol, and coffee consumption preceding Parkinson's disease: a case-control study. *Neurology.* 2000;55:1350-1358.

43. Elbaz A, Manubens-Bertran JM, Balderischi M, et al. Parkinson's disease, smoking, and family history. EUROPARKINSON Study Group. *J Neurol.* 2000;247:793-798.

44. Tanner CM, Goldman SM, Aston DA, et al. Smoking and Parkinson's disease in twins. *Neurology.* 2002;58:581-588.

45. Langston JW, Irwin I, Ricaurte GA. Neurotoxins, parkinsonism and Parkinson's disease. *Pharmacol Ther.* 1987;32(1):19-49.

46. Abbott RD, Ross GW, White LR, et al. Environmental, life-style, and physical precursors of clinical Parkinson's disease: recent findings from the Honolulu-Asia Aging Study. *J Neurol.* 2003;250:30-39.

47. Ascherio A, Chen H, Schwarzschild MA, Zhang SM, Colditz GA, Speizer FE. Caffeine, postmenopausal estrogen, and risk of Parkinson's disease. *Neurology.* 2003;60:790-795.

48. Ross GW, Petrovitch H. Current evidence for neuroprotective effects of nicotine and caffeine against Parkinson's disease. *Drugs Aging.* 2001;18:797-806.

49. Schwarzschild MA, Chen JF, Ascherio A. Caffeinated clues and the promise of adenosine A(2A) antagonists in PD. *Neurology.* 2002;58:1154-1160.

50. German DC, Manaye K, Smith WK, Woodward DJ, Saper CB. Midbrain dopaminergic cell loss in Parkinson's disease: computer visualization. *Ann Neurol.* 1989;26:507-514.

51. Graybiel AM, Hirsch EC, Agid Y. The nigrostriatal system in Parkinson's disease. *Adv Neurol.* 1990;53:17-29.

52. Wakabayashi K, Takahashi H. Neuropathology of autonomic nervous system in Parkinson's disease. *Eur Neurol.* 1997;38(suppl):2-7.

53. Micieli G, Tosi P, Marcheselli S, Cavallini A. Autonomic dysfunction in Parkinson's disease. *Neurol Sci.* 2003;24(suppl):S32-34.

54. Zarow C, Lyness SA, Mortimer JA, Chui HC. Neuronal loss is greater in the locus coeruleus than nucleus basalis and substantia nigra in Alzheimer and Parkinson diseases. *Arch Neurol.* 2003;60:337-341.

55. Bosboom JL, Stoffers D, Wolters EC. Cognitive dysfunction and dementia in Parkinson's disease. *J Neural Transm.* 2004;111:1303-1315.

56. Jellinger KA. Lewy body-related alpha-synucleinopathy in the aged human brain. *J Neural Transm.* 2004;111:1219-1235.

57. Jellinger KA. Morphological substrates of mental dysfunction in Lewy body disease: an update. *J Neural Transm.* 2000;59(suppl):185-212.

58. Wolters EC. Psychiatric complications in Parkinson's disease. *J Neural Transm.* 2000;60(suppl):291-302.

59. Marsden CD, Obeso JA. The functions of the basal ganglia and the paradox of stereotaxic surgery in Parkinson's disease. *Brain.* 1994;117:877-897.

60. Gibb WR. Functional neuropathology in Parkinson's disease. *Eur Neurol.* 1997;38 (suppl):21-25.

61. Blandini F, Nappi G, Tassorelli C, Martignoni E. Functional changes of the basal ganglia circuitry in Parkinson's disease. *Prog Neurobiol.* 2000;62:63-88.

62. Obeso JA, Rodriguez-Oroz MC, Rodriguez M, et al. Pathophysiologic basis of surgery for Parkinson's disease. *Neurology.* 2000;55(suppl):S7-12.

63. Silkis I. The cortico-basal ganglia-thalamocortical circuit with synaptic plasticity. II. Mechanism of synergistic modulation of thalamic activity via the direct and indirect pathways through the basal ganglia. *Biosystems.* 2001;59:7-14.

64. Lee CS, Schulzer M, Mak E, Hammerstad JP, Calne S, Calne DB. Patterns of asymmetry do not change over the course of idiopathic parkinsonism: implications for pathogenesis. *Neurology.* 1995;45:435-439.

65. Hughes AJ, Ben-Shlomo Y, Daniel SE, Lees AJ. What features improve the accuracy of clinical diagnosis in Parkinson's disease: a clinicopathologic study. *Neurology.* 2001;57(suppl):S34-38.

66. Oppel F, Umbach WU. A quantitative measurement of tremor. *Electroencephalogr Clin Neurophysiol.* 1977;43:885-888.

67. Griffiths RA, Dalziel JA, Sinclair KG, Dennis PD, Good WR. Tremor and senile parkinsonism. *J Gerontol.* 1981;36:170-175.

68. Findley LJ, Gresty MA, Halmagyi GM. Tremor, the cogwheel phenomenon and clonus in Parkinson's disease. *J Neurol Neurosurg Psychiatry.* 1981;44:534-546.

69. Jankovic J, Schwartz KS, Ondo W. Re-emergent tremor of Parkinson's disease. *J Neurol Neurosurg Psychiatry.* 1999;67:646-650.

70. Weintraub D, Stern MB. Psychiatric complications in Parkinson disease. *Am J Geriatr Psychiatry.* 2005;13:844-851.

71. Pollock M, Hornabrook RW. The prevalence, natural history and dementia of Parkinson's disease. *Brain.* 1966;89:429-448.

72. Rippon GA, Marder KS. Dementia in Parkinson's disease. *Adv Neurol.* 2005;96:95-113.

73. Rajput AH, Rozdilsky B, Rajput A. Alzheimer's disease and idiopathic Parkinson's disease coexistence. *J Geriatr Psychiatry Neurol.* 1993;6:170-176.

74. Brown DF, Dababo MA, Bigio EH, et al. Neuropathologic evidence that the Lewy body variant of Alzheimer disease represents coexistence of Alzheimer disease and idiopathic Parkinson disease. *J Neuropathol Exp Neurol.* 1998;57:39-46.

75. Bertrand E, Lechowicz W, Szpak GM, Lewandowska E, Dymecki J, Wierzba-Bobrowicz T. Limbic neuropathology in idiopathic Parkinson's disease with concomitant dementia. *Folia Neuropathol.* 2004;42:141-150.

76. Iseki E. Dementia with Lewy bodies: reclassification of pathological subtypes and boundary with Parkinson's disease or Alzheimer's disease. *Neuropathology.* 2004;24:72-78.

77. Alexander GE, DeLong MR, Strick PL. Parallel organization of functionally segregated circuits linking basal ganglia and cortex. *Annu Rev Neurosci.* 1986;9:357-381.
78. Rippon GA, Marder KS. Dementia in Parkinson's disease. *Adv Neurol.* 2005;96:95-113.
79. Cooper B, Holmes C. Previous psychiatric history as a risk factor for late-life dementia: a population-based case-control study. *Age Ageing.* 1998;27:181-188.
80. Haugarvoll K, Aarsland D, Wentzel-Larsen T, Larsen JP. The influence of cerebrovascular risk factors on incident dementia in patients with Parkinson's disease. *Acta Neurol Scand.* 2005;112:386-390.
81. Fenelon G, Mahieux F, Huon R, Ziegler M. Hallucinations in Parkinson's disease: prevalence, phenomenology and risk factors. *Brain.* 2000;123:733-745.
82. Miyasaki JM, Shannon K, Voon V, et al. Quality Standards Subcommittee of the American Academy of Neurology. Practice Parameter: evaluation and treatment of depression, psychosis, and dementia in Parkinson disease (an evidence-based review): report of the Quality Standards Subcommittee of the American Academy of Neurology. *Neurology.* 2006;66:996-1002.
83. Habermann-Little B. An analysis of the prevalence and etiology of depression in Parkinson's disease. *J Neurosci Nurs.* 1991;23:165-169.
84. Kostic VS, Filipovic SR, Lecic D, Momcilovic D, Sokic D, Sternic N. Effect of age at onset on frequency of depression in Parkinson's disease. *J Neurol Neurosurg Psychiatry.* 1994;57:1265-1267.
85. Hantz P, Caradoc-Davies G, Caradoc-Davies T, Weatherall M, Dixon G. Depression in Parkinson's disease. *Am J Psychiatry.* 1994;151:1010-1014.
86. Veazey C, Aki SO, Cook KF, Lai EC, Kunik ME. Prevalence and treatment of depression in Parkinson's disease. *J Neuropsychiatry Clin Neurosci.* 2005;17:310-323.
87. Menza MA, Robertson-Hoffman DE, Bonapace AS. Parkinson's disease and anxiety: comorbidity with depression. *Biol Psychiatry.* 1993;34:465-470.
88. Menza MA, Sage J, Marshall E, Cody R, Duvoisin R. Mood changes and "on-off" phenomena in Parkinson's disease. *Mov Disord.* 1990;5:148-151.
89. Nissenbaum H, Quinn NP, Brown RG, Toone B, Gotham AM, Marsden CD. Mood swings associated with the 'on-off' phenomenon in Parkinson's disease. *Psychol Med.* 1987;17:899-904.
90. Siemers ER, Shekhar A, Quaid K, Dickson H. Anxiety and motor performance in Parkinson's disease. *Mov Disord.* 1993;8:501-506.
91. Maricle RA, Nutt JG, Carter JH. Mood and anxiety fluctuation in Parkinson's disease associated with levodopa infusion: preliminary findings. *Mov Disord.* 1995;10:329-332.
92. Santamaria J, Tolosa ES, Valles A, Bayes A, Blesa R, Masana J. Mental depression in untreated Parkinson's disease of recent onset. *Adv Neurol.* 1987;45:443-446.
93. Rye DB. Excessive daytime sleepiness and unintended sleep in Parkinson's disease. *Curr Neurol Neurosci Rep.* 2006;6:169-176.
94. Garcia-Borreguero D, Odin P, Serrano C. Restless legs syndrome and PD: a review of the evidence for a possible association. *Neurology.* 2003;61(suppl):S49-55.
95. Rye DB. Parkinson's disease and RLS: the dopaminergic bridge. *Sleep Med.* 2004;5:317-328.
96. Poewe W, Hogl B. Akathisia, restless legs and periodic limb movements in sleep in Parkinson's disease. *Neurology.* 2004;63(suppl):S12-16.
97. Onofrj M, Thomas A, D'Andreamatteo G, et al. Incidence of RBD and hallucination in patients affected by Parkinson's disease: 8-year follow-up. *Neurol Sci.* 2002;23(suppl): S91-94.
98. Lauterbach EC. The neuropsychiatry of Parkinson's disease and related disorders. *Psychiatr Clin North Am.* 2004;27:801-825.
99. Postuma RB, Lang AE, Massicotte-Marquez J, Montplaisir J. Potential early markers of Parkinson disease in idiopathic REM sleep behavior disorder. *Neurology.* 2006;66:845-851.
100. Dewey RB Jr. Autonomic dysfunction in Parkinson's disease. *Neurol Clin.* 2004;22(suppl):S127-139.
101. Adler CH. Nonmotor complications in Parkinson's disease. *Mov Disord.* 2005;20(suppl):S23-29.
102. Goldstein DS. Orthostatic hypotension as an early finding in Parkinson's disease. *Clin Auton Res.* 2006;16:46-54.
103. Ueki A and Otsuka M. Life style risks of Parkinson's disease: association between decreased water intake and constipation. *J Neurol.* 2004;251(suppl)18-23.
104. Winge K, Skau AM, Stimpel H, Nielsen KK, Werdelin L. Prevalence of bladder dysfunction in Parkinsons disease. *Neurourol Urodyn.* 2006;25:116-122.
105. Papatsoris AG, Deliveliotis C, Singer C, Papapetropoulos S. Erectile dysfunction in Parkinson's disease. *Urology.* 2006;67:447-451.
106. Fahn S, Elton R, Members of the UPDRS Development Committee. In: Fahn S, Marsden CD, Calne DB, Goldstein M, eds. *Recent Developments in Parkinson's Disease*, Vol 2. Florham Park, NJ: Macmillan Health Care Information; 1987;153-163;293-304.
107. Hoehn MM, Yahr MD. Parkinsonism: onset, progression and mortality. *Neurology.* 1967;17:427-442.

108. McRae C, Diem G, Vo A, O'Brien C, Seeberger L. Schwab & England: standardization of administration. *Mov Disord.* 2000;15:335-336.
109. Becker G, Muller A, Braune S, et al. Early diagnosis of Parkinson's disease. *J Neurol.* 2002;249(suppl):40-48.
110. Jankovic J. Parkinson's disease therapy: tailoring choices for early and late disease, young and old patients. *Clin Neuropharmacol.* 2000;23:252-261.
111. Diederich NJ, Moore CG, Leurgans SE, Chmura TA, Goetz CG. Parkinson disease with old-age onset: a comparative study with subjects with middle-age onset. *Arch Neurol.* 2003;60:529-533.
112. Schrag A, Ben-Shlomo Y, Brown R, Marsden CD, Quinn N. Young-onset Parkinson's disease revisited-clinical features, natural history, and mortality. *Mov Disord.* 1998;13:885-894.
113. Colcher A, Simuni T. Clinical manifestations of Parkinson's disease. *Med Clin North Am.* 1999;83:327-347.
114. Witjas T, Kaphan E, Azulay JP, et al. Nonmotor fluctuations in Parkinson's disease: frequent and disabling. *Neurology.* 2002;59:408-413.
115. Marras C, Rochon P, Lang AE. Predicting motor decline and disability in Parkinson disease: a systematic review. *Arch Neurol.* 2002;59:1724-1728.
116. Weintraub D, Moberg PJ, Duda JE, Katz IR, Stern MB. Effect of psychiatric and other nonmotor symptoms on disability in Parkinson's disease. *J Am Geriatr Soc.* 2004;52:784-788.
117. de Jong GJ, Meerwaldt JD, Schmitz PI. Factors that influence the occurrence of response variations in Parkinson's disease. *Ann Neurol.* 1987;22:4-7.
118. Hauser RA, Deckers F, Lehert P. Parkinson's disease home diary: further validation and implications for clinical trials. *Mov Disord.* 2004;19:1409-1413.
119. Larsen JP, Karlsen K, Tandberg E. Clinical problems in non-fluctuating patients with Parkinson's disease: a community-based study. *Mov Disord.* 2000;15:826-829.
120. Ahlskog JE, Muenter MD. Frequency of levodopa-related dyskinesias and motor fluctuations as estimated from the cumulative literature. *Mov Disord.* 2001;16:448-458.
121. Bonnet AM, Loria Y, Saint-Hilaire MH, Lhermitte F, Agid Y. Does long-term aggravation of Parkinson's disease result from nondopaminergic lesions? *Neurology.* 1987;37:1539-1542.
122. Schaafsma JD, Giladi N, Balash Y, Bartels AL, Gurevich T, Hausdorff JM. Gait dynamics in Parkinson's disease: relationship to Parkinsonian features, falls and response to levodopa. *J Neurol Sci.* 2003;212:47-53.
123. Hausdorff JM, Schaafsma JD, Balash Y, Bartels AL, Gurevich T, Giladi N. Impaired regulation of stride variability in Parkinson's disease subjects with freezing of gait. *Exp Brain Res.* 2003;149:187-194.
124. Gorell JM, Johnson CC, Rybicki BA. Parkinson's disease and its comorbid disorders: an analysis of Michigan mortality data, 1970 to 1990. *Neurology.* 1994;44:1865-1868.
125. de Rijk MC, Rocca WA, Anderson DW, Melcon MO, Breteler MM, Maraganore DM. A population perspective on diagnostic criteria for Parkinson's disease. *Neurology.* 1997;48:1277-1281.
126. Jankovic J, McDermott M, Carter J, et al. Variable expression of Parkinson's disease: a base-line analysis of the DATATOP cohort. The Parkinson Study Group. *Neurology.* 1990;40:1529-1534.
127. Goetz CG, Pappert EJ, Blasucci LM, et al. Intravenous levodopa in hallucinating Parkinson's disease patients: high-dose challenge does not precipitate hallucinations. *Neurology.* 1998;50:515-517.
128. Borghammer P, Kumakura Y, Cumming P. Fluorodopa F. 18 positron emission tomography and the progression of Parkinson disease. *Arch Neurol.* 2005;62:1480.
129. Fischman AJ. Role of [18F]-dopa-PET imaging in assessing movement disorders. *Radiol Clin North Am.* 2005;43:93-106.
130. Filippi L, Manni C, Pierantozzi M, et al. 123I-FP-CIT semi-quantitative SPECT detects preclinical bilateral dopaminergic deficit in early Parkinson's disease with unilateral symptoms. *Nucl Med Commun.* 2005;26:421-426.
131. Wang J, Jiang YP, Liu XD, et al. 99mTc-TRODAT-1 SPECT study in early Parkinson's disease and essential tremor. *Acta Neurol Scand.* 2005;112:380-385.
132. Zweig RM, Lilien DL, Tainter K, Patterson J. The role of radiotracer imaging in Parkinson disease. *Neurology.* 2005;65:1144-1145.
133. Butkovic-Soldo S, Tomic S, Stimac D, et al. Patients review: drug-induced movement disorders. *Coll Antropol.* 2005;29:579-582.
134. Sachdev PS. Neuroleptic-induced movement disorders: an overview. *Psychiatr Clin North Am.* 2005;28:255-274.
135. Weiner WJ. A differential diagnosis of Parkinsonism. *Rev Neurol Dis.* 2005;2:124-131.
136. Tolosa E, Wenning G, Poewe W. The diagnosis of Parkinson's disease. *Lancet Neurol.* 2006;5:75-86.
137. Pearce JM. Neurodegeneration with brain iron accumulation: a cautionary tale. *Eur Neurol.* 2006;56:66-68.
138. Ahlskog JE. Diagnosis and differential diagnosis of Parkinson's disease and parkinsonism. *Parkinsonism Relat Disord.* 2000;7:63-70.
139. Demirkiran M, Bozdemir H, Sarica Y. Vascular parkinsonism: a distinct, heterogeneous clinical entity. *Acta Neurol Scand.* 2001;104:63-67.

140. Rascol O. The pharmacological therapeutic management of levodopa-induced dyskinesias in patients with Parkinson's disease. *J Neurol.* 2000;247(suppl):51-57.

141. Lees AJ, Katzenschlager R, Head J, Ben-Shlomo Y. Ten-year follow-up of three different initial treatments in de-novo PD: a randomized trial. *Neurology.* 2001;57:1687-1694.

142. Holloway RG, Shoulson I, Fahn S, et al. Pramipexole vs. levodopa as initial treatment for Parkinson disease: a 4-year randomized controlled trial. The Parkinson Study Group. *Arch Neurol.* 2004;61:1044-53. Erratum in: *Arch Neurol.* 2005;62:430.

143. Noyes K, Dick AW, Holloway RG. Pramipexole vs. levodopa as initial treatment for Parkinson's disease: a randomized clinical-economic trial. The Parkinson Study Group. *Med Decis Making.* 2004;24:472-485.

144. Vokaer M, Azar NA, de Beyl DZ. Effects of levodopa on upper limb mobility and gait in Parkinson's disease. *J Neurol Neurosurg Psychiatry.* 2003;74:1304-1307.

145. Nyholm D. Pharmacokinetic optimisation in the treatment of Parkinson's disease: an update. *Clin Pharmacokinet.* 2006;45:109-136.

146. Tai CH, Wu RM. Catechol-O-methyltransferase and Parkinson's disease. *Acta Med Okayama.* 2002;56:1-6.

147. Walters C. Other pharmacological treatments for motor complications and dyskinesias. *Mov Disord.* 2005;20(suppl):S38-44.

148. Widnell KL, Comella C. Role of COMT inhibitors and dopamine agonists in the treatment of motor fluctuations. *Mov Disord.* 2005;20(suppl):S30-37.

149. Kumar N, Van Gerpen JA, Bower JH, Ahlskog JE. Levodopa-dyskinesia incidence by age of Parkinson's disease onset. *Mov Disord.* 2005;20:342-344.

150. Mazzella L, Yahr MD, Marinelli L, Huang N, Moshier E, Di Rocco A. Dyskinesias predict the onset of motor response fluctuations in patients with Parkinson's disease on L-dopa monotherapy. *Parkinsonism Relat Disord.* 2005;11:151-155.

151. Rascol O, Brooks DJ, Korczyn AD, De Deyn, PP, Clarke CE, Lang AE. A five year study of the incidence of dyskinesia in patients with early Parkinson's disease who were treated with ropinirole or levodopa. 056 Study Group. *N Engl J Med.* 2000;342:1484-1491.

152. Agid Y, Bonnet AM, Ruberg M, Javoy-Agid F. Pathophysiology of L-dopa-induced abnormal involuntary movements. *Psychopharmacology.* 1985;2(suppl):145-159.

153. Ebadi M, Hama Y. Dopamine, GABA, cholecystokinin and opioids in neuroleptic-induced tardive dyskinesia. *Neurosci Biobehav Rev.* 1988;12:179-187.

154. Piccini P, Weeks RA, Brooks DJ. Alterations in opioid receptor binding in Parkinson's disease patients with levodopa-induced dyskinesias. *Ann Neurol.* 1997;42:720-726.

155. Block G, Liss C, Reines S, Irr J, Nibbelink D. Comparison of immediate-release and controlled release carbidopa/levodopa in Parkinson's disease. A multicenter 5-year study. The CR First Study Group. *Eur Neurol.* 1997;37:23-27.

156. Dupont E, Andersen A, Boas J, et al. Sustained-release Madopar HBS compared with standard Madopar in the long-term treatment of de novo parkinsonian patients. *Acta Neurol Scand.* 1996;93:14-20.

157. Koch G, Brusa L, Caltagirone C, et al. rTMS of supplementary motor area modulates therapy-induced dyskinesias in Parkinson disease. *Neurology.* 2005;65:623-625.

158. Michel PP, Hefti F. Toxicity of 6-hydroxydopamine and dopamine for dopaminergic neurons in culture. *J Neurosci Res.* 1990;26:428-435.

159. Mytilineou C, Han SK, Cohen G. Toxic and protective effects of L-dopa on mesencephalic cell cultures. *J Neurochem.* 1993;61:1470-1478.

160. Mena MA, Pardo B, Paino CL, De Yebenes JG. Levodopa toxicity in foetal rat midbrain neurones in culture: modulation by ascorbic acid. *Neuroreport.* 1993;4:438-440.

161. Mena MA, Davila V, Sulzer D. Neurotrophic effects of L-DOPA in postnatal midbrain dopamine neuron/cortical astrocyte cocultures. *J Neurochem.* 1997;69:1398-1408.

162. Quinn N, Parkes D, Janota I, Marsden CD. Preservation of the substantia nigra and locus coeruleus in a patient receiving levodopa (2 kg) plus decarboxylase inhibitor over a four-year period. *Mov Disord.* 1986;1:65-68.

163. Rajput AH, Fenton M, Birdi S, Macaulay R. Is levodopa toxic to human substantia nigra? *Mov Disord.* 1997;12(5):634-638.

164. Agid Y, Ahlskog E, Albanese A, et al. Levodopa in the treatment of Parkinson's disease: a consensus meeting. *Mov Disord.* 1999;14:911-913.

165. The Parkinson Study Group. Levodopa and the Progression of Parkinson's Disease *NEJM.* 2004;351:2498-2508.

166. Suchowersky O, Gronseth G, Perlmutter J, Reich S, Zesiewicz T, Weiner WJ. Quality Standards Subcommittee of the American Academy of Neurology. Practice Parameter: neuroprotective strategies and alternative therapies for Parkinson disease (an evidence-based review): report of the Quality Standards Subcommittee of the American Academy of Neurology. *Neurology.* 2006;66:976-982.

167. Stacy M. Apomorphine: North American clinical experience. *Neurology.* 2004;62(suppl):S18-21.

168. Watts RL, Jankovic J, Waters C, Rajput A, Boroojerdi B, Rao J. Randomized, blind, controlled trial of transdermal rotigotine in early Parkinson disease. *Neurology.* 2007;68:272-276.

169. Whone AL, Watts RL, Stoessl AJ, et al. REAL-PET Study Group. Slower progression of Parkinson's disease with ropinirole versus levodopa: The REAL-PET study. *Ann Neurol.* 2003;54:93-101.

170. Navan P, Findley LJ, Jeffs JA, Pearce RK, Bain PG. Randomized, double-blind, 3-month parallel study of the effects of pramipexole, pergolide, and placebo on Parkinsonian tremor. *Mov Disord.* 2003;18:1324-1331.

171. Navan P, Findley LJ, Jeffs JA, Pearce RK, Bain PG. Double-blind, single-dose, cross-over study of the effects of pramipexole, pergolide, and placebo on rest tremor and UPDRS part III in Parkinson's disease. *Mov Disord.* 2003;18:176-180.

172. Van Camp G, Flamez A, Cosyns B, Goldstein J, Perdaens C, Schoors D. Heart valvular disease in patients with Parkinson's disease treated with high-dose pergolide. *Neurology.* 2003;61:859-861.

173. Van Camp G, Flamez A, Cosyns B, et al. Treatment of Parkinson's disease with pergolide and relation to restrictive valvular heart disease. *Lancet.* 2004;363:1179-1183.

174. Olanow CW, Obeso JA. Preventing levodopa-induced dyskinesias. *Ann Neurol.* 2000; 47(suppl):S167-176.

175. Rinne UK, Bracco F, Chouza C, et al. Early treatment of Parkinson's disease with cabergoline delays the onset of motor complications. Results of a double-blind levodopa controlled trial. The PKDS009 Study Group. *Drugs.* 1998;55(suppl):23-30.

176. Albin RL, Frey KA. Initial agonist treatment of Parkinson disease: a critique. *Neurology.* 2003;60:390-394.

177. Olanow CW, Stocchi F. Why delaying levodopa is a good treatment strategy in early Parkinson's disease. *Eur J Neurol.* 2000;7(suppl):3-8.

178. Stacy M. Apomorphine: North American clinical experience. *Neurology.* 2004 Mar 23;62(6 Suppl 4):S18-21.

179. LeWitt PA. Subcutaneously administered apomorphine: pharmacokinetics and metabolism. *Neurology.* 2004;62(suppl):S8-11.

180. Koller W, Stacy M. Other formulations and future considerations for apomorphine for subcutaneous injection therapy. *Neurology.* 2004;62(suppl):S22-26.

181. Guldberg HC, Marsden CA. Catechol-O-methyl transferase: pharmacological aspects and physiological role. *Pharmacol Rev.* 1975;27:135-206.

182. Guay DR. Tolcapone, a selective catechol-O-methyltransferase inhibitor for treatment of Parkinson's disease. *Pharmacotherapy.* 1999;19:6-20.

183. Micek ST, Ernst ME. Tolcapone: a novel approach to Parkinson's disease. *Am J Health Syst Pharm.* 1999;56:2195-205.

184. Ahlskog JE. Parkinson's disease: new treatment strategies. *Compr Ther.* 1990;16:41-46.

185. Hauser RA. Levodopa/carbidopa/entacapone (Stalevo). *Neurology.* 2004;62(suppl): S64-71.

186. Wessel K, Szelenyi I. Selegiline—an overview of its role in the treatment of Parkinson's disease. *Clin Investig.* 1992;70:459-462.

187. Yu PH. Pharmacological and clinical implications of MAO-B inhibitors. *Gen Pharmacol.* 1994;25:1527-1539.

188. Gotez ME, Dirr A, Burger R, Rausch WD, Riederer P. High dose selegiline augments striatal ubiquinol in mouse: an indication of decreased oxidative stress or of interference with mitochondrial respiration? A pilot study. *J Neural Transm.* 1995;46(suppl):149-156.

189. Thiffault C, Aumont N, Quirion R, Poirier J. Effect of MPTP and L-deprenyl on antioxidant enzymes and lipid peroxidation levels in mouse brain. *J Neurochem.* 1995;65:2725-2733.

190. Muralikrishnan D, Samantaray S, Mohanakumar KP. D-deprenyl protects nigrostriatal neurons against 1-methyl-4-phenyl-1,2,3,6-tetrahydropyridine-induced dopaminergic neurotoxicity. *Synapse.* 2003;50:7-13.

191. de la Cruz CP, Revilla E, Steffen V, Rodriguez-Gomez JA, Cano J, Machado A. Protection of the aged substantia nigra of the rat against oxidative damage by (-)-deprenyl. *Br J Pharmacol.* 1996;117:1756-1760.

192. Thomas CE, Huber EW, Ohlweiler DF. Hydroxyl and peroxyl radical trapping by the monoamine oxidase-B inhibitors deprenyl and MDL 72,974A: implications for protection of biological substrates. *Free Radic Biol Med.* 1999;22:733-737.

193. LeWitt PA. Deprenyl's effect at slowing progression of parkinsonian disability: the DATATOP study. The Parkinson Study Group. *Acta Neurol Scand.* 1991;136(suppl):79-86.

194. LeWitt P, Oakes D, Cui L. The need for levodopa as an end point of Parkinson's disease progression in a clinical trial of selegiline and alpha-tocopherol. The Parkinson Study Group. *Mov Disord.* 1997;12:183-189.

195. Shoulson I. DATATOP: a decade of neuroprotective inquiry. The Parkinson Study Group. Deprenyl And Tocopherol Antioxidative Therapy Of Parkinsonism. *Ann Neurol.* 1998;44(suppl):S160-166.

196. Goetz CG, Schwid SR, Eberly SW, Oakes D, Shoulson I. Safety of rasagiline in elderly patients with Parkinson disease. *Neurology.* 2006;66:1427-1429.

197. Chen JJ, Ly AV. Rasagiline: a second-generation monoamine oxidase type-B inhibitor for the treatment of Parkinson's disease. *Am J Health Syst Pharm.* 2006;63:915-928.

198. Pahwa R, Factor SA, Lyons KE, et al. Quality Standards Subcommittee of the American Academy of Neurology. Practice Parameter: treatment of Parkinson disease with motor fluctuations and dyskinesia (an evidence-based review): report of the Quality Standards Subcommittee of the American Academy of Neurology. *Neurology.* 2006;66:983-995.

199. Brocks DR. Anticholinergic drugs used in Parkinson's disease: An overlooked class of drugs from a pharmacokinetic perspective. *J Pharm Pharm Sci.* 1999;2:39-46.

200. Kishore A, Snow BJ. Drug management of Parkinson's disease. *Can Fam Physician.* 1996;42:946-952.

201. Verhagen Metman L, Del Dotto P, van den Munckhof P, Fang J, Mouradian MM, Chase TN. Amantadine as treatment for dyskinesias and motor fluctuations in Parkinson's disease. *Neurology.* 1998;50:1323-1326.

202. Snow BJ, Macdonald L, Mcauley D, Wallis W. The effect of amantadine on levodopa-induced dyskinesias in Parkinson's disease: a double-blind, placebo-controlled study. *Clin Neuropharmacol.* 2000;23:82-85.

203. Silver DE, Sahs AL. Livedo reticularis in Parkinson's disease patients treated with amantadine hydrochloride. *Neurology.* 1972;22:665-669.

204. Goetz CG, Poewe W, Rascol O, Sampaio C. Evidence-based medical review update: pharmacological and surgical treatments of Parkinson's disease: 2001 to 2004. *Mov Disord.* 2005;20:523-539.

205. Metman LV, O'Leary ST. Role of surgery in the treatment of motor complications. *Mov Disord.* 2005;20 Suppl 11:S45-56.

206. Paul G. Cell transplantation for patients with Parkinson's disease. *Handb Exp Pharmacol.* 2006:361-388.

207. Jankovic J, Cardoso F, Grossman RG, Hamilton WJ. Outcome after stereotactic thalamotomy for parkinsonian, essential, and other types of tremor. *Neurosurgery.* 1995;37:680-686.

208. Laitinen LV, Bergenheim AT, Hariz MI. Ventroposterolateral pallidotomy can abolish all parkinsonian symptoms. *Stereotact Funct Neurosurg.* 1992;58:14-21.

209. Laitinen LV. Pallidotomy for Parkinson's disease. *Neurosurg Clin N Am.* 1995;6:105-112.

210. Lang AE. Surgery for levodopa-induced dyskinesias. *Ann Neurol.* 2000;47(suppl):S193-199.

211. Lozano AM, Lang AE. Pallidotomy for Parkinson's disease. *Adv Neurol.* 2001;86:413-420.

212. Baron MS, Vitek JL, Bakay RA, et al. Treatment of advanced Parkinson's disease by unilateral posterior GPi pallidotomy: 4-year results of a pilot study. *Mov Disord.* 2000;15:230-237.

213. Fine J, Duff J, Chen R, et al. Long-term follow-up of unilateral pallidotomy in advanced Parkinson's disease. *N Engl J Med.* 2000;342:1708-1714.

214. Higuchi Y, Iacono RP. Surgical complications in patients with Parkinson's disease after posteroventral pallidotomy. *Neurosurgery.* 2003;52:558-571.

215. Bronstein JM, DeSalles A, DeLong MR. Stereotactic pallidotomy in the treatment of Parkinson disease: an expert opinion. *Arch Neurol.* 1999;56:1064-1069.

216. Andy OJ, Jurko MF, Sias FR Jr. Subthalamotomy in treatment of Parkinsonian tremor. *J Neurosurg.* 1963;20:860-870.

217. Hullay J, Velok J, Gombi R, Boczan G. Subthalamotomy in Parkinson's disease. *Confin Neurol.* 1970;32(2):345-348.

218 Diederich N, Goetz CG, Stebbins GT, et al. Blinded evaluation confirms long-term asymmetric effect of unilateral thalamotomy or subthalamotomy on tremor in Parkinson's disease. *Neurology.* 1992;42:1311-1314.

219. Alvarez L, Macias R, Lopez G, et al. Bilateral subthalamotomy in Parkinson's disease: initial and long-term response. *Brain.* 2005;128:570-583.

220. Montgomery EB Jr, Baker KB. Mechanisms of deep brain stimulation and future technical developments. *Neurol Res.* 2000;22:259-266.

221. Israel Z, Hassin-Baer S. Subthalamic stimulation for Parkinson's disease. Isr Med Assoc J. 2005;7:458-463.

222. Schuurman PR, Bosch DA, Bossuyt PM, et al. A comparison of continuous thalamic stimulation and thalamotomy for suppression of severe tremor. *N Engl J Med.* 2000;342:461-468.

223. Kumar R, Lozano AM, Sime E, Halket E, Lang AE. Comparative effects of unilateral and bilateral subthalamic nucleus deep brain stimulation. *Neurology.* 1999;53:561-566.

224. Kumar R, Lozano AM, Kim YJ, et al. Double-blind evaluation of subthalamic nucleus deep brain stimulation in advanced Parkinson's disease. *Neurology.* 1998;51:850-855.

225. Martinez-Martin P, Valldeoriola F, Tolosa E, et al. Bilateral subthalamic nucleus stimulation and quality of life in advanced Parkinson's disease. *Mov Disord.* 2002;17:372-377.

226. Burchiel KJ, Anderson VC, Favre J, Hammerstad JP. Comparison of pallidal and subthalamic nucleus deep brain stimulation for advanced Parkinson's disease: results of a randomized, blinded pilot study. *Neurosurgery.* 1999;45:1375-1382.

227. Molinuevo JL, Valldeoriola F, Tolosa E, et al. Levodopa withdrawal after bilateral subthalamic nucleus stimulation in advanced Parkinson disease. *Arch Neurol.* 2000;57:983-988.

228. Krack P, Poepping M, Weinert D, Schrader B, Deuschl G. Thalamic, pallidal, or subthalamic surgery for Parkinson's disease? *J Neurol.* 2000;247(suppl)122-134.

229. Krack P, Pollak P, Limousin P, Benabid AL. Levodopa-inhibiting effect of pallidal surgery. *Ann Neurol.* 1997;42:129-130.

230. Bejjani BP, Damier P, Arnulf I, et al. Deep brain stimulation in Parkinson's disease: opposite effects of stimulation in the pallidum. *Mov Disord.* 1998;13:969-970.

231. Volkmann J, Sturm V, Weiss P, et al. Bilateral high-frequency stimulation of the internal globus pallidus in advanced Parkinson's disease. *Ann Neurol.* 1998;44:953-961.

232. Krause M, Fogel W, Kloss M, Rasche D, Volkmann J, Tronnier V. Pallidal stimulation for dystonia. *Neurosurgery.* 2004;55:1361-1368.

233. Vidailhet M, Vercueil L, Houeto JL, et al. French Stimulation du Pallidum Interne dans la Dystonie (SPIDY) Study Group. Bilateral deep-brain stimulation of the globus pallidus in primary generalized dystonia. *N Engl J Med.* 2005;352:459-467.

234. Limousin P, Krack P, Pollak P, et al. Electrical stimulation of the subthalamic nucleus in advanced Parkinson's disease. *N Engl J Med.* 1998;339:1105-1111.

235. Madrazo I, Drucker-Colin R, Diaz V, Martinez-Mata J, Torres C, Becerril JJ. Open microsurgical autograft of adrenal medulla to the right caudate nucleus in two patients with intractable Parkinson's disease. *N Engl J Med.* 1987;316:831-834.

236. Madrazo I, Leon V, Torres C, et al. Transplantation of fetal substantia nigra and adrenal medulla to the caudate nucleus in two patients with Parkinson's disease. *N Engl J Med.* 1988;318:51.

237. Freed CR, Greene PE, Breeze RE, et al. Transplantation of embryonic dopamine neurons for severe Parkinson's disease. *N Engl J Med.* 2001;344:710-719.

238. Greene PE, Fahn S. Status of fetal tissue transplantation for the treatment of advanced Parkinson disease. *Neurosurg Focus.* 2002;13:3.

239. Schumacher JM, Ellias SA, Palmer EP, et al. Transplantation of embryonic porcine mesencephalic tissue in patients with PD. *Neurology.* 2000;54:1042-1050.

240. Stover NP, Bakay RA, Subramanian T, Raiser CD, Cornfeldt ML, Schweikert AW, Allen RC, Watts RL. Intrastriatal implantation of human retinal pigment epithelial cells attached to microcarriers in advanced Parkinson disease. *Arch Neurol.* 2005; 62:1833-1837.

241. Pisani A, Centonze D, Bernardi G, Calabresi P. Striatal synaptic plasticity: implications for motor learning and Parkinson's disease. *Mov Disord.* 2005;20:395-402.

242. Ueki Y, Mima T, Kotb MA, et al. Altered plasticity of the human motor cortex in Parkinson's disease. *Ann Neurol.* 2006;59:60-71.

243. Harburn KL, Hill KM, Kramer JF, Noh S, Vandervoort AA, Matheson JE. An overhead harness and trolly system for balance and ambulation assessment and training. *Arch Phys Med Rehabil.* 1993;74:220-223.

244. Gauthier L, Dalziel S, Gauthier S. The benefits of group occupational therapy for patients with Parkinson's disease. *Am J Occup Ther.* 1987;41:360-365.

245. Gaudet P. Measuring the impact of Parkinson's disease: an occupational therapy perspective. *Can J Occup Ther.* 2002;69:104-113.

246. Hammen VL, Yorkston KM. Speech and pause characteristics following speech rate reduction in hypokinetic dysarthria. *J Commun Disord.* 1996;29:429-444.

247. Clarke CE, Gullaksen E, Macdonald S, Lowe F. Referral criteria for speech and language therapy assessment of dysphagia caused by idiopathic Parkinson's disease. *Acta Neurol Scand.* 1998;97:27-35.

248. Ramig LO, Countryman S, O'Brien C, Hoehn M, Thompson L. Intensive speech treatment for patients with Parkinson's disease: short-and long-term comparison of two techniques. *Neurology.* 1996;47:1496-1504.

249. Ramig LO, Fox C, Sapir S. Parkinson's disease: speech and voice disorders and their treatment with the Lee Silverman Voice Treatment. *Semin Speech Lang.* 2004;25:169-180.

250. Eisenberg DM, Davis RB, Ettner SL, et al. Trends in alternative medicine use in the United States, 1990-1997: results of a follow-up national survey. *JAMA.* 1998;280:1569-1575.

251. Ishikawa T, Funahashi T, Kudo J. Effectiveness of the Kampo kami-shoyo-san (TJ-24) for tremor of antipsychotic-induced parkinsonism. *Psychiatry Clin Neurosci.* 2000;54:579-582.

252. Shults CW, Flint Beal M, Song D, Fontaine D. Pilot trial of high dosages of coenzyme Q10 in patients with Parkinson's disease. *Exp Neurol.* 2004;188:491-494.

253. Etminan M, Gill SS, Samii A. Intake of vitamin E, vitamin C, and carotenoids and the risk of Parkinson's disease: a meta-analysis. *Lancet Neurol.* 2005;4:362-365.

254. Blindauer K, Shoulson I, Oakes D, et al. A randomized controlled trial of etilevodopa in patients with Parkinson disease who have motor fluctuations. The Parkinson Study Group. *Arch Neurol.* 2006;63:210-216.

255. Zareba G. Rotigotine: a novel dopamine agonist for the transdermal treatment of Parkinson's disease. *Drugs Today* (Barcelona). 2006;42:21-28.

256. Blandini F. Neuroprotection by rasagiline: a new therapeutic approach to Parkinson's disease? *CNS Drug Rev.* 2005;11:183-194.

257. Pinna A, Wardas J, Simola N, Morelli M. New therapies for the treatment of Parkinson's disease: adenosine A2A receptor antagonists. *Life Sci.* 2005;77:3259-3267.

258. Hadaczek P, Kohutnicka M, Krauze MT, et al. Convection-enhanced delivery of adeno-associated virus type 2 (AAV2) into the striatum and transport of AAV2 within monkey brain. *Hum Gene Ther.* 2006;17:291-302.

259. Dowd E, Monville C, Torres EM, et al. Lentivector-mediated delivery of GDNF protects complex motor functions relevant to human Parkinsonism in a rat lesion model. *Eur J Neurosci.* 2005;22:2587-2595.

260. Fjord-Larsen L, Johansen JL, Kusk P, et al. Efficient in vivo protection of nigral dopaminergic neurons by lentiviral gene transfer of a modified Neurturin construct. *Exp Neurol.* 2005;195:49-60.

261. Correia AS, Anisimov SV, Li JY, Brundin P. Stem cell-based therapy for Parkinson's disease. *Ann Med.* 2005;37:487-498.

262. Moriyasu K, Yamazoe H, Iwata H. Induction dopamine releasing cells from mouse embryonic stem cells and their long-term culture. *J Biomed Mater Res A.* 2006;77:136-147.

263. Shimizu K, Yamada M, Matsui Y, Tamura K, Moriuchi S, Mogami H. Neural transplantation in mouse Parkinson's disease. *Stereotact Funct Neurosurg.* 1990;54-55:353-357.

264. Gordon PH, Yu Q, Qualls C, et al. Reaction time and movement time after embryonic cell implantation in Parkinson disease. *Arch Neurol.* 2004;61:858-861.

2

NEUROPLASTICITY: IMPLICATIONS FOR PARKINSON'S DISEASE

Sheila Mun-Bryce, OTR, PhD

BRAIN PLASTICITY ACROSS THE LIFESPAN

Neuroplasticity, the nervous system's normal capacity to change in response to a stimulus, is prevalent throughout the human lifespan. Nervous system plasticity is the basis of learning, as in a toddler first identifying colors; the basis of relearning, as in an American driving on the left side of the road in England; and the basis of adaptation, as in a high altitude long distance runner having to compete in the subtropical Florida Everglades.[1] Each of these behavioral experiences stimulates and modifies the nervous system. The ability of the nervous system to change in response to a stimulus is the fundamental premise of occupational therapy, physical therapy, and speech-language therapy; it is the physiological mechanism underlying rehabilitation in the clinic and developmental readiness in the classroom. Plastic changes within the nervous system are crucial for treatment goals to be achieved.

Biochemical, structural, and physiological alterations occur in the nervous system in response to behavioral experience and learning.[2] Long-term functional changes resulting from behavioral experience and learning are associated with the modification and strengthening of synaptic connections. Classically, this synaptic junction includes the pre-synaptic terminal of one neuron, the post-synaptic region of another neuron, and the synaptic cleft that separates the two neurons (Figure 2-1). Inhibitory or excitatory signals are propagated from one cell to the next by the release of a chemical molecule or neurotransmitter, from vesicles in the pre-synaptic terminal into the synaptic cleft. The neurotransmitter binds to the post-synaptic receptors of the second neuron and signal transmission results.

Figure 2-1. Anatomy of a simple synaptic junction. Signal transmission from one neuron to another occurs at the synapse. Action potentials propagate toward the axon terminal of the pre-synaptic neuron, triggering synaptic vesicles to release a chemical neurotransmitter into the synaptic cleft. The neurotransmitter diffuses across the minute space that separates the two neuronal cells and binds to receptors on the post-synaptic neuron. This receptor binding activates cellular events and signal transmission in the post-synaptic neuron.

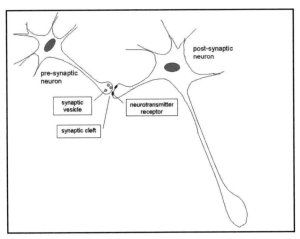

Figure 2-2. Evidence of neuroplastic changes as a result of behavioral experience and learning in neuron on right as compared to neuron on left in illustration. Evidence of structural changes in the post-synaptic dendritic region and the pre-synaptic axon terminal region of neurons have been detected, including: A) increased dendritic branching, B) increased dendritic spine density, C) increased number of perforated synapses, and D) increased number of multiple synaptic connections per neuron.

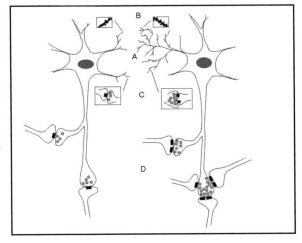

Behavioral experience and learning have been associated with the anatomical modification of existing neural circuitry. Structural changes in the post-synaptic dendritic region and in the pre-synaptic axon terminal region of neurons have been repeatedly quantified as a result of environmental enrichment and motor learning experiments. As depicted in Figure 2-2, morphological alterations include increases in branching and spine density in dendrites and increased number of perforated synapses and number of multiple synaptic connections per neuron.[3-5] The persistence of a neuronal change has also been delineated biochemically by measuring changes in neurotransmitters such as glutamate, acetylcholine, and dopamine.

Although the word *neuroplasticity* implies that plastic processes occur only in neurons, evidence of plasticity has also been found in non-neuronal cells such as astrocytes, glia, and oligodendrocytes. Myelination of neuronal axons by oligodendrocytes and Schwann cells is a form of neural plasticity that is responsive to behavioral experience and learning environments. This process has been shown to continue well into the adult years and plays a critical role in neural tissue repair following injury. The morphological changes observed in astrocytes appear to parallel alterations seen in neurons in response to increased activity. Scientific evidence has demonstrated that these non-neuronal cells can modulate the local environment to optimize synaptic efficacy.[6] Normal nervous system development and recovery from injury stimulate a plastic environment that promotes change in neuronal and non-neuronal cells.

Early neurophysiological studies used recording electrodes to delineate the receptive fields of neurons in the somatosensory cortex representing different parts of the body. Similarly, maps of the motor cortex were generated by stimulating neural fields to elicit movement of various skeletal muscles. Research in cortical plasticity has furthered the understanding of how these cortical maps are readily altered as a result of peripheral nerve denervation or loss of a specific body part.[7]

Behavioral experience can also modify these cortical maps. Multiple neuroplastic mechanisms are involved in the functional reorganization of cortical brain regions. The *use-dependent hypothesis* of cortical plasticity postulates that neural activity or use of specific sensory and motor pathways can produce plastic changes in the brain. Repetitive, use-dependent behavior generates plasticity and cortical reorganization in an organism. Modification of local synaptic processes underlies the use-dependent alterations of motor output.

As an extension of the use-dependent hypothesis, the *learning-dependent hypothesis* specifies that changes in cortical map representation require the acquisition of a novel sensory, motor, or perceptual skill. Repetitive use-dependent behavior alone does not underlie the modification of cortical maps. The learning-dependent hypothesis is based on experimental results demonstrating an expansion of the corresponding motor representation fields only when specific muscle movements required to achieve the task were successfully learned. Task-related functional reorganization occurs only when accompanied by skill learning.[8]

Human studies that map the receptive fields of neurons in the somatosensory and motor cortices have demonstrated that representations of the hand can be altered by sensory experience and repetitive practice of a specific sensorimotor skill. The cortical representation of the digits of the skilled hand in the sensorimotor cortex is expanded in string musicians and blind Braille readers as compared to the unskilled hand.[9]

Evidence of plasticity has been demonstrated in subcortical brain regions, such as the basal ganglia and substantia nigra, which are susceptible to the degenerative processes of Parkinson's disease (PD).[10] This chapter will review how the central nervous system adapts following a lesion, and therapeutic approaches that enhance neuroplasticity and recovery of function. New research in neuroimaging techniques and constraint induced movement therapy will also be explored, as well as how reorganization of cortical networks affect motor control, particularly in PD rehabilitation. We will also examine how rehabilitative therapy can enhance nervous system plasticity such that effective interventions can be developed in neurodegenerative diseases such as PD.

NEURAL REORGANIZATION FOLLOWING BRAIN INJURY

Cortical regions of the brain are functionally silent shortly after brain injury or stroke.[11] The brain's responsiveness to external stimulation, as measured electrophysiologically by event-related potentials, is reduced or absent. Functional mapping of brain activity indicates a decrease in the cortical representation of body regions that were affected by injury. Motor paresis and loss of consciousness or cognitive functioning are prominent clinical manifestations during this critical period. Early neuroplastic changes that manifest as a result of brain injury or neurodegeneration can be due in part to a disinhibition of intact brain regions, deafferentation and degeneration of structural inputs, and the loss of neurotransmitters (Figure 2-3).

Neuroplastic changes that occur during normal development are time-, location-, and activity-dependent. Scientific studies have shown how deprivation of visual stimuli to kittens during a critical period in development can lead to the absence of sight. The lack of

Figure 2-3. Neuroplastic changes that result from neurodegeneration or injury can be due to: 1) disinhibition of intact brain regions. The inhibitory input from Neuron A has a modulatory pre-synaptic effect on Neuron B. This inhibitory influence can be lost when the nervous system is damaged. As a result, disinhibition of Neuron B causes an increase in excitatory input post-synaptically and a net hyperactivity can result. 2) Damage to the nervous system often results in deafferentation and degeneration of structural inputs, as depicted by Neuron C. The reduction or absence of neurotransmitter input from Neuron C results as these neurons become metabolically compromised.

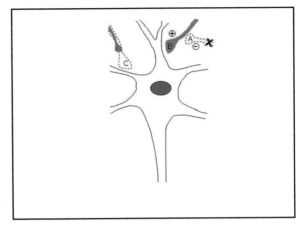

afferent input to cells of the visual system during this period of neural development hindered neuroplastic processes that were crucial for the acquisition of vision. Just as neuroplastic changes during development are time- and activity-dependent, so are plasticity changes that result from injury to the nervous system. Critical periods exist across the lifespan in which injury to the nervous system during this period will result in maladaptive to no recovery. Behavioral outcome studies in both animals and humans demonstrate how functional recovery is different at the various developmental ages. Good behavioral outcome and functional recovery were seen in rats who received a unilateral brain injury 10 days after birth, as compared to adult animals who displayed less behavioral improvement following unilateral brain injury. Poor behavioral outcome was observed when brain damage occurred at birth.[12]

Animal studies have also shown how changes in brain cell morphology resulting from nervous system injury are similar to those resulting from learning.[12,13] Injury-induced cellular reorganization occurs primarily in dendrites and synapses, and requires protein synthesis. The nervous system environment after injury is sensitive to adaptive and plasticity processes, similar to the nervous system environment during development. Trophic and remodeling factors that promote neuronal maturation and growth during normal development have been detected in the nervous system following injury. These factors seem to play a role in protecting and preventing further damage to neural cells as well as promote repair. Physiological events induced by injury to the nervous system create an environment that is sensitive to reorganization and regeneration. This presents a potential therapeutic window for optimizing functional recovery.

The effects of injury to the nervous system are far reaching; pathophysiological events not only affect the primary damage site but also adjacent tissue areas and functionally connected remote neural regions. Altered function is detected in nervous system regions that show no evidence of damage but are directly and indirectly connected to the damaged area. Time- and activity-dependent dendritic arborization occurs in both the affected and intact contralesional brain hemispheres following brain damage. These changes in dendritic morphology have been used as indicators of synaptic plasticity in experimental studies of cortical injury. In particular, the number of dendrite branches and spines was associated with recovery time following unilateral brain injury. Within a week after lesion induction, a decrease in dendrite branches was detected in interneurons adjacent to the lesion site of adult and infant rats. At 1 month post-injury, dendritic branching gradually increased over the duration of the 6-month study and correlated with behavioral improvement.[12] Concurrently, an initial rise in dendritic branching of pyramidal cells was observed in the intact contralesional hemisphere following unilateral brain injury. This was followed by a gradual decline in branching in this intact hemisphere and associated with the recovered use of the affected forelimb.[14] These studies suggest that adaptive changes in both injured and intact brain regions may play a role in recovery following a unilateral injury to the brain.

Recovery processes continue beyond the 6 months to 1 year period after nervous system injury. This expanded therapeutic window of functional recovery was underscored by recent reports of improved motor functioning following intense training of the affected extremity of humans and animals. Use-dependent change is the basis of constraint induced (CI) therapy that has been successfully used on individuals who were 2 years post acute stroke. Traditionally, minimal to no improvement in motor recovery was expected during this chronic period. CI therapy has been shown to induce a recruitment of neurons and increase the area of excited cortex in response to movement of the stroke affected body side.[15,16] The expansion of cortical representation measured in animal and human studies is evidence of the neural basis for this intense use-dependent therapy.[17]

How intact, functionally connected neural regions contribute to the processes of reorganization and recovery after acute nervous system insult is yet to be understood. Clinical recovery of language skills following aphasic stroke has been associated not only with the functional restoration of neural networks in the left brain hemisphere, but also the recruitment of neuronal systems in the right hemisphere.[18] Similar recruitment effects have been noted in motor and sensory function. Damage to the primary motor cortex resulted in an increased activation of secondary motor areas during the recovery period. Whether activation of associated brain regions as a result of neural injury underlies the clinical presence of unwanted extraneous movements warrants further study.

Neuroscientists attribute much of the functional recovery seen in individuals following brain injury and stroke to the reconnecting and reorganizing of brain areas. Researchers examined activation patterns of the brain in individuals with good recovery from paretic stroke using functional magnetic resonance imaging (fMRI). The most chronic subject in this study was 15 months post stroke. A larger area of the motor cortices was activated, and an increased degree of activation occurred in these motor areas during finger movements.[11] The plastic changes that were observed in these recovered stroke subjects most likely reflect a reorganization of cortical maps and the activation of alternate motor representation sites. As the ability to measure functional reorganization improves, effective assessment of clinical outcome following nervous system damage should also progress.

BRAIN PLASTICITY IN PARKINSON'S DISEASE

The degenerative processes of PD lead to a milieu of neuroplastic changes that are pathological in nature. One of the most notable pathological indicators of PD is the loss of dopamine producing cells in the substantia nigra, which send dopaminergic projections to the basal ganglia, often referred to as the *striatum*. This centrally located brain structure is involved in movement control due to the role of dopamine in regulating incoming excitatory signals from cortical motor regions. In addition, the striatum is instrumental in forming select motor memories and the removal of extraneous motor information. The long-term potentiation (LTP) process of memory formation involves the modification and strengthening of synaptic connections. With LTP, repeated activation of excitatory pathways results in long-lasting plastic changes at the synapse that are associated with gene transcription and protein synthesis. Removing unnecessary motor information therefore requires reversing this synaptic strengthening to a pre-potentiated state and is called *long-term depression* (LTD) of synaptic transmission.[19]

A recent theory of synaptic plasticity in the striatum suggests that this bidirectional process may underlie motor memory storage in the basal ganglia. The loss of dopamine input prevents the long-term potentiation and depression of synaptic transmission and results in impaired striatal plasticity. Experimental studies of PD have supported this theory by showing a deficit in striatal plasticity as a result of decreased dopamine levels. Striatal plasticity could be restored with levodopa (L-dopa) treatment.[19] In addition, dendritic spine density, a marker of synaptic plasticity, was significantly lower in the affected striatum of an animal model of PD. Researchers also report alterations in synaptic reorganization in postmortem examination of striatal tissue from individuals diagnosed with PD.[19]

For over 50 years, anecdotal studies have documented the benefits of physical activity and exercise for persons diagnosed with PD.[20-22] Improved motor ability and a slowing of the degenerative process were observed when exercise therapy was incorporated into the clinical treatment program. These early clinical findings have recently been validated in the basic science laboratory, reversing the translational benchtop to bedside mode of scientific research.

Research evidence supporting the effectiveness of activity-dependent therapy in PD has been collected from two widely used experimental models of Parkinson's disease, the 6-hydroxydopamine (6-OHDA) model in the rat and the 1-methyl-4-phenyl-1,2,3,6-tetrahydropyridine (MPTP) model in the mouse. A single dose of 6-OHDA infused unilaterally into the medial forebrain bundle of the rat brain results in the loss of dopaminergic neurons in that brain hemisphere. In comparison, dopamine depletion occurs in both hemispheres following the systemic administration of MPTP in the second animal model of PD. Both of these models result in classical symptoms of Parkinson's including abnormal synaptic plasticity, and the loss of behavioral functioning and dopamine substrates.[23]

Studies using these two animal models have confirmed the significance of physical activity in preventing the loss of motor ability in PD. In one notable study, daily treadmill running, initiated on the day of dopamine depletion injury, ameliorated motor function and protected dopamine systems in both models of PD.[23] Researchers assessed motor function with a battery of behavioral tests including asymmetric forelimb use, forelimb akinesia in which forelimb movement is absent, and impaired forelimb placing in response to an external stimulus in the 6-OHDA lesioned rat. Behavioral tests that analyzed forepaw stride length and forepaw use on an inverted grid were conducted on the MPTP mouse. Less behavioral impairment was observed in 6-OHDA or MPTP animals following 10 days of moderate treadmill running as compared to sedentary dopamine depleted animals. Neurochemical analysis revealed a sparing of dopamine and its metabolites in the basal ganglia of exercised animals in comparison to their sedentary counterparts. Moreover, behavioral recovery was complete in both the 6-OHDA and MPTP groups when exercise was made part of the treatment regime. In comparison, sedentary dopamine depleted animals showed persistent behavioral deficits. Physically active PD animals continued to show no behavioral deficits as long as the twice a day exercise period was maintained.

Decreased physical activity is an early symptom of PD, often occurring years before the first appearance of clinical parkinsonian signs.[24] Theoretically, this decrease in activity may also contribute to the degenerative process rather than just be a symptom of dopaminergic damage. The early implementation of motor therapy has been shown to markedly improve functional outcome in both the clinical and laboratory settings. In rat models of PD, motor symptoms are not evident until dopamine levels are depleted by 80%.[25] A mild, early PD animal has a 20% drop in dopamine levels and displays no behavioral abnormalities. However, when researchers casted the impaired limb of a mild, early PD animal for 7 days after 6-OHDA lesion, creating disuse of the affected limb, they noted significant motor impairment as well as a 60% loss of nigrostriatal dopamine projections. This finding supports the theory that decreased physical activity during the early stages of PD can lead to the progressive worsening of motor dysfunction and dopamine deficits.[23]

Evidence for functional improvement in individuals with severe PD symptoms has been promising in recent experimental studies. A higher 6-OHDA dose created 90% dopamine depletion and severe symptoms of PD in the affected limb.[26] These severely impaired animals needed to rely on their affected limb after their unaffected limb was casted for the first 7 days after lesion. Assessment of motor function in these casted animals showed an absence of behavioral asymmetry and akinesia in the affected limb. The cast was then removed from the unaffected limb and placed on the affected limb for the next 7 days. Behavior gains that resulted from casting the non-affected limb during the initial period of dopamine depletion injury were lost when a period of disuse was subsequently introduced by casting the impaired limb.

Animal studies have shown that movement therapy targeting impaired motor patterns promotes neuroplastic changes and induces the production of neurotrophic factors including brain derived neurotrophic factor (BDNF)[27] and glial derived neurotrophic factor (GDNF).[28] These neurotrophic factors nurture neuronal growth and other regenerative processes. The presence of these neuroprotective compounds prevent or slow the degenerative process of PD. Exercise incorporated in the daily regime of a patient with early stage PD can protect the nervous system from further degeneration. However, these effects are not permanent and are lost if the patient adopts a sedentary lifestyle. Investigators also detected marked neurochemical losses as a result of this delayed period of non-use in the impaired limb.[26] In summary, these findings suggest that movement therapy and exercise regimens for PD need to be continuous to maintain a functional and neurochemical quality of life.

THERAPEUTIC ENHANCEMENT OF BRAIN PLASTICITY AND FUNCTIONAL RECOVERY IN PD

As described earlier in the chapter, much of the neuroplastic changes that occur during normal development and as a result of injury to the nervous system are time- and activity-dependent. This also seems to apply to brain plasticity in PD. Investigators demonstrated the importance of timing in therapeutic intervention in a constraint use experiment in the 6-OHDA animal. They placed the non-affected forelimb of a 6-OHDA animal in a cast, forcing the animal to use its affected limb.[26] Casting of the non-affected limb was performed during different periods following dopamine depletion to determine whether therapeutic intervention was time-dependent. The forced use of the affected limb during the first week after 6-OHDA lesion prevented movement pattern deficits and curtailed the amount of dopamine loss. They observed the absence of behavioral impairments throughout the 60-day duration of the experiment. In contrast, partial sparing of behavioral impairments was reported when casting of the unimpaired limb was performed 3 days after dopamine depletion. Abnormal movement patterns and dopamine loss were not prevented, however, when the non-impaired limb was casted during the second week after lesion. Full impairment, movement asymmetry, and no sparing of striatal dopamine resulted when casting of the unaffected limb was delayed to day 14. As summarized in

Figure 2-4. Improvements in motor function and dopamine sparing are time- and use-dependent. Casting of the unaffected limb causes an animal to rely on the affected limb in this dopamine depletion study. When the unaffected limb was casted for the first 7 days after injury, an absence of behavior impairment was coupled with increased levels of dopamine in striatal tissue. Partial behavior impairments and some striatal dopamine sparing were observed when casting of the unaffected limb was delayed for 3 days after dopamine depletion, whereas no sparing of behavior functioning or dopamine stores was seen when casting was delayed for 14 days. (Adapted from Tillerson JL, Miller GW. Forced limb-use and recovery following brain injury. *Neuroscientist.* 2002;8(6):574-585.)

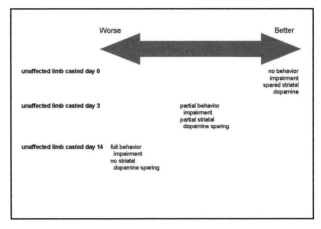

Figure 2-4, experimental models of PD have shown that improvements in motor ability and dopamine sparing are time- and use-dependent. These experiments also reconfirm that movement therapy targeting affected motor patterns of PD can slow the progression of neurodegeneration.

Experimental evidence has also demonstrated how rehabilitation training that focuses on a simplified movement pattern can result in improved motor performance in the 6-OHDA model.[29] These animals displayed impairment in successfully retrieving food pellets using the limb ipsilateral to the dopamine depleted brain hemisphere. This impairment was attributed to a failure in paw supination and in releasing the food pellet to the mouth. Following daily training on a simpler skilled-reaching task, animals with the 6-OHDA lesion performed equally as well as their control counterparts. These rehabilitation benefits were retained over a few weeks even though histological examination revealed complete dopamine loss in these animals. Findings from this study suggest that analyzing the components of a dysfunctional movement pattern in order to develop appropriate rehabilitative training protocols can lead to effective restoration of function in PD.

Deterioration of dopaminergic nigrostriatal nerve fibers has been associated with excessive inhibition of thalamic and frontal lobe functioning, and impaired activation of the supplementary motor area.[30] Difficulty initiating and executing movements, two defining features of PD, may be due in part to deficits in this supplementary motor area, which is involved in generating preparatory strategies and learned motor patterns. Anatomical connectivity and cellular responsiveness are altered in brain regions such as the subthalamic nucleus, basal ganglia, and substantial nigra, all of which are affected by the degenerative nature of PD. The viability of these functional connections plays a key role in the beneficial effects of recently developed treatment modalities that use electric current to alleviate the clinical symptoms of PD.

Deep brain stimulation (DBS) therapy uses high-frequency stimulation to modulate the activity of the subthalamic nucleus, one of the key targets of this treatment approach.[31] Although there are several theories as to how DBS affects the nervous system, they all seem to focus on modulation of the neuronal synapse and implicate plastic changes.[31] These changes take place locally within the thalamus and in the more distant globus pallidus interna and the substantial nigra compacta due to the connective pathways between these structures.

Other brain stimulation techniques have shown similar improvement in motor function in PD individuals as DBS. The electrical stimulation used in these techniques targets the primary motor cortex and is based on the premise that parkinsonian motor deficits are associated with excess excitability or reduced inhibition at the motor cortex level.[32] One of these stimulation techniques is called *transcranial direct current stimulation* (tDCS). Weak anode and cathode electrical currents are delivered through the scalp to enhance or dampen cerebral excitability. Data from a recent clinical research study showed functional improvement trends that were associated with increased motor evoked potentials (MEP) in PD individuals following anodal stimulation of the primary motor cortex.[32]

The cortical stimulation technique, which applies epidural electric current to the motor cortex, has also relieved PD symptoms comparable with DBS.[33] Electrodes are implanted on the dura overlying the primary motor cortex so that low-frequency cortical stimulation can be administered over an extended period. Initially used to reduce central pain that is often secondary to brain infarction or nerve injury, cortical stimulation of the primary motor cortex reportedly alleviates rigidity and tremor of PD after several minutes of stimulation.[33] The subthreshold stimulation provided by tDCS and cortical stimulation apparently modulates inhibitory and excitatory activity of the primary motor cortex.

A third stimulation technique is transcranial magnetic stimulation (TMS), which has been used in many PD studies to both identify pathological alterations in cortical motor function and as a potential treatment modality. This non-invasive technique theoretically activates the primary motor cortex by depolarizing neurons. At least one TMS coil is used to produce rapidly varying magnetic fields that penetrate the scalp and skull. This magnetic stimulation induces electrical currents that result in MEP responses that can be recorded over the scalp or a target muscle such as the thenar muscle in the hand or forearm flexors in the upper extremity.[11] Evidence from TMS studies has revealed that the MEP amplitude is larger at rest in patients with PD as compared to non-PD patients, and therefore less of an increase in MEP amplitude occurs during voluntary contraction. This finding suggests that the presence of elevated tonic activity in the motor cortex at rest underlies the clinical rigidity of PD, and is coupled with poor neuron recruitment during voluntary movement, which manifests as bradykinesia and muscle weakness in PD.[34]

The therapeutic role of TMS in PD continues to be debated. Early clinical studies using repetitive TMS suggest that motor cortex stimulation may be effective in improving motor performance.[35] According to these studies, TMS affects motor function by exciting corticospinal neurons,[36] which suggests that the presence of MEPs may impede PD degenerative processes. However, results from clinical studies have been difficult to interpret and reproduce, due in part to the wide variability in TMS protocol parameters.[34] Repetitive TMS treatment has reportedly long-lasting effects for at least 30 days. These benefits were prolonged with maintenance TMS treatments. Physiologically, repetitive TMS in humans has been shown to induce a selective increase in DA.[19,31] Elevated DA in intact corticostriatal terminals may optimize the signal-to-noise ratio at corticostriatal glutamatergic synapses, which then improves the efficacy of signal transmission and synaptic connectivity.[37,38] Adequately controlled clinical studies are needed to determine whether a combined repetitive TMS treatment with drug therapy can hinder or ameliorate the progression of PD.

In summary, the effectiveness of DBS and other stimulation therapies are due in part to the inherent plasticity of brain cells and on the functional connections that exist among key brain structures.[31,39]

Traditionally, scientists have quantified changes in the brain that result from learning or recovery from damage by manually counting the number of synapses and the dendritic branching on a neuron, measuring the size of the pre- and post-synaptic terminal, and counting the terminal perforations and the synaptic boutons. Recent advances in neuroimaging technology have enhanced the feasibility of examining nervous system plasticity and mapping nervous system changes in humans at a more dynamic level. In particular, positron emission tomography (PET), single photon emission computed tomography (SPECT), and fMRI techniques have enabled researchers to construct multiple brain maps in the same subject without implanting electrodes or other invasive instruments.

Several brain function studies using functional imaging techniques are based in part on the premise that activation of neuronal and non-neuronal cells is coupled with an increase in energy demand leading to a local increase in blood flow. The rise in blood delivery to tissues in this active brain region results in an increase in the ratio of oxygen bound hemoglobin (oxyhemoglobin) to unbound hemoglobin (deoxyhemoglobin) producing the fMRI signal. One widely used fMRI technique in human studies measures the blood oxygenation level-dependent (BOLD) signal of the brain while a subject performs a predetermined task. Brain maps that define the spatial and temporal dynamics of neural function can then be generated by incorporating the fMRI data onto anatomical MRIs of the brain.[40] Researchers have garnered much insight on brain function in PD by examining task-related changes in BOLD signal in the same subject before and after pharmacological intervention.[41] In one clinical study, there was less activation of the bilateral supplementary motor areas and the primary motor cortex contralateral to the affected hand as compared with the unaffected extremity in early hemi-parkinsonian individuals who had not started drug therapy. An increase in BOLD signal was observed in these motor related cortices after L-dopa administration, suggesting that modulation of functional motor circuits had occurred.[41]

Cerebral blood flow and regional metabolism can be measured with PET, which uses radioactively labeled tracers having relatively short half-lives (minutes to hours). PET is often preferred over fMRI in speech and language studies due to the swallowing and other speech-related movement artifacts created during fMRI acquisitions. A recent study used PET to demonstrate the significant impact of therapeutic treatment on the adult human brain. Individuals with idiopathic PD who had voice and speech symptoms participated in an intense voice treatment program.[42] PET scan images showed increased neural activity in specific brain regions of PD subjects who displayed improved speech and voice function following this voice therapy. These activated sites included the basal ganglia, which have been shown to be involved in the automatic initiation of movement. Whether this functional reorganization of the brain persists with continued voice therapy and whether maintenance of this therapy slows the degenerative processes of PD are important questions for future studies.

Neuroimaging of fluorine-18 labeled dopa (^{18}F-dopa) using PET has been instrumental in evaluating the effects of dopamine replacement therapies, including the functional viability of human fetal cells grafted into the striatum of PD patients. After the neural tissues are transplanted, the survival of the graft can be monitored by detecting the storage and release of dopamine. Whether neural connections have been made with the host brain can also be determined with this radioisotope and PET.[43] In addition, ^{18}F-dopa has shown to be a reliable indicator of the effectiveness of neurotrophic infusion treatment on dopamine restoration. Experimental findings have indicated that neurotrophic factor GDNF prevents the degeneration of dopamine neurons in experimental models of PD. Clinical researchers have since conducted studies in which GDNF is infused into the striatal putamen of patients with PD.[44-46] The uptake of ^{18}F-dopa is used to calculate dopamine concentration changes in the putamen and dopamine storage in nigral tissue.

Outcome results from studies of these two dopamine restorative therapies have been promising but variable. Moreover, unwanted side effects including dyskinesia have been reported in the transplantation studies.

The production of radiolabeled molecules specific for measuring deficits in the dopaminergic and other neurotransmitter systems have advanced the use of PET and SPECT techniques in PD studies.[47] SPECT measures tissue radioactivity following the injection of compounds that are bound to a relatively long half (hours to a few days) single photon emitting radionuclide. PET and SPECT have been used as complementary modalities to calculate neurotransmitter concentrations and receptor binding at the pre- and post-synaptic level. These two radiotracer-based functional imaging tools have furthered the understanding of the pathological mechanism underlying PD not only in the area of motor function but also the depression and cognitive deficits that are often associated with this neurodegenerative disease. PET and SPECT are used to monitor dopamine system dysfunction in specific brain structures, assess neurotransmitter fluctuations, and measure the loss of dopamine terminal function in PD.[48] Therapeutically, these molecular imaging techniques have provided a way to measure the effectiveness of pharmacological interventions that target dopamine loss. In particular, researchers can establish the efficacy of novel drugs that are similar to L-dopa but lack adverse side effects by calculating dopamine concentration and binding in the brain following drug delivery.[49]

NEUROREHABILITATION: POTENTIAL FOR IMPROVED FUNCTIONAL OUTCOMES IN PD

The human brain maintains the ability to make physiological changes and reorganize neuronal networks throughout life. Sensory and motor representations in the cortex can reorganize rapidly in response to different stimuli and as a result of nervous system damage. Abnormal brain plasticity may underlie the symptoms related to movement disorders. However, this injury-induced neuroplastic environment is sensitive to reorganization and regeneration and provides for optimizing functional recovery.[12,13,17] Advancement in the treatment of movement disorders such as PD may conceivably require innovative approaches that combine molecular, pharmacological, neural stimulation, and rehabilitation therapies. The combined use of these therapies can be directed toward the prevention of clinical PD, improving function in patients with PD, and slowing the degenerative processes of PD.

Gains in motor recovery of stroke have been demonstrated in clinical studies where investigators implemented a combination of therapeutic modalities. One promising study examined the effect of combined cortical stimulation and rehabilitation therapies on functional recovery in chronic stroke.[50] Epidural cortical stimulation was applied to the motor cortex of a stroke patient in conjunction with a daily program of occupational therapy. The investigators attributed improvement in motor performance seen following 3 weeks of therapy to the combination of the two treatment modalities. This anecdotal report has since led to subsequent clinical studies intent on examining whether concurrent cortical stimulation and rehabilitation treatment enhances motor representation maps that manifest as improved functional outcome.[51] It is highly feasible that similar innovative approaches can be developed as successful intervention strategies for the PD population.

Although researchers often measure the effectiveness of their proposed intervention with motor assessment tools such as grip strength and reaction time, few studies incorporate rehabilitative treatment components into their protocol. A recent study used standard motor tests to demonstrate the beneficial effects of tDCS on motor function in individuals with chronic stroke. In their discussion, the authors conceded that combining tDCS with motor training could possibly have further enhanced the observed improvements in motor function.[52]

Scientific evidence of the impact of rehabilitative treatment on recovery of the nervous system following injury or damage continues to expand. Rehabilitation professionals are in an ideal position to take active roles in developing effective therapies that target specific functional outcomes. Understanding nervous system plasticity and reorganization enables us to develop effective therapies that are based on the principles of plasticity and target individuals with neurodegenerative diseases.

REFERENCES

1. Teich AF, Qian N. Learning and adaptation in a recurrent model of V1 orientation selectivity. *J Neurophysiol.* 2003; 89(4):2086-2100.
2. Grossman AW, Churchill JD, Bates KE, Kleim JA, Greenough WT. A brain adaptation view of plasticity: is synaptic plasticity an overly limited concept? *Prog Brain Res.* 2002; 138:91-108.
3. Greenough WT, Black JE, Wallace CS. Experience and brain development. *Child Dev.* 1987;58(3):539-559.
4. Mollgaard K, Diamond MC, Bennett EL, Rosenzweig MR, Lindner B. Quantitative synaptic changes with differential experience in rat brain. *Int J Neurosci.* 1971;2(3):113-127.
5. Turner AM, Greenough WT. Differential rearing effects on rat visual cortex synapses. I. Synaptic and neuronal density and synapses per neuron. *Brain Res.* 1985;329(1-2):195-203.
6. Churchill JD, Grossman AW, Irwin SA, Galvez R, Klintsova AY, Weiler IJ et al. A converging-methods approach to fragile X syndrome. *Dev Psychobiol.* 2002;40(3):323-338.
7. Merzenich MM, Nelson RJ, Stryker MP, Cynader MS, Schoppmann A, Zook JM. Somatosensory cortical map changes following digit amputation in adult monkeys. *J Comp Neurol.* 1984;224(4):591-605.
8. Plautz EJ, Milliken GW, Nudo RJ. Effects of repetitive motor training on movement representations in adult squirrel monkeys: role of use versus learning. *Neurobiol Learn Mem.* 2000;74(1):27-55.
9. Elbert T, Pantev C, Wienbruch C, Rockstroh B, Taub E. Increased cortical representation of the fingers of the left hand in string players. *Science.* 1995; 270(5234):305-307.
10. Hirsch EC. Nigrostriatal system plasticity in Parkinson's disease: effect of dopaminergic denervation and treatment. *Ann Neurol.* 2000; 47(4 Suppl 1):S115-S120.
11. Cramer SC, Nelles G, Benson RR, Kaplan JD, Parker RA, Kwong KK et al. A functional MRI study of subjects recovered from hemiparetic stroke. *Stroke.* 1997;28(12):2518-2527.
12. Kolb B, Gibb R. Environmental enrichment and cortical injury: behavioral and anatomical consequences of frontal cortex lesions. *Cereb Cortex.* 1991;1(2):189-198.
13. Ivanco TL, Greenough WT. Physiological consequences of morphologically detectable synaptic plasticity: potential uses for examining recovery following damage. *Neuropharmacology.* 2000;39(5):765-776.
14. Jones TA, Schallert T. Overgrowth and pruning of dendrites in adult rats recovering from neocortical damage. *Brain Res.* 1992;581(1):156-160.
15. Liepert J, Bauder H, Wolfgang HR, Miltner WH, Taub E, Weiller C. Treatment-induced cortical reorganization after stroke in humans. *Stroke.* 2000;31(6):1210-1216.
16. Miltner WH, Bauder H, Sommer M, Dettmers C, Taub E. Effects of constraint-induced movement therapy on patients with chronic motor deficits after stroke: a replication. *Stroke.* 1999;30(3):586-592.
17. Taub E, Uswatte G. Constraint-induced movement therapy: bridging from the primate laboratory to the stroke rehabilitation laboratory. *J Rehabil Med.* 2003;(41 Suppl):34-40.
18. Cao Y, Vikingstad EM, George KP, Johnson AF, Welch KM. Cortical language activation in stroke patients recovering from aphasia with functional MRI. *Stroke.* 1999; 30(11):2331-2340.
19. Picconi B, Centonze D, Hakansson K, Bernardi G, Greengard P, Fisone G et al. Loss of bidirectional striatal synaptic plasticity in L-DOPA-induced dyskinesia. *Nat Neurosci.* 2003;6(5):501-506.
20. Namen JM, Ettinger H, Lowe PJ. Parkinsonism and rehabilitation. *Geriatrics.* 1955; 10(9):405-410.
21. Knott M. Report of a case of parkinsonism treated with proprioceptive facilitation technics. *Phys Ther Rev.* 1957;37(4):229.
22. Szekely BC, Kosanovich NN, Sheppard W. Adjunctive treatment in Parkinson's disease: physical therapy and comprehensive group therapy. *Rehabil Lit.* 1982;43(3-4):72-76.
23. Tillerson JL, Caudle WM, Reveron ME, Miller GW. Exercise induces behavioral recovery and attenuates neurochemical deficits in rodent models of Parkinson's disease. *Neuroscience.* 2003;119(3):899-911.
24. Hristova AH, Koller WC. Early Parkinson's disease: what is the best approach to treatment. *Drugs Aging.* 2000;17(3):165-181.

25. Spirduso WW, Gilliam PE, Schallert T, Upchurch M, Vaughn DM, Wilcox RE. Reactive capacity: a sensitive behavioral marker of movement initiation and nigrostriatal dopamine function. *Brain Res.* 1985;335(1):45-54.

26. Tillerson JL, Miller GW. Forced limb-use and recovery following brain injury. *Neuroscientist.* 2002;8(6):574-585.

27. Bezard E, Dovero S, Belin D, Duconger S, Jackson-Lewis V, Przedborski S et al. Enriched environment confers resistance to 1-methyl-4-phenyl-1,2,3,6-tetrahydropyridine and cocaine: involvement of dopamine transporter and trophic factors. *J Neurosci.* 2003; 23(35):10999-11007.

28. Cohen AD, Tillerson JL, Smith AD, Schallert T, Zigmond MJ. Neuroprotective effects of prior limb use in 6-hydroxydopamine-treated rats: possible role of GDNF. *J Neurochem.* 2003;85(2):299-305.

29. Vergara-Aragon P, Gonzalez CL, Whishaw IQ. A novel skilled-reaching impairment in paw supination on the "good" side of the hemi-Parkinson rat improved with rehabilitation. *J Neurosci.* 2003;23(2):579-586.

30. Thobois S, Guillouet S, Broussolle E. Contributions of PET and SPECT to the understanding of the pathophysiology of Parkinson's disease. *Neurophysiol Clin.* 2001; 31(5):321-340.

31. Andrews RJ. Neuroprotection for the new millennium. Matchmaking pharmacology and technology. *Ann N Y Acad Sci.* 2001;939:114-125.

32. Fregni F, Boggio PS, Santos MC, Lima M, Vieira AL, Rigonatti SP et al. Noninvasive cortical stimulation with transcranial direct current stimulation in Parkinson's disease. *Mov Disord.* 2006;21(10):1693-1702.

33. Canavero S, Paolotti R, Bonicalzi V, Castellano G, Greco-Crasto S, Rizzo L et al. Extradural motor cortex stimulation for advanced Parkinson disease. Report of two cases. *J Neurosurg.* 2002;97(5):1208-1211.

34. Cantello R, Tarletti R, Civardi C. Transcranial magnetic stimulation and Parkinson's disease. *Brain Res Brain Res Rev.* 2002;38(3):309-327.

35. Pascual-Leone A, Valls-Sole J, Brasil-Neto JP, Cammarota A, Grafman J, Hallett M. Akinesia in Parkinson's disease. II. Effects of subthreshold repetitive transcranial motor cortex stimulation. *Neurology.* 1994;44(5):892-898.

36. Amassian VE, Cracco RQ, Maccabee PJ, Cracco JB, Henry K. Some positive effects of transcranial magnetic stimulation. *Adv Neurol.* 1995;67:79-106.

37. Nicola SM, Woodward HF, Hjelmstad GO. Contrast enhancement: a physiological effect of striatal dopamine? *Cell Tissue Res.* 2004;318(1):93-106.

38. Strafella AP, Paus T, Fraraccio M, Dagher A. Striatal dopamine release induced by repetitive transcranial magnetic stimulation of the human motor cortex. *Brain.* 2003; 126(Pt 12):2609-2615.

39. McIntyre CC, Savasta M, Walter BL, Vitek JL. How does deep brain stimulation work? Present understanding and future questions. *J Clin Neurophysiol.* 2004;21(1):40-50.

40. Cramer SC, Bastings EP. Mapping clinically relevant plasticity after stroke. *Neuropharmacology.* 2000;39(5):842-851.

41. Buhmann C, Glauche V, Sturenburg HJ, Oechsner M, Weiller C, Buchel C. Pharmacologically modulated fMRI—cortical responsiveness to levodopa in drug-naive hemiparkinsonian patients. *Brain.* 2003;126(Pt 2):451-461.

42. Liotti M, Ramig LO, Vogel D, New P, Cook CI, Ingham RJ et al. Hypophonia in Parkinson's disease: neural correlates of voice treatment revealed by PET. *Neurology.* 2003;60(3):432-440.

43. Lindvall O, Hagell P. Clinical observations after neural transplantation in Parkinson's disease. *Prog Brain Res.* 2000;127:299-320.

44. Gill SS, Patel NK, Hotton GR, O'Sullivan K, McCarter R, Bunnage M et al. Direct brain infusion of glial cell line-derived neurotrophic factor in Parkinson disease. *Nat Med.* 2003; 9(5):589-595.

45. Slevin JT, Gash DM, Smith CD, Gerhardt GA, Kryscio R, Chebrolu H et al. Unilateral intraputaminal glial cell line-derived neurotrophic factor in patients with Parkinson disease: response to 1 year each of treatment and withdrawal. *Neurosurg Focus.* 2006; 20(5):E1.

46. Lang AE, Gill S, Patel NK, Lozano A, Nutt JG, Penn R et al. Randomized controlled trial of intraputamenal glial cell line-derived neurotrophic factor infusion in Parkinson disease. *Ann Neurol.* 2006;59(3):459-466.

47. Cropley VL, Fujita M, Innis RB, Nathan PJ. Molecular imaging of the dopaminergic system and its association with human cognitive function. *Biol Psychiatry.* 2006; 59(10):898-907.

48. Brooks DJ, Piccini P. Imaging in Parkinson's disease: the role of monoamines in behavior. *Biol Psychiatry.* 2006;59(10):908-918.

49. Whone AL, Watts RL, Stoessl AJ, Davis M, Reske S, Nahmias C et al. Slower progression of Parkinson's disease with ropinirole versus levodopa: the REAL-PET study. *Ann Neurol.* 2003;54(1):93-101.

50. Brown JA, Lutsep H, Cramer SC, Weinand M. Motor cortex stimulation for enhancement of recovery after stroke: case report. *Neurol Res.* 2003;25(8):815-818.

51. Brown JA, Lutsep HL, Weinand M, Cramer SC. Motor cortex stimulation for the enhancement of recovery from stroke: a prospective, multicenter safety study. *Neurosurgery.* 2006;58(3):464-473.

52. Hummel F, Cohen LG. Improvement of motor function with noninvasive cortical stimulation in a patient with chronic stroke. *Neurorehabil Neural Repair.* 2005;19(1):14-19.

Suggested Reading

Cantello R, Tarletti R, Civardi C. Transcranial magnetic stimulation and Parkinson's disease. *Brain Research Reviews*. 2002;38:309-327.

Cramer SC, Bastings EP. Mapping clinically relevant plasticity after stroke. *Neuropharmacology*. 2000;39:842-851.

Piccini P. Neurodegenerative movement disorders: the contribution of functional imaging. *Current Opinion Neurology*. 2004;17:459-466.

Picconi B, Pisani A, Barone I, Bonsi P, Centonze D, Bernardi G, Calabresi. Pathological synaptic plasticity in the striatum: implications for Parkinson's disease. *Neurotoxicity*. 2005;26:779-783.

Woodlee MT, Schallert T. The interplay between behavior and neurodegeneration in rat models of Parkinson's disease and stroke. *Restorative Neurology and Neuroscience*. 2004;22:153-161.

van der Lee JH. Constraint-induced movement therapy: some thoughts about theories and evidence. *J Rehabil Med*. 2003;Supplement 41:41-45.

Assessments and Outcome Measures for Parkinson's Disease

Aliya I. Sarwar, MD; Marilyn Trail, MOT, OTR; Eugene C. Lai, MD, PhD

Introduction

The field of medicine continues to evolve into a more scientific, evidence-based discipline due to increased requirements for quantifiable evidence on the efficacy of treatment, mounting health care costs, and the desire of health care providers to improve the quality of care offered to consumers of health services. Measurement tools provide a valid means for health care professionals to determine the effect and outcome of treatment.[2]

Parkinson's disease (PD) is a progressive multi-system neurodegenerative disorder with accumulating disability and evolving physical, emotional, and social repercussions.[3,4] Accurate assessment of the functional and psychosocial status of the patient at a given stage of the disease is essential to formulate an appropriate treatment plan. Such assessments are also integral to scientific studies focused either on tracking the evolution of the disease and/or studying the effects of therapeutic interventions. Reliable and valid instruments that are easy to administer and that comprehensively reflect the patient's disease status are invaluable to both research and practice.[5]

Some scales specific to PD were developed to provide an accurate and standardized profile of overall disability, whereas others present a broad overview of the patient's functional limitations. The choice of a particular measure depends on the clinical and research needs at hand.[2]

Particularly challenging for the examiner are the fluctuating symptoms experienced by patients with PD due to both side effects of medications and the disease itself, which can dramatically alter the patient's functional status throughout the day and affect the validity and reliability of test scores.[6] Given the broad range of symptoms involved, there is presently no single measure that comprehensively assesses the full spectrum of disease manifestations. Such an all-inclusive instrument would hardly be practical to administer in most clinical or home-based settings.[6] Most of the instruments used at the time of this writing focus only on specific aspects of the disease such as motor function, activities of daily living, and quality of life.

Parkinson's disease imposes both motor (ie, gait dysfunction, postural instability, tremor, dyskinesia) and non-motor symptoms (ie, depression, anxiety, pain, sleep disturbances), and its pharmacological treatment is associated with life-impacting side effects. Clinicians and researchers can evaluate outcomes using a range of assessment strategies including elemental assessments (ie, magnetic resonance imaging [MRI] of the brain following deep brain stimulation [DBS]), functional evaluations (ie, activities of daily living [ADL]), and measurement of quality of life variables (ie, well-being). Outcomes data may be obtained by a clinician or other expert rater, self-report, or proxy report.[7]

A scale or score defines and records the degree or severity of a clinical deficit.[6] "Scales and scores systematize information by assigning numbers to certain conditions. These conditions are usually classes of phenomena that are similar to one another but different from those in other such classes as to quantity and quality. The numbers correspond to categories in a ranking system, an ordinal scale whereby the dimensions of the categories and the intervals separating them are unequal."[6] Staging systems, such as the Hoehn and Yahr,[8] can indicate severity and usually focus on the evolution of a disease over time. Generally, an illness such as PD that affects large numbers of people will have more scales and scores to describe it than an illness that has a low incidence.[6]

CHARACTERISTICS OF SCALES AND SCORES

Herndon and Cutter[2] have listed and defined the characteristics that should be contained in a scale.

1. It should be *appropriate* to the task—A measure should be used for the purpose for which it was designed. For instance, it would be inadvisable to use an impairment scale to assess rehabilitation.

2. The instrument must be *valid*, ie, it should measure what it purports to measure. An instrument validated for adults and subsequently used to test children is no longer valid. For an detailed description of the different types of validity, see Herndon and Cutter.[2]

3. It must be *accurate*. Results should correlate with other measures of the same impairment or disability.

4. It must be precise, ie, reproducible or *reliable*. The patient should receive the same score from either the same or a different examiner. Instruments that only use categories such as mild, moderate, and severe usually have lower reliability than more continuous variables.

5. It should be *efficient* and easy to use, with little special training.

6. It should be *sensitive* to change in the underlying condition yet relatively insensitive to symptom fluctuation. This is particularly important when assessing patients with PD. Care should be taken to distinguish between mere symptom fluctuation and change in the underlying disease.

7. It should be *consistent* over time.

TYPES OF ASSESSMENTS USED TO MEASURE PARKINSON'S DISEASE

Motor disability, such as problems with gait and coordination, is one of the most dramatic and clinically challenging aspects of PD.[3] Traditionally, the majority of the scales and measures developed have focused on this aspect of the disease. Some, such as the Unified Parkinson's Disease Rating Scale (UPDRS), comprehensively measure individual motor and non-motor signs and symptoms.[9] Other measures in this category are designed to provide a broad overview of the disease, such as Hoehn and Yahr.[8]

Cognitive dysfunction has been increasingly understood as a significant contributor of disability in PD.[10-12] Several standardized instruments are available to assess and quantify cognitive functioning in PD, although none are disease-specific. There remains a challenge from the scientific standpoint to select, develop, and employ standardized, valid, reliable measures uniquely sensitive to PD dementia and associated emotional states.

Assessment of the patient's overall functional status is usually a key element in most clinical- and research-based evaluations because improvement in this area forms the basis of most therapeutic endeavors.[13] It is even more relevant for rehabilitation specialists involved in assessing and quantifying the patient's ability to perform both simple and complex everyday tasks. Accurate assessment forms the basis of effective planning to improve the problem areas, in turn allowing the patient to regain or retain independent living skills. Because functional status reflects "practical disability," it is also a useful gauge to assess the patient's disease progression and response to therapeutic interventions, including medications.

Quality of life (QOL), a global construct comprising the patient's health status, medical treatment, and intervention outcomes, also includes the patient's reflections and reactions to nonmedical aspects of his or her life, such as finances, work, family, friends, and other life circumstances. *Health-related QOL* refers to the patient's physical health and functioning without emphasis on his or her experiences and perceptions of illness.[14] Researchers frequently employ QOL as an outcome measure in clinical trials. In a systematic review of PD specific QOL instruments, Marinus et al[15] found that the Parkinson's Disease Questionnaire-39 (PDQ39)[16-18] had undergone the most extensive psychometric evaluation, and it is the QOL instrument most commonly used in clinical and research trials.

Although there are a number of instruments available to assess the various dimensions of PD (Table 3-1), this chapter will discuss only the most commonly used scoring, scaling, and staging systems used by movement disorder specialists and the ones the authors deem most appropriate for physical therapists, occupational therapists, and speech-language pathologist to draw upon when assessing this patient population. We will describe the UPDRS,[9] the Hoehn and Yahr Staging Scale,[8,19] the Schwab and England Activities of Daily Living Scale,[20] and the PDQ39[16-18] as well as a less commonly used measure but one useful to allied health professionals, the Self-Reported Disability Scale in Patients with Parkinsonism.[21,22] The measures described in this chapter are particularly advantageous for rehabilitation specialists because they can be used both in the hospital and community settings and most can be administered in a fairly short amount of time.

Unified Parkinson's Disease Rating Scale (UPDRS)

Developed in 1987, the UPDRS,[9] the best known and most widely used scale and the gold standard for the assessment of parkinsonism, was designed to follow the clinical course of PD over time. The UPDRS consists of four parts that measure: 1) mentation, behavior, and mood (ie, cognition, motivation); 2) ADL (ie, speech, handwriting, dress-

TABLE 3-1

An Abbreviated List of Outcome Measures for Parkinson's Disease

Abbreviated Columbia Scale according to Montgomery et al.	Montgomery GK, Reynolds C, Warren RM. Qualitative assessment of Parkinson's disease: study of reliability and data reduction with an abbreviated Columbia scale. *Clin Neuropharmacol*. 1985;8:83-92.
Columbia Rating Scale	Martilla RJ, Rinne UK. Disability and progression in Parkinson's disease. *Acta Neurol Scan*. 1977;56:159-169.
Depression and ADL Scale according to Brown et al.	Brown RG, MacCarthy B, Gotham AM, Der GJ, Marsden CD. Depression and disability in Parkinson's disease. a follow up of 132 cases. *Psychol Med*. 1988;18(1):49-55.
Disability Rating Scale according to Alba et al. (New York Rating Scale)	Alba A, Trainor FS, Ritter W, Dasco MM. A clinical disability rating for Parkinson patients. *J Chron Dis*. 1968;21:507-522.
Extrapyramidal Disorder Profile according to Lakke et al.	Barbeau A, Duvoisin RC, Gerstenbrand F, Lakke JPWF, Marsden CD, Stern G. Classification of extrapyramidal disorders. *J Neurol Sci*. 1981;51:311-327.
Movement Profile according to Lakke et al.	Barbeau A, Duvoisin RC, Gerstenbrand F, Lakke JPWF, Marsden CD, Stern G. Classification of extrapyramidal disorders. *J Neurol Sci*. 1981;51:311-327.
New York University Parkinson's Disease Disability Scale	Lieberman AN. Parkinson's disease: a clinical review. *Am J Med Sci*. 1974;267:66-80.
Northwestern University (NWU) Disability Scale	Canter CJ, de la Torre R, Mier M. A method of evaluating disability in patients with Parkinson's disease. *J Nerv Ment Dis*. 1961;133:143-147.
The Parkinson's Disease Questionnaire (PDQ-39)	Jenkinson C, Fitzpatrick R, Peto V, Greenhall R, Hyman N. The Parkinson's Disease Questionnaire (PDQ-39): development and validation of a Parkinson's disease summary index score. *Age Ageing*. 1997;26(5):353-357.
Parkinsonism Scale according to Schacter et al.	Schacter M, Marsden CD, Parkes JD, Jenner P, Testa B. Deprenyl in the management of response fluctuations in patients with Parkinson's disease on levodopa. *J Neurol Neurosurg Psych*. 1980;43:1016-1021.

TABLE 3-1, CONTINUED
An Abbreviated List of Outcome Measures for Parkinson's Disease

Parkinson's Disease Scale according to Sutcliffe et al.	Sutcliffe RLG, Prior R, Mawby B, McQuilan WJ. Parkinson's disease in the district of the Northampton Health Authority, United Kingdom. A study of prevalence and disability. *Acta Neurol Scand.* 1985;72:363-379.
Parkinson's Disease Score according to Schwab	Schwab RS. Progressing and prognosis in Parkinson's disease. *J Nerv Ment Dis.* 1960;130:556-566.
Parkinson's Score according to Weiner et al.	Weiner WJ, Koller WC, Perlik S, Nausieda PA, Klawans HL. Drug holiday and management of Parkinson's disease. *Neurology.* 1980;30:1257-1261.
Self-Reported Disability Scale in Patients with Parkinsonism	Brown RG, MacCarthey B, Jahanshahi M, Marsden CD. Accuracy of self-reported disability in patients with parkinsonism. *Arch Neurol.* 1989;46(9):955-959.
Staging of Parkinsonism according to Hoehn and Yahr	Hoehn MM, Yahr MD. Parkinsonism: onset, progression, and mortality. *Neurology.* 1967;17:427-422.
Staging in Parkinsonism according to Schwab and England	Schwab RS, England AC. Projection technique for evaluating surgery in Parkinson's disease. In: Gillingham FJ, Donaldson MC, eds. *Third symposium on Parkinson's disease.* Edinburgh: ES Livingston; 1969.
UCLA Parkinsonism Scale	McDowell F, Lee JE, Swift T, Sweet RD, Ogsbury JS, Kessler JT. Treatment of Parkinson's syndrome with L Dihydroxyphenylalanine (Levodopa). *Ann Intern Med.* 1970:72;29-35.
Unified Parkinson's Disease Rating Scale (UPDRS)	Fahn S, Elton RL, and Members of the UPDRS Development Committee. Unified Parkinson's disease rating scale. In: Fahn S, Marsden CD, Goldstein M, et al, eds. *Recent Developments in Parkinson's Disease II.* New York: Macmillan; 1987;153-163.
University of British Columbia (UBC) Parkisonism Scale	Larsen TA, Calne S, Calne DB. Assessment of Parkinson's disease. *Clin Neuropharmacol.* 1984;7:165-169.
Webster Score	Webster DD. Critical analysis of the disability in Parkinson's disease. *Mod Treat.* 1968;5:257-282.

Source: Masur H, Papke K, Althoff S. *Scales and Scores in Neurology: Quantification of Neurological Deficits in Research and Practice.* Stuttgart: Thieme; 2004.

ing); 3) motor skills (ie, tremor, rigidity, posture, gait); and 4) complications of therapy (ie, dyskinesia, motor fluctuations). Physical therapists, occupational therapists, and speech-language pathologists may find the motor and ADL portions of the UPDRS particularly useful.

The Movement Disorder Society (MDS) Task Force for Rating Scales for Parkinson's Disease's critique of the UPDRS sums up the instrument's strengths and weaknesses.[1] Strengths include its application across the clinical spectrum of PD and its nearly comprehensive coverage of motor symptoms. From a clinometric standpoint, it is the most tested of the PD scales, and its standardized ratings allow for clinicians and researchers to use summary scores to communicate globally regarding the severity and impairment of disability. Siderowf et al[23] and other researchers[24] have found the UPDRS to have excellent test-retest reliability. Another unique feature is that a videotape can be ordered to train raters and to enhance its inter-rater reliability.[25]

Shortcomings of the present version include "floor effects," which limit the sensitivity in the mild disease stage when "0.5" ratings are used in the absence of corresponding scale validation to capture subtle motor signs; ambiguous wording of instructions; and failure to cover symptoms such as anxiety, sexual dysfunction, and fatigue.[26] The ADL scale of the UPDRS has been critiqued as "conceptually unclear" because it contains items that measure impairment such as salivation, falls, and sensory complaints.[27] The items assessing depression, motivation/initiative, and tremor have been shown to poorly associate with other domains measured by the UPDRS.[28] Martinez-Martin et al[28] propose that features of PD such as depression, motivation, and tremor are better evaluated with scales developed to measure these specific aspects. The Task Force recommended that the MDS sponsor the development of a new version of the UPDRS and encourage efforts to establish its clinometric properties, especially addressing the need to define a minimal clinically relevant difference and a minimal clinically relevant incremental difference, as well as testing its correlation with the current UPDRS[1] (see Appendices).

Hoehn and Yahr Staging Scale

Hoehn and Yahr developed their scale after collecting and analyzing data on 802 patients with confirmed PD.[8] The HY Scale quantifies the severity of PD by classifying the disease into six stages: 0 = "no clinical signs evident," 1 = "unilateral involvement only," 2 = "bilateral involvement only," 3 = "first evidence of impaired postural and righting reflexes by examination or a history of poor balance, falls, and so on; disability is mild to moderate," 4 = "fully developed severe disease; disability marked," and 5 = "confinement to bed or wheelchair." The HY is a useful tool for allied health professionals. It takes only a short time to score and can be administered in any setting.

The Movement Disorder Society Task Force for rating scales for PD prepared a critique of the HY Scale.[19] Strengths include its wide utilization and acceptance. Progressively higher stages correlate with neuroimaging studies of dopaminergic loss, and a higher correlation exists between the HY Scale and some standardized scales of motor impairment, disability, and quality of life. Weaknesses include the scale's mixing of impairment and disability and its nonlinearity. Because the scale is weighted heavily toward postural instability as the primary index of disease severity, it does not completely capture impairments or disability from other motor features of PD and does not address non-motor problems.

Direct clinometric testing of the HY Scale has been limited, but the scale fulfills at least some criteria for reliability and validity, especially for the mid-ranges of the scale (stages 2 to 4). Although a "modified HY Scale" that includes 0.5 increments has been adopted widely, no clinometric data are available on this adaptation. The Task Force recommends that the original five-point scale be maintained[19] (see Appendices).

Schwab and England Activities of Daily Living Scale

The Schwab and England[20] is a disability scale commonly used by neurologists and clinicians involved in the care of patients with PD. It rates the patient's ability to perform ADL from 100% (essentially normal) to 0% (vegetative). The score, however, is significantly influenced by co-morbid medical conditions, the patient's mental state, and the effect of medications.[6]

The Schwab and England enables the clinician to categorize a patient's functional ability. It is not intended as a comprehensive assessment. Because categories are broad, there may be some overlap. The objective of the scale is to represent an overall average functional capacity of the patient rather than a momentary state.

In their review of clinical evaluation tools for PD, Ramaker et al[27] noted that there have not been many studies to evaluate the characteristics of the Schwab and England scale. However, based on their review of existing studies, they concluded that there was evidence that the scale has "good reliability" and "substantial validity" (see Appendices).

Parkinson's Disease Questionnaire—PDQ-39

The PDQ-39, developed to assess health-related quality of life in PD, reflects the patient's perception of life domains.[16-18] It is comprised of 39 items and 8 subscales that measure quality of life dimensions related to PD—mobility, ADL, emotional well-being, stigma, social support, cognition, communication, and bodily discomfort. These quality of life domains were identified through in-depth interviews with patients diagnosed with PD. The content and construct validity of the PDQ-39 scores used as measures of therapeutic outcomes have been well established.[17]

The data from the PDQ-39 can be presented either in a profile form or as a single index figure.[17] The profile is of potential value in research aimed at studying the effect of therapeutic interventions on specific aspects of functioning. The PDQ-39 provides an additional tool for allied health professionals to measure treatment outcomes as well as supplying information on meaningful life issues that are pertinent to therapy (see Appendices).

Self-Reported Disability Scale in Patients With Parkinsonism

The Self-Reported Disability Scale in Patients with Parkinsonism addresses a wide range of daily activities.[21] The scale encompasses (directly and indirectly) essentially all major areas of everyday function and allows the patient to rate his or her ability to perform ADL (ie, bed mobility, hygiene, dressing) and IADL (ie, dialing a telephone, pouring milk, using public transportation). The 25-item questionnaire asks the patient to indicate how much assistance he or she needs for different tasks and rates the answers on a 5-point scale ranging from 1 = "able to do alone without difficulty" to 5 = "unable to do at all."[22] Eleven items test mobility and 14 test use of the hands.[6]

Brown and colleagues[21] found that the self-reported disabilities are similar to disabilities reported by the patient's partner or a neutral observer. In another study Biemans et al[22] found the internal consistency to be high. Although the questionnaire has limitations that are inherent in all subjective measures, it is a helpful tool for the therapist to obtain the patient's perception of his or her functional ability (see Appendices).

Other outcome measures are listed in Table 3-2.

TABLE 3-2

An Abbreviated List of Other Outcome Measures Used for Assessment of Patients With Parkinson's Disease

Berg Balance Scale	Berg KO, Wood-Dauphinee SL, Williams JI, Maki B. Measuring balance in the elderly: validation of an instrument. *Can J Public Health*. 1992;83(Suppl2):27-11.
Functional Reach Test	Duncan PW, Weiner DK, Chandler J, Studenski S. Functional reach: a new clinical measure of balance. *J Gerontol*. 1990;45:M192-M197.
The Multidimensional Fatigue Inventory (MFI)	Smets EM, Garssen B, Bonke B, DeHaes JC. The Multidimensional Fatigue Inventory (MFI): psychometric qualities of an instrument to assess fatigue. *J Psychosom Res*. 1995;39(3):315-325.
Mini-Mental Status Exam (MMSE)	Folstein MF, Folstein SE, McHugh PR. "Mini-mental state."
Purdue Pegboard Test	Buddenberg LA, Davis C. Test-retest reliability of the Purdue Pegboard Test. *Am J Occup Ther*. 2000;54(5):555-558.
Safety Assessment of Function and the Environment for Rehabilitation (SAFER)	Oliver R, Blathwayt J, Brackley C, Tamaki T. Development of the Safety Assessment of Function and the Environment for Rehabilitation (SAFER) tool. *Can J Occup Ther*. 1993;60(2):78-82.
The Timed Get Up and Go (TUG) Test	Podsiadlo D, Richardson S. The timed "Up & Go": a test of basic functional mobility for frail elderly persons. *J Am Geriatr Soc*. 1991;39:142-148.
Voice Handicap Index (VHI)	Jacobson, Johnson, Grywalski, Silbergleit, Jacobson, Benninger, Newman. The Voice Handicap Index (VHI). *Am J Speech Lang Pathol*. 1997;6:66-70.

ADDITIONAL MEASURES REQUIRING DATA FROM APPARATUS-BASED PROCEDURES

Some highly sophisticated apparatus-based measures have also been developed to quantify the various symptoms of PD. This includes tremor quantification using electromagnetic tracking systems,[29] or high resolution laser simultaneously with an accelerometer.[30] Quantitative digitography (QDG) quantitatively assesses digital motor control using a computer-interfaced musical keyboard.[31,32]

Taylor Tavares et al[31] reported that kinematics of a repetitive alternating finger tapping (RAFT) task using QDG correlated with UPDRS motor scores, particularly with the bradykinesia subscore, in 33 PD patients. A similar BRAIN TEST[33] is a computerized alternating finger tapping test that generates the following variables: 1) kinesia score— number of keystrokes/min, 2) akinesia time—cumulative time that keys are depressed, 3) dysmetria score—a weighted score generated from incorrectly hit keys and corrected for speed, and 4) arrhythmia score—variance of the time interval between individual keystrokes. The authors reported a significant correlation between the four test parameters and PD rating scores of the Hoehn and Yahr, Schwab and England, and the UPDRS.

Computerized dynamic posturography (CDP) can quantify balance and related sensory processing in parkinsonism.[34,35] Surface EMG has been used to study the recruitment pattern of distal muscles and to quantify distal muscle activation timing to evaluate slowness in PD.[36]

A quantitative procedure using a Purdue Pegboard–like apparatus for objective assessment of PD-related fine motor impairment was reported by Muller et al.[37] Twenty-eight PD patients were assessed before and during a levodopa challenge test. A Purdue Pegboard–like apparatus measured the total time taken to insert 25 pegs from a rack into a series of appropriate holes by a computer to 100 millisecond accuracy. Simultaneous rating with the Motor Section of the UPDRS was also performed. The authors noted significant correlations to the rated severity of PD. Additionally, subject comparisons and correlation analysis demonstrated the potential of this tool to reflect scored motor improvement levadopa intake.[37]

The use of the aforementioned measures has been limited to small groups of patients. Although promising, much remains to be seen regarding their practical utility in routine clinical and research settings.

TIME AND FREQUENCY OF ASSESSMENT

Choosing the appropriate frequency and time of administration is an important part of optimal assessment in the clinical and research settings. The frequency of administration should depend on the examiner's previous experience or available data regarding the expected rate of change of the attribute in response to a particular intervention. The timing of administration should take into account the "on" and "off" phenomenon experienced by PD patients (see Chapter 1). Using the same valid, reliable measure in both on and off states is a better way to assess symptoms of disability than a random assessment. Off state disability or on state functional status can vary at different times of the day, depending on the level of fatigue, emotional status, and the effect of medications and meals. Valid measures like the UPDRS provide an opportunity to capture the patient's disability in both states. Implementing such a measure at a specific time improves the accuracy of data by minimizing the relative time-locked variability of symptoms.

LIMITATIONS OF CURRENTLY AVAILABLE INSTRUMENTS

The major limitations of currently used PD-related rating scales are similar to those inherent in other such instruments (ie, inter-rater variability, subjective impressions, insensitivity of subtle modification). Additionally, the instruments currently available do not comprehensively capture the broad range of symptoms and disabilities experienced by patients with PD.[26] The multitude of symptoms involved and their variability renders the task of developing a comprehensive rating scale extremely challenging.

Another limitation is the lack of accommodation for fluctuations in symptoms inherent in all aspects of the disease and the side effects of the medications. The fluctuations can occur throughout the day in association with or independent of certain events, eg, medication intake. Hence, the measured disability at one particular point in time is hardly a reflection of overall disability unless the time distribution factors and specific event changing the clinical picture are incorporated into the scoring system. The broad variety of parkinsonian symptoms and their unique relationship to each other can be a pitfall for cumulative scores. In most measuring systems, each symptom is assessed separately, requiring highly differentiated weighting and thus fails to capture inter-relationships between the symptoms. The cumulative score of a particular scale may not accurately represent nor parallel the change in clinical status. In an extreme case scenario, the score may reflect worsening, whereas the clinical status improves or vice versa.

DEVELOPMENT OF NEW ASSESSMENT AND QUANTIFICATION SCALES FOR PARKINSON'S DISEASE

The role of neurorehabilitation specialists in the management of Parkinson's disease is multidimensional.[38] The goal of intervention is to help maximize the patient's ability to live independently. However, when independence is no longer feasible, intervention is geared to facilitate the patient's acceptance and adaptation to new physical and social circumstances and to develop new roles and activities.

Several valid and reliable measures exist to evaluate motor disability in PD. However, other aspects of the disease affecting the patient's overall quality of life are not always a standard component of the neurorehabilitation assessment. This includes assessment of subtle cognitive changes, especially frontal lobe impairment and associated executive dysfunction, and quantification of subtle mood changes (subclinical depression), anxiety state, sexual dysfunction, and other aspects of autonomic system dysfunction, eg, posturally related hypotension causing dizziness and sweating abnormalities.

Assessment of and strategies to manage mild frontal lobe dysfunction cannot be over-emphasized. Its associated behavioral manifestations (ie, apathy, loss of initiative, difficulty with working memory) can mimic depression but do not improve with depression management strategies alone.[11]

These behavioral changes are an independent risk factor for poor QOL and can be a significant hindrance towards achieving therapy goals. Postural dizziness can cause imbalance and worsening gait and contribute to generalized body bradykinesia (patient tries to minimize the "dizzy feeling" by moving cautiously and slower than normal). Modifications of existing scales or development of newer ones to incorporate these symptoms can improve the quality of assessment and the usefulness of the management plan.

Assessment of fatigue as an independent contributor to overall disability is also lacking.[26] Visual difficulty, described as "impaired depth perception" stemming from visual fixation and ocular motility impairment, is also an under-recognized symptom with broad functional consequences, the most noteworthy being its effect on the patient's gait, balance, and driving ability.[39]

Measures developed to objectively assess the patient's potential to adapt (physically and emotionally) to changing living and social situations (eg, relocating to an assisted living facility or a nursing home) would also be beneficial. Such a measure could also be used to plan and follow the progress of interventions in a non-compliant or demented patient.

The aforementioned is by no means a comprehensive coverage of the evolving needs of patients with PD. The idea, however, is that development of valid and reliable quantification measures should keep pace with new discoveries and enhanced understanding of the disease.

CONCLUSIONS

Measurement of disability in PD is a challenging task. The disability is multidimensional, complex, and fluctuating. The available instruments, although useful, are still often either too cumbersome to implement and/or of limited utility. At times, some of the most disabling aspects of the disease are not addressed by the available measures. A truly comprehensive scale is likely to be impractical in most clinical- and research-based settings, and individual measures focusing on one or several aspects of PD will continue to have a wide utility. Thus, the true focus should be on developing valid and reliable measures that effectively capture the neglected PD symptoms, that is, non-motor dysfunction, and their impact on the overall disease disability in specific relation to the clinical "on" and "off" state.

The Movement Disorders Society's Task Force is actively engaged in modifying the currently available, validated, reliable, widely used instruments, namely the UPDRS and HY Scales to reflect much needed changes.[1,19]

REFERENCES

1. The Unified Parkinson's Disease Rating Scale (UPDRS): status and recommendations. *Mov Disord.* 2003;18(7):738-750.
2. Herndon RM, Cutter G. Introduction to clinical neurologic scales. In: Herndon RM, ed. *Handbook of Neurologic Rating Scales.* New York: Demos Medical Publishing; 2006:1-7.
3. Nutt JG, Wooten GF. Clinical practice. Diagnosis and initial management of Parkinson's disease. *N Engl J Med.* 2005;353(10):1021-1027.
4. Marttila RJ, Rinne UK. Disability and progression in Parkinson's disease. *Acta Neurol Scand.* 1977;56(2):159-169.
5. Baas H, Stecker K, Fischer PA. Value and appropriate use of rating scales and apparative measurements in quantification of disability in Parkinson's disease. *J Neural Transm Park Dis Dement Sect.* 1993;5(1):45-61.
6. Masur H, Papke K, Althoff S. *Scales and Scores in Neurology: Quantification of Neurological Deficits in Research and Practice.* Stuttgart: Thieme, 2004.
7. Cook KF. Assessments and outcome measures for Parkinson's disease. *PADRRECC Bulletin.* 2003;1(2):3-8.
8. Hoehn MM, Yahr MD. Parkinsonism: onset, progression and mortality. *Neurology.* 1967;17(5):427-442.
9. Fahn S, Elton TL, & members of the UPDRS Development Committee. Unified Parkinson's Disease Rating Scale. In: Fahn S, Marsden CD, Goldstein Metal, eds. *Recent Developments in Parkinson's Disease.* New York: MacMillan;1987:153-163.
10. Weintraub D, Stern MB. Psychiatric complications in Parkinson disease. *Am J Geriatr Psychiatry.* 2005;13(10):844-851.
11. Stocchi F, Brusa L. Cognition and emotion in different stages and subtypes of Parkinson's disease. *J Neurol.* 2000;247 Suppl 2:II114-II121.
12. Locascio JJ, Corkin S, Growdon JH. Relation between clinical characteristics of Parkinson's disease and cognitive decline. *J Clin Exp Neuropsychol.* 2003; 25(1):94-109.
13. Larsen TA, Calne S, Calne DB. Assessment of Parkinson's disease. Clin Neuropharmacol. 1984;7(2):165-169.
14. Nelson ND, Trail M, Van JN, Appel SH, Lai EC. Quality of life in patients with amyotrophic lateral sclerosis: perceptions, coping resources, and illness characteristics. *J Palliat Med.* 2003;6(3):417-424.
15. Marinus J, Ramaker C, van Hilten JJ, Stiggelbout AM. Health related quality of life in Parkinson's disease: a systematic review of disease specific instruments. *J Neurol Neurosurg Psychiatry.* 2002;72(2):241-248.
16. Peto V, Jenkinson C, Fitzpatrick R, Greenhall R. The development and validation of a short measure of functioning and well being for individuals with Parkinson's disease. *Qual Life Res.* 1995;4(3):241-248.
17. Jenkinson C, Fitzpatrick R, Peto V, Greenhall R, Hyman N. The Parkinson's Disease Questionnaire (PDQ-39): development and validation of a Parkinson's disease summary index score. *Age Ageing.* 1997;26(5):353-357.
18. Peto V, Jenkinson C, Fitzpatrick R. PDQ-39: a review of the development, validation and application of a Parkinson's disease quality of life questionnaire and its associated measures. *J Neurol.* 1998;245 Suppl 1:S10-S14.
19. Goetz CG, Poewe W, Rascol O, Sampaio C, Stebbins GT, Counsell C et al. Movement Disorder Society Task Force report on the Hoehn and Yahr staging scale: status and recommendations. *Mov Disord.* 2004;19(9):1020-1028.

20. Schwab RS. Progression and prognosis in Parkinson's disease. *J Nerv Ment Dis.* 1960;130:556-566.
21. Brown RG, MacCarthy B, Jahanshahi M, Marsden CD. Accuracy of self-reported disability in patients with parkinsonism. *Arch Neurol.* 1989;46(9):955-959.
22. Biemans MA, Dekker J, van der Woude LH. The internal consistency and validity of the Self-Assessment Parkinson's Disease Disability Scale. *Clin Rehabil.* 2001; 15(2):221-228.
23. Siderowf A, McDermott M, Kieburtz K, Blindauer K, Plumb S, Shoulson I. Test-retest reliability of the unified Parkinson's disease rating scale in patients with early Parkinson's disease: results from a multicenter clinical trial. *Mov Disord.* 2002;17(4):758-763.
24. Metman LV, Myre B, Verwey N, Hassin-Baer S, Arzbaecher J, Sierens D et al. Test-retest reliability of UPDRS-III, dyskinesia scales, and timed motor tests in patients with advanced Parkinson's disease: an argument against multiple baseline assessments. *Mov Disord.* 2004;19(9):1079-1084.
25. Goetz CG, Stebbins GT, Chmura TA, Fahn S, Klawans HL, Marsden CD. Teaching tape for the motor section of the unified Parkinson's disease rating scale. *Mov Disord.* 1995;10(3):263-266.
26. Ebersbach G, Baas H, Csoti I, Mungersdorf M, Deuschl G. Scales in Parkinson's disease. *J Neurol.* 2006; 253 Suppl 4:iv32-iv35.
27. Ramaker C, Marinus J, Stiggelbout AM, Van Hilten BJ. Systematic evaluation of rating scales for impairment and disability in Parkinson's disease. *Mov Disord.* 2002;17(5):867-876.
28. Martinez-Martin P, Gil-Nagel A, Gracia LM, Gomez JB, Martinez-Sarries J, Bermejo F. Unified Parkinson's Disease Rating Scale characteristics and structure. The Cooperative Multicentric Group. *Mov Disord.* 1994;9(1):76-83.
29. O'Suilleabhain PE, Dewey RB, Jr. Validation for tremor quantification of an electromagnetic tracking device. *Mov Disord.* 2001;16(2):265-271.
30. Duval C, Jones J. Assessment of the amplitude of oscillations associated with high-frequency components of physiological tremor: impact of loading and signal differentiation. *Exp Brain Res.* 2005;163(2):261-266.
31. Taylor Tavares AL, Jefferis GS, Koop M, Hill BC, Hastie T, Heit G et al. Quantitative measurements of alternating finger tapping in Parkinson's disease correlate with UPDRS motor disability and reveal the improvement in fine motor control from medication and deep brain stimulation. *Mov Disord.* 2005; 20(10):1286-1298.
32. Bronte-Stewart HM, Ding L, Alexander C, Zhou Y, Moore GP. Quantitative digitography (QDG): a sensitive measure of digital motor control in idiopathic Parkinson's disease. *Mov Disord.* 2000;15(1):36-47.
33. Homann CN, Suppan K, Wenzel K, Giovannoni G, Ivanic G, Horner S et al. The Bradykinesia Akinesia Incoordination Test (BRAIN TEST), an objective and user-friendly means to evaluate patients with parkinsonism. *Mov Disord.* 2000; 15(4):641-647.
34. Jagielski J, Kubiczek-Jagielska M, Sobstyl M, Koziara H, Blaszczyk J, Zabek M et al. [Posturography as objective evaluation of the balance system in Parkinson's disease patients after neurosurgical treatment. A preliminary report]. *Neurol Neurochir Pol.* 2006;40(2):127-133.
35. Soto A, Labella T, Santos S, Rio MD, Lirola A, Cabanas E et al. The usefulness of computerized dynamic posturography for the study of equilibrium in patients with Meniere's disease: correlation with clinical and audiologic data. *Hear Res.* 2004;196(1-2):26-32.
36. Bishop M, Brunt D, Pathare N, Ko M, Marjama-Lyons J. Changes in distal muscle timing may contribute to slowness during sit to stand in Parkinsons disease. *Clin Biomech.* (Bristol, Avon) 2005;20(1):112-117.
37. Muller T, Benz S. Quantification of the dopaminergic response in Parkinson's disease. *Parkinsonism Relat Disord.* 2002;8(3):181-186.
38 Trend P, Kaye J, Gage H, Owen C, Wade D. Short-term effectiveness of intensive multidisciplinary rehabilitation for people with Parkinson's disease and their carers. *Clin Rehabil.* 2002;16(7):717-725.
39. Davidsdottir S, Cronin-Golomb A, Lee A. Visual and spatial symptoms in Parkinson's disease. *Vision Res.* 2005;45(10):1285-1296.

Cognitive Impairments Associated With Parkinson's Disease

Michele K. York, PhD; Julie A. Alvarez, PhD

Introduction

Although Parkinson's disease (PD) is a progressive motor disorder, cognitive changes have been reported at all stages of the disease process.[1,2] The characteristics associated with cognitive decline and its progression in PD have been studied extensively. Although the cognitive decline reported in early stage PD is subtle and does not often interfere with daily functioning, PD patients have been shown to demonstrate cognitive slowing and executive functioning problems at early stages.[3] Furthermore, longitudinal research has described PD-related cognitive deficits in language, visuospatial functioning, long-term memory, and executive functioning that are greater than what would be expected to occur as a result of normal aging.[4] Although the prevalence of dementia in patients with PD continues to be debated with estimates ranging from 10% to 40%, a review of prevalence studies by Rajput[5] suggests that approximately 29% of patients are diagnosed with PD-related dementia.

A consensus has not been reached on how to define the criteria for PD-related mild cognitive changes. Mild cognitive impairment (MCI) is recognized as the intermediate classification that occurs between the cognitive statuses of "within normal limits" to "demented." Individuals with a diagnosis of MCI are impaired in one cognitive domain but continue to be independent with their daily functioning.[6] Specific criteria for MCI in PD have not been adequately defined.

Several criteria have been proposed for diagnosing dementia in Parkinson's disease patients. *The Diagnostic and Statistical Manual of Mental Disorders—Fourth Edition* (DSM-IV)[7] provides general criteria that can be used as a guideline for diagnosing dementia

> ## SIDEBAR 4-1: DSM-IV[7] DIAGNOSTIC CRITERIA FOR DEMENTIA
>
> 1. Memory impairment (impaired ability to learn new information or to recall previously learned information)
> 2. At least one of the following cognitive disturbances:
>   a. aphasia (language disturbance)
>   b. apraxia (impaired ability to carry out motor activities despite intact motor function)
>   c. agnosia (failure to recognize or identify objects despite intact sensory function)
>   d. disturbance in executive functioning (ie, planning, organizing, sequencing, abstracting)
> 3. Significant impairment in social or occupational functioning
> 4. Significant decline from previous level of functioning

in PD patients (Sidebar 4-1). Cummings and Benson[8] proposed an alternate criterion for a diagnosis of dementia in patients with PD. They defined dementia as an acquired persistent decline in intellectual functioning with significant impairment in at least three of the following domains: language, memory, visuospatial skills, personality or mood, and executive functions (Sidebar 4-2). Recently, a task force organized by the Movement Disorder Society proposed clinical diagnostic criteria for dementia associated with PD (Sidebar 4-3). These criteria were based on a systematic review of the literature and a group consensus of Movement Disorder specialists.[9]

> ## SIDEBAR 4-2: CUMMINGS AND BENSON[8] CRITERIA FOR DEMENTIA
>
> Persistent decline in intellectual functioning and significant impairments in at least three of the following cognitive domains:
>
> 1. Language
> 2. Memory
> 3. Visuospatial skills
> 4. Personality/mood
> 5. Executive functions

PD-related cognitive changes follow a pattern of decline that is clinically and pathophysiologically different from Alzheimer's disease (AD). This difference originally was classified as a distinction between subcortical and cortical dementias.[10] Cortical dementia describes a clinical syndrome that affects language, memory, and visuospatial functioning early in the course of the disease, including the presence of aphasia, agnosia, and

Sidebar 4-3: Parkinson's Disease Dementia (PD-D) Clinical Diagnostic Criteria[9]

I. Core Features

   1. Diagnosis of Parkinson's disease-Queens Square Brain Bank criteria

   2. Dementia with insidious onset, slow progression, develops within the context of established Parkinson's disease and diagnosed by history, clinical and mental examination, defined as:

     a. Impairment in more than one cognitive domain

     b. Representing a decline from premorbid level

     c. Deficit severe enough to impair daily life (independent of motor or autonomic impairment)

II. Associated Clinical Features

   1. Cognitive features:

     a. Attention-Impaired, may fluctuate

     b. Executive functions-Impaired

     c. Visuospatial functions-Impaired

     d. Memory-Impaired, free recall which usually improves with cueing

     e. Language-Largely preserved, impaired word finding

   2. Behavioral features:

     a. Apathy

     b. Personality and mood changes, including depression and anxiety

     c. Hallucinations

     d. Delusions

     e. Excessive daytime sleepiness

III. Features which do not exclude PD-D, but make the diagnosis uncertain

   1. Co-existence of any other abnormality, which may by itself cause cognitive impairment, but judged not to be the cause of dementia (e.g., white matter changes on imaging)

   2. Time interval between the development of motor and cognitive symptoms not known

IV. Features suggesting other conditions or diseases as cause of mental impairment, which, when present make it impossible to reliably diagnose PD-D

   1. Cognitive and behavioral symptoms appearing solely in the context of other conditions such as acute confusion due to systemic diseases or drug intoxication or Major Depression according to DSM-IV

   2. Features compatible with "Probable Vascular dementia" criteria according to NINDS-AIREN

SIDEBAR 4-3, CONTINUED

Probable PD-D

  A. Core features: Both must be present

  B. Associated Clinical features:

      1. Typical profile of cognitive deficits including impairment in at least 2/4 core cognitive domains

      2. Presence of at least one behavioral symptom supports diagnosis of Probable PD-D; however, lack of behavioral symptom does not exclude the diagnosis

  C. None of the group III features present

  D. None of the group IV features present

Possible PD-D

  A. Core features: Both must be present

  B. Associated clinical features:

      1. Atypical profile of cognitive impairment in one or more domains

      2. Behavioral symptoms may or may not be present

  OR

  C. One or more of the group III features present

  D. None of the group IV features present

Adapted from Emre M, Aarsland D, Brown R, et al. Clinical diagnostic criteria for dementia associated with Parkinson's disease. *Mov Disord.* 2007;22:1689-1707

---

apraxia. Cortical dementias arise from impairments in interconnections between different areas of the cortex.[11] In contrast, subcortical dementias encompass the clinical symptoms of cognitive slowing, impaired memory recall and retrieval, and executive deficits, which arise from dysfunction between subcortical areas (eg, thalamus, striatum) and cortical areas. PD-related dementia is considered a subcortical dementia because the neuronal death that causes the primary motor symptoms of PD is in the substantia nigra pars reticulata, a subcortical brain structure that is highly interconnected with the frontal and prefrontal cortices.

This chapter begins by briefly reviewing the neural circuitry believed to be responsible for PD-related cognitive changes and by discussing the role of neuropsychology in the evaluation of PD patients. We then describe nine cognitive domains: orientation, intelligence, executive functioning, memory, attention, language, visuospatial functioning, information processing speed, and psychomotor functions/motor sequencing, evaluated by a comprehensive neuropsychological assessment, specific measures used to assess these cognitive areas, and the literature on the performance of PD patients in these areas. We also discuss briefly the most common neurobehavioral disturbances in PD. The chapter also describes cognitive rehabilitation methods for remediation and compensation of memory deficits. We focus on the memory strategies that have been shown to have empirical efficacy with patients with various neurological disorders. The chapter concludes with a case study of a PD patient who was evaluated several times over a 2-year period and a discussion of how his neuropsychological findings were able to assist his physical and occupational therapists in addressing his needs.

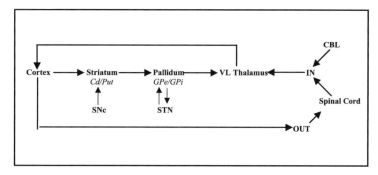

Figure 4-1. Current model of cortical–subcortical motor function. CBL = cerebellum, Cd = caudate, Put = putamen, SNc = substantia nigra pars compacta, GPe = globus pallidus externus, GPi = globus pallidus internus, STN = subthalamic nucleus, VL = ventrolateral.

NEURAL CIRCUITRY OF COGNITION IN PARKINSON'S DISEASE

PD patients demonstrate loss of neurons in the pars compacta of the substantia nigra and subsequent dopamine (DA) depletion in the striatum.[12-14] Disturbed function of the basal ganglia-thalamocortical "motor" circuit is thought to be responsible for hypokinetic (decreased motor activity) and hyperkinetic (increased motor activity) states depending on the specific neural pathways involved (Figure 4-1). Evidence suggests that the striatum is connected to the frontal cortex by several independent but parallel pathways, including but not limited to the "motor" circuit.[13,14] Specifically, DA depletion in the lateral orbitofrontal and the dorsolateral prefrontal circuits has been suggested as a possible mechanism of cognitive impairment in PD.[12] However, DA depletion in PD is not believed to be limited to nigrostriatal pathways, but also may be a consequence of direct depletion of DA in the ascending pathways from the ventromedial tegmentum.[12-14] The complex nature of these parallel pathways suggests that cognitive dysfunction in PD may be a consequence of disruption not only in the primary motor circuit but also in a number of interconnected pathways from the basal ganglia to the cortex.

NEUROPSYCHOLOGICAL EVALUATIONS

Neuropsychological assessments can provide an accurate and unbiased estimate of various aspects of a patient's behavioral capacity throughout the progression of a disease. The task of the neuropsychologist is to dissect an observed test performance into its components in order to identify the abilities (or disabilities) underlying it. The neuropsychological examination provides a profile of the cognitive strengths and weaknesses of a patient. This information can serve as an aid in diagnosis, a guide to management, a basis for deciding whether a patient should be advised to return to work, and a baseline for plotting future changes in status. Specific indications for neuropsychological assessment in PD are to:

1. Identify the presence and nature of early or mild disturbances in cognitive function.

Figure 4-2. PD patient performing standard neuropsychological evaluation.

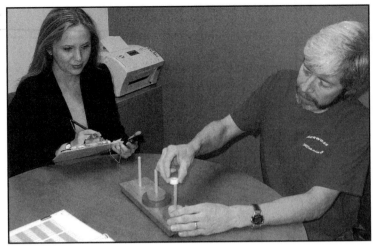

2. Aid in the differentiation of depression or other causes of behavioral impairment from brain disease.
3. Elucidate the natural progression of PD-related cognitive changes or dementia through repeated administration of standardized tests.
4. Assist in planning for rehabilitation.
5. Evaluate the effects of new medications or surgical interventions (eg, pallidotomy, Deep Brain Stimulation [DBS]).
6. Aid in making decisions regarding a patient's ability to make his or her own health and financial decisions as well as future living planning.

Strategies of neuropsychological assessment may be categorized broadly as fixed battery (ie, administration of a comprehensive, invariant series of tests) or as flexible or adjustive (selection of tests according to the reason for referral, pertinent clinical data, information obtained during an interview, and the patient's ability to cooperate). In general, neuropsychological test batteries can take between 3 to 20 hours to administer depending on the level of neurologic impairment and the referral question, with the average clinical neuropsychological outpatient evaluation taking between 4 to 6 hours (Figure 4-2). However, due to numerous disease-related factors, including fatigue, on/off medication periods, and disabling motor problems, PD patient evaluations are usually limited to 1 to 4 hours. Consequently, such fixed batteries as the Halstead-Reitan,[15] which require considerable amounts of time to administer, are rarely used for PD patients.

COGNITION IN PARKINSON'S DISEASE

Orientation and Brief Testing Batteries

Orientation is a basic cognitive capacity that typically must be attained before rehabilitation of other cognitive skills. The Mini-Mental Status Examination (MMSE) of Folstein and associates[16] is the most routinely administered orientation measure used by neurologists to screen for orientation and cognitive impairments informally. The test, which is comprised of 11 questions and yields a maximum of 30 points, combines orientation questions along with assessment of attention/concentration, cognitive flexibility, language, constructional ability, and immediate and brief delayed recall. MMSE scores of 24 to 30 are considered to indicate cognitive status within the normal range.[17] In a longitudinal study comparing 77 patients with PD to 43 controls, 19% of the PD patients performed significantly poorer on the MMSE during a 2-year period compared to none of the controls.[18] In another longitudinal study, 17% of PD patients significantly declined in mental status (ie, ≥4-point difference on the MMSE) over a 2-year period.[19] However, the MMSE has been criticized for being insensitive to differences between dementing disorders, and particularly insensitive to cognitive decline in subcortical dementias. For example, Jefferson et al[20] found no differences in MMSE summary scores between patients with PD, AD, and vascular dementia, indicating that this test should not be used as a diagnostic tool. Furthermore, in a study examining PD patients with dementia, only 46% of demented PD patients scored below the traditional cutoff score of 24 on the MMSE.[21] Moreover, in a study defining cognitive dysfunction as impaired performance on at least three neuropsychological tests, there was no difference found in MMSE scores between cognitively intact and cognitively impaired PD patients.[22] Huber and Bornstein[23] noted that the MMSE "is insensitive to mild cognitive deficits in PD because more than half of the points are derived from measures of orientation and language, which are typically spared even in PD patients with moderately severe cognitive impairment."[23(p42)]

In response to the criticisms of the MMSE and the need for rapid cognitive evaluation (screening), many brief test batteries (10 to 30 minutes in length) have been designed to assess early cognitive impairment or to assess the course of mental decline in dementing illnesses. The Dementia Rating Scale (DRS)[24] and Neurobehavioral Cognitive Status Examination[25] incorporate brief, easily administered measures that tap many of the cognitive domains into a single measure of cognitive function. In general, these measures are more useful for staging the progress or severity of PD, rather than for diagnostic classification or diagnosis of dementia.[26] When used for their stated purpose—namely, to identify cases that warrant more detailed study—these procedures have proved to be fairly successful. For example, the DRS, which yields five subscale scores (Attention, Initiation/Perseveration, Construction, Conceptualization, and Memory) as well as an assessment of the patient's overall level of cognitive functioning, accounted for more variation in PD patients' level of cognitive functioning than either the MMSE or a battery of tests selected to assess specific cognitive deficits associated with PD.[27] The results of this study suggest that the DRS can be a valid mental status screening test of cognitive functioning for individuals with PD.

The Repeatable Battery for the Assessment of Neuropsychological Status (RBANS) is a slightly longer assessment battery that takes approximately 30 minutes to administer.[28] It provides a brief assessment of a patient's cognitive status and can be used to measure change over time in five cognitive domains (Immediate Memory, Visuospatial/Constructional, Language, Attention, and Delayed Memory) using 12 subtests (List Learning, Story Memory, Figure Copy, Line Orientation, Digit Span, Coding, Picture Naming, Semantic Fluency, List Recall, List Recognition, Story Recall, and Figure Recall). A study by Beatty et al[29] examined the classification accuracy of the RBANS for diagnosing the subcortical dementia syndrome of PD. They found that the RBANS correctly classified 78% of their sample of PD patients with dementia using an algorithm proposed by Randolph et al.[30] Despite its usefulness in discriminating patterns of impairment in PD, the authors recommended that a diagnosis of dementia in patients with PD should not be based solely on RBANS results.[31]

Intelligence

The Wechsler Adult Intelligence Scale—Third Edition (WAIS-III) is the most widely used test for assessment of overall level of cognitive functioning.[32] Even though the Wechsler procedures originally were not designed to assess cognitive impairment associated with cerebral disease, they have the advantage of standardization on large normative populations and yield reliable results when the findings of different examiners are compared.

Standardization of the Wechsler scales across a wide span of age in normal subjects permits conversion of raw scores to standardized scores that yield a mean intelligence quotient (IQ) of 100, with a standard deviation of 15, at any age in the normal population. Accordingly, IQs range from 85 to 115 in 68% of the population (within one standard deviation of the mean), and 95% of the population have IQs of 70 to 130 (within two standard deviations of the mean). The WAIS comprises two major scales—Verbal and Performance. In contrast to the Verbal Scale, which largely reflects retention of previously acquired (and frequently overlearned) factual information, the Performance Scale emphasizes visuospatial capacity and visuomotor speed on relatively novel problems. The Performance Scale is less dependent on formal education and appears to be more vulnerable to the effects of normal aging and neurologic conditions that disproportionately impair perceptual motor skills and speed such as PD. The motor impairments associated with PD may necessitate modification of standard testing procedures or substitution of other cognitive tests. The WAIS-III Matrix Reasoning subtest, however, is an untimed test that is more suitable for examinees whose response speed may be slowed, and it provides a relatively culture-fair and language-free assessment on the Performance Scale. In addition, tests such as the Leiter Scale, Raven's Progressive Matrices, and Peabody Picture Vocabulary Test require less reliance on timing and motor performance than the WAIS-III Performance subtests, thereby circumventing these limitations.[33-35]

The Wechsler Abbreviated Scale of Intelligence (WASI) was developed in 1999 to offer a brief (15 to 30 minutes) and reliable estimate of general intellectual functioning.[36] This standardized test is designed for use in individuals aged 6 to 89 years and yields Verbal, Performance, and Full-Scale IQ scores. Norms are provided for the administration of variations of four WAIS-III subtests (Vocabulary, Block Design, Similarities, and Matrix Reasoning) and an even shorter version using only the Vocabulary and Matrix Reasoning subtests. The WASI should be used only as an estimate of general intellectual functioning.

Eighty-five percent of PD patients, compared to 15% of the general population, have WAIS Verbal IQ–Performance IQ discrepancies of greater than 10 points and 36.5% of PD patients have a 25-point VIQ–PIQ difference, which is found in less than 1% of the general population.[37] As expected, the VIQ–PIQ discrepancy is due to PD patients consistently performing better on verbal, as compared to performance, measures.[37] In a meta-analytic review comparing the neuropsychological profiles of 2,730 patients with PD (2,134 nondemented, 596 demented) to 2,464 normal controls, demented PD patients demonstrated significantly large deficits in WAIS-R Performance IQ as compared to controls (d = –3.40) whereas nondemented PD patients demonstrated more modest deficits (d = –0.63).[38] Of note, there is less than 5% overlap between demented PD patients and controls in the distribution of Performance IQ scores, suggesting that this index can discriminate virtually all demented PD patients from controls.[38] In addition, the Performance IQ deficits for demented and nondemented PD patients are considerably larger than the effect sizes obtained for Verbal IQ deficits in comparison to controls (d = –1.58 and d = –0.11, respectively).

Executive Functioning

In general, executive functions refer to "higher-level" cognitive processes involved in the control and regulation of "lower-level" cognitive processes such as reasoning, decision making, and problem solving. Research suggests that there are three component factors underlying executive functions: (1) inhibition and switching,[39-43] (2) working memory,[44-49] and (3) sustained and selective attention.[48,50-52] The dorsolateral prefrontal cortex has been linked to a variety of executive functions, including verbal and design fluency, response inhibition, working memory, organizational skills, maintaining and shifting set, planning, reasoning, problem solving, and abstract thinking.[53-59] Frontostriatal functioning is vital for the execution of more complex tasks such as decision making, problem solving, behavioral adaptation, everyday social interactions, and management of occupational demands (eg, switching from one task to another). Safety, financial planning, driving, and occupational performance, which are areas that physicians and allied health professionals are often asked to address for their patients, can be of concern in patients who demonstrate impairments in these cognitive domains. Given the frontostriatal pathology implicated in PD, patients with PD have been found to be impaired on a variety of executive function tasks.[60-71]

The Wisconsin Card Sorting Test (WCST)[72] is the most widely employed executive function procedure for evaluating the capacity for abstract reasoning and flexibility in problem solving.[44,73-78] Stimulus cards differing in color, form, and number are presented to the patient for sorting into groups according to a principle pre-established by the examiner. As the patient sorts the cards, he or she is told whether his or her responses are correct or incorrect. The number of trials required to achieve 10 consecutive correct responses is recorded. When (or if) the patient has mastered the task, the principle of sorting is changed by the examiner, and once again the number of trials required to achieve correct sorting is recorded. Measures of the capacity for abstract thinking (ie, the number of trials required to achieve a solution) and of flexibility in problem solving (ie, perseverative errors on successive sorting) are derived from the patient's performance. PD patients demonstrate deficits on the WCST,[38,79-82] which may be attributable to an interruption of frontostriatal neural circuitry.[83] A meta-analytic review found that the magnitude of effect for the number of perseverative errors on the WCST was twofold in demented (d = 1.50) versus nondemented (d = 0.68) PD patients.[38]

Many other tests have been employed to assess executive functions. The Categories Test of the Halstead-Reitan battery requires the patient to solve novel problems by selecting a relevant dimension such as color or shape in response to stimuli that are presented in a visual display.[15] The Trail Making Test Part B requires the patient to alternate between a series of numbers and letters in order.[15] This test also requires intact visual tracking, motor skills, and visuomotor integration for optimal performance and, thus, it is not considered a test of specific frontal lobe integrity.[84] The Stroop test is one of the most widely employed measures of selective attention,[48,85-87] and it is regularly used by approximately 50% of neuropsychologists.[74] The Stroop test consists of three sets of stimuli: (1) color words printed in black ink, (2) color patches or colored Xs, and (3) color words printed in incongruous colored ink (eg, the word "RED" printed in blue ink). The patient must read the color words on the first sheet, the colors on the second sheet, and the color of the ink (ie, not the words) on the third sheet. In the latter task, the normal tendency to read the words, rather than the color of the ink in which the words are printed, elicits a significant slowing in reaction time (RT) called the "Stroop effect" or "interference effect." Stroop[88] found that healthy college students' mean RT increased by 74% from naming color patches to naming the incongruous colored ink in which color words were printed. A meta-analytic review found that the Stroop test was the least sensitive executive function task in discriminating nondemented PD patients (d = –0.13) and demented PD patients (d = –0.72) from controls.[38]

Memory

Disturbances of memory are such a frequent consequence of cerebral disease that their assessment can be considered to be one of the most important components of the neuropsychological examination. Several distinctions are made between various contrasting forms of memory, each of which may be differentially impaired in patients with brain damage. These contrasting forms of memory (ie, short-term versus long-term; verbal versus nonverbal; declarative versus procedural; recall versus recognition) will be discussed in the following sections.

Short-Term and Long-Term Memory

Short-term memory (STM), also known as immediate memory, usually is compared with long-term memory (LTM). STM, which operates within a time period of 45 seconds or less and with minimal opportunity for rehearsal, largely depends on attentional processes, processing speed, and the accurate perception of incoming information. STM is divided into primary memory (the ability to retain information in memory for a short time) and working memory (the ability to maintain and manipulate the information held in primary memory). Working memory is a limited-capacity cognitive process involved in the temporary maintenance, manipulation, and transformation of verbal or spatial material. PD patients demonstrate reduced working memory spans when compared to control patients.[89-92] LTM, which involves the temporary or permanent storage of information, is divided into "recent memory" for events occurring hours or days before recall and "remote memory" for events that occurred further back in time. Evaluation of recent memory for information presented by the examiner over days or weeks is usually impractical in clinical testing. In a clinical setting, assessment of recent memory is typically limited to a memory delay of 30 minutes to 1 hour. LTM is dependent on the integrity of the mesial temporal region of the brain,[93] an area of the brain generally spared by PD. Thus, patients with PD typically do not demonstrate deficits in memory for remote events.[38,94]

Verbal and Nonverbal Memory

Another important distinction in neuropsychology is that between verbal and nonverbal memory. Defects in the learning and retention of verbal material (names or sentences) typically are found in patients with left hemisphere disease, whereas corresponding defects in the learning and retention of nonverbal material (abstract figures and faces) typically are found in patients with right hemisphere lesions.[95] PD-related declines have been found for both verbal and nonverbal memory[95]; however, a meta-analytic review found that PD patients generally exhibit greater deficits on verbal versus nonverbal memory measures.[38]

Declarative and Procedural Memory

Another distinction is the differentiation between declarative and procedural memory. Declarative memory involves the retention of factual information, or "knowing that" for both verbal (eg, names) and nonverbal (eg, faces) information, whereas procedural memory involves the retention of motor skills and overlearned operations, or "knowing how" for tasks such as tying shoelaces. Declarative memory comprises both episodic and semantic memory. Episodic memory is involved in the "where" and "when" relationships among events and the temporal sequence, whereas semantic memory is defined as the knowledge of facts and concepts. In a meta-analytic review, Zakzanis and Freedman[38] found that nondemented PD patients displayed a large impairment (d = 1.82) on the Tower of Toronto, a test of rule learning, suggesting impaired procedural memory. Other studies also have found that PD patients are impaired on procedural tasks involving implicit learning of new rule-based responses (eg, Tower of Hanoi) and complex motor skills (eg, pursuit rotor tracking).[96-99]

Recall and Recognition Memory

Recognition memory, or memory paradigms that provide a forced-choice format, offer additional information compared with a free recall format. The recognition format provides cues to retrieve the information more easily. The Warrington Recognition Memory Test offers a verbal and nonverbal measure of recognition memory with the presentation of a series of 50 words and 50 faces followed individually by a two–forced-choice format.[100] Patients who are unable to communicate orally are able to perform this task by pointing to their choices. PD patients typically have problems with free recall but not with recognition memory,[38,101-105] suggesting that PD patients have difficulty with retrieval of information rather than encoding. In contrast to this widely accepted view, a recent meta-analysis found that recognition memory impairments do occur in patients with PD, with the largest deficits occurring in those PD patients with dementia.[106] Nevertheless, PD patients generally have more difficulty with recall, as compared to recognition, which is consistent with a subcortical pattern of memory impairment as opposed to the cortical pattern found in dementing processes such as AD.[107]

Assessment of Memory Functions

Wechsler Memory Scales

The Wechsler Memory Scale (WMS), which is the most widely used test battery for the evaluation of memory functions, is a composite of verbal and nonverbal tests that probes immediate memory, delayed memory, and attention.[108,109] It provides an overall memory score as well as scores for verbal, visual, and delayed memory. The WMS-III takes approximately 2 hours to complete. This extended period of time is not realistic for PD patients. Consequently, many neuropsychologists choose to administer a limited portion of the subtests such as Logical Memory, Verbal Paired Associates, Faces, and Visual Reproduction. Several studies have found that PD patients perform worse than controls on immediate and delayed recall of verbal and nonverbal WMS subtests.[38,110,111]

Verbal Memory Tests

Other tests have been devised to measure specific forms of memory. The Buschke Selective Reminding Test allows for assessment of long-term storage and continuous long-term retrieval of verbal material.[112] The Rey Auditory-Verbal Learning Test (RAVLT),[113] California Verbal Learning Test-II,[114] and Hopkins Verbal Learning Test,[115] which measure the ability to learn and recall lists of words, are widely employed procedures of proven clinical utility. PD patients consistently have demonstrated deficits on immediate and delayed recall of word lists.[38,104,116-118]

Nonverbal Memory Tests

Visual stimuli (objects, faces, geometric figures, abstract designs) have been employed to assess nonverbal memory.[95] The Rey-Osterrieth Complex Figure Test[119] requires the patient to copy a complex abstract design and to reproduce the design without forewarning following a brief delay (30 seconds to 3 minutes) and a long delay (20 to 45 minutes). The Brief Visual Memory Test[120] incorporates a serial design learning paradigm over three trials and assesses delayed free recall and recognition memory. The Benton Visual Retention Test[121] utilizes a three-figure design format. Studies have found that PD patients exhibit deficits on a variety of nonverbal memory tests such as complex figure drawings and the visual reproduction subtest of the WMS.[38,122-125]

Attention

"Attention" is not a unitary concept. Several more or less independent types (eg, simple, selective, divided, shifting) have been identified. It is clear that attentional deficit can be completely or partially responsible for observed impairment in learning, retention, perception, and problem solving.[95]

Attentional processes currently are evaluated by a variety of examination procedures, including the Arithmetic, Digit Symbol-Coding, Digit Span, and Letter-Number Sequencing subtests of the WAIS-III, the Reitan Trail Making Test, and cancellation tests in which the patient marks only designated target letters interspersed with other nontarget letters or distractor items in lengthy sequences.[15,32,95] Auditory information processing tasks include the Paced Auditory Serial Addition Test[126] and the serial subtraction of sevens from the MMSE.[127] Covert selective attention can be assessed by means of a chronometric procedure called the Covert Orienting of Visuospatial Attention Task (COVAT), which is a computer-administered reaction time (RT) task involving simple target detection.[128] Visual attention is manipulated by providing cues, in advance of target presentation, which indicate that a target is about to appear. Although visual attention is generally associated with overt eye movements, Posner's task measures covert orienting, which is attention to a location that is not foveated. Choice reaction time (response to a button or key corresponding to a specific imperative stimulus) and continuous performance tasks provide additional measures of selective and sustained attention.[95] The Conners' Continuous Performance Task (CPT-II) is a computer-based RT task that is frequently used in clinical assessments of attentional disorders.[129] The CPT-II is designed to measure sustained attention, or vigilance. It has a greater number of target trials than alternate CPT paradigms, circumventing the problem of ceiling and floor effects and resulting in more reliable statistics. Patients are required to press the spacebar as quickly as possible whenever any letter of the alphabet appears on the computer screen, except the target letter "X." The CPT-II records omission errors (failure to respond after any letter, except X, appears) and commission errors (pressing the spacebar after the letter X appears). Omission errors may reflect inattention, whereas commission errors may reflect impulsivity. Theoretically, the CPT-II is more sensitive to errors of commission because the frequency of responding over the 14-minute task to non-target letters creates a tendency to respond to the target letter X when inhibition is required.

Although there have been mixed findings regarding the presence of attentional deficits in patients with PD,[130] a meta-analytic review found that PD patients generally demonstrate intact performance on simple measures of attention and concentration (eg, Digit Span) relative to other neuropsychological domains.[38] However, demented PD patients demonstrate impairment on more complex measures of attention such as Trail Making, Digit Symbol-Coding, and Arithmetic.[38] PD patients also have demonstrated RT impairment on covert orienting tasks.[131-133]

Language

Previous models of language function suggested that language impairments were the result of primary damage to the cortex (eg, AD, Korsakoff's disease).[134] However, more recent findings have incorporated subcortical brain structures (such as those implicated in PD) into these models of language, providing more flexibility and a deeper understanding of the neural circuitry responsible for communication.[135] One distinction in language performance is made between receptive language (the awareness and comprehension of language) and expressive language (the formulation and production of appropriate language). Impairments in the perceptual integration or recognition of language are known as *agnosias*, which fall within the domain of receptive language impairments, whereas impairments in the expression of language are classified as *aphasias*. *Paraphasias*, or misspoken words, frequently are found during the middle and late stages of AD, but rarely are demonstrated in PD, whereas patients with PD demonstrate impairments in speech fluency, word-finding, and speech initiation.[95]

Assessment of naming ability, which is the most frequently impaired linguistic function in patients with brain disease, is assessed by procedures that require the naming of line drawings of objects on visual confrontation, such as the Boston Naming Test.[136] Standardized aphasia test batteries provide profiles of percentile scores for a variety of language functions, such as word association, repetition, naming, and receptive ability.[137-139] A meta-analytic review found that language was the least impaired cognitive domain in nondemented PD patients and only mild language deficits were found in demented PD patients.[38] Thus, although language functions are relatively spared throughout the progression of PD, demented PD patients do show declines in verbal skills as compared to nondemented PD patients.

Verbal fluency is the ability to generate words beginning with a specified letter (phonemic fluency) or to generate exemplars of a specified category (semantic fluency). Impaired verbal fluency performance is correlated with subsequent development of dementia in PD.[140] A large body of empirical evidence has found that PD patients generate fewer words on both phonemic and semantic verbal fluency tasks than demographically matched controls.[38,141-145]

Visuospatial Functioning

Visuospatial performance comprises a variety of abilities, such as visual form discrimination, complex visual discrimination, color discrimination, visuoperceptual organization, visual matrices, constructional praxis, and visual neglect. A variety of visuospatial tasks have been developed to tap each of these abilities, including identification of the slope of visually presented lines or pairs of lines, complex visual discrimination, integration of visual information into meaningful percepts, differentiation between figure and background, and completion of visual matrices that progressively get more difficult.[32,35,146] Impairment in spatial thinking, as found in defective localization of objects in space, judgment of distance and direction, and geographic orientation, has long been regarded as a specific sign of disease of the right hemisphere.[147] Visuoconstructive deficit is commonly present in patients with posterior lesions, but right frontal lesion sites also have been reported in affected cases.[95,148] Furthermore, inattention or neglect of the left visual field is a frequent consequence of right posterior lesions. Failure to search for and manipulate stimuli in the left visual field may produce a defective level of performance. The presence of neglect may be obvious by observing the patient performing daily activities, but the degree of inattention can be assessed by line bisection, drawing a clock, geographic localization using a map, a test of crossing lines scattered throughout a page, or a paragraph reading test in which the indentation of sentences is variable.[95] Although clock face drawing[138] originally was used to assess neglect,[149] it is now also used as a screening procedure for other neurological conditions including dementia.[95] The patient first is asked to draw a clock to command ("set the time for 10 after 11") and, depending on his or her performance on the freehand drawing portion of the test, the patient may be asked to copy a clock drawing with the hands already set at 10 after 11 (Figure 4-3).

Figure 4-3. Example of a visuospatial deficit in a patient with Parkinson's disease.

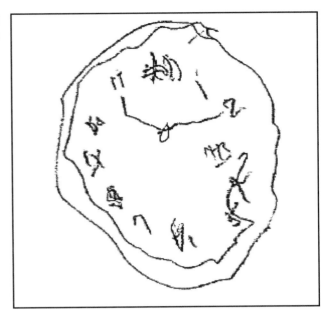

Impairment of visuospatial function frequently has been found in PD patients, including deficits in visual discrimination, visuoperceptual and visuospatial processing, visuomotor abilities, visual attention, visuospatial cognition (eg, mental rotation), and body-spatial orientation.[150-155] However, many visuospatial abilities are not affected and may remain intact throughout the course of the disease such as visual sensory functions and visual recognition skills. A meta-analytic review found that visuospatial deficits are minimal in nondemented PD patients when effect sizes are taken into consideration; however, the magnitude of effect was larger in demented PD patients, which "may be an artifact of timing rules and slowed performance rather than a higher level disturbance in visuoperceptual and visuospatial processes."[38(p140)]

Information Processing Speed

Information processing speed generally is measured by speed-dependent and mental tracking tests. Several factors have been found to influence response speed. Younger individuals, men, well-educated persons, and individuals without a history of head injury tend to process information faster than their counterparts.[95] Reaction time tests are relatively direct measures of processing speed; however, these tests are not used frequently in clinical settings. Information processing speed typically is evaluated clinically by the following examination procedures: Trail Making Test, Digit Symbol-Coding, and Symbol Search.[15,32] The Trail Making Test has two parts—the patient first must draw lines to connect numbered circles in order (Part A) and then the patient must connect numbered and lettered circles alternating between numbers and letters in order (Part B). The patient is encouraged to connect the circles "as fast as possible" without lifting the pencil from the paper and without making any errors. The Processing Speed Index (PSI) of the WAIS-III comprises two subtests—Digit Symbol-Coding and Symbol Search. The PSI correlates strongly with Trail Making ($r = -.49$),[156] which supports the notion that these three tests (Trail Making, Digit Symbol-Coding, and Symbol Search) are valid convergent measures of processing speed.

The term *bradyphrenia*, which describes a syndrome characterized by slowing of cognitive processing, commonly is discussed in the literature on cognitive impairment in PD.

Although there have been some mixed findings regarding the presence of bradyphrenia in patients with PD,[157] cognitive slowing often has been demonstrated in PD patients.[158-161] Furthermore, a meta-analytic review found that demented PD patients demonstrate large deficits compared to controls on certain processing speed measures (eg, WAIS-R Digit Symbol, d = –2.16), while they display milder impairments on other measures of processing speed (eg, Trail Making Test, d = 0.80).[38]

Psychomotor Functions and Motor Sequencing

Motor impairment is the hallmark feature of PD and will be discussed in detail in several chapters. Consequently, this chapter will focus only briefly on the evaluation of motor function from a neuropsychological perspective. Bradykinesia is described as motor slowness both in initiating behavior and in responding to external stimuli. PD patients demonstrate bradykinesia from an early stage of disease progression and it is considered to be a core deficit in PD.[162] Neuropsychological examinations provide a brief evaluation of motor functioning using measures that tap speed of either fine or gross motor skills, particularly in the hands and fingers. Measures of speed of movement that have been employed clinically are finger tapping and quickness in placing pegs in a board.[148,163,164] Some evidence suggests that the value of these simple speed tasks as indexes of the presence of brain damage compares favorably with that of other types of clinical tests.[148,165] Manual dexterity and fine motor speed are impaired in both demented and nondemented patients with PD.[38,166] A meta-analytic review found that there is less than 5% overlap between demented PD patients and normal controls in the distribution of scores on manual dexterity measures, suggesting that this index can discriminate virtually all demented PD patients from controls.[38]

Neuropsychological evaluations also can encompass several additional assessments of motor ability, including apraxia, impersistence, and perseveration. Apraxia is an inability to carry out a skilled motor activity, despite having the physical ability to perform the action. There are many types of apraxia affecting facial movements (buccofacial), arms and legs (limb-kinetic), verbal commands (ideomotor), and sequential movements (ideational). PD patients generally perform within normal limits on measures of apraxia.[167] Motor impersistence is the inability to sustain a movement that has been asked of the patient. Motor perseveration refers to an inflexible or "sticky" motor response caused by a failure of automatic regulatory mechanisms.[95] Motor sequencing involves complex coordination of different movements in a predetermined order. However, motor sequencing is not dependent entirely on a primary motor ability. Cognitive abilities that tap prefrontal cortex functioning, such as set shifting, temporal ordering, and cognitive sequencing can affect an individual's ability to perform motor sequences. In PD, despite the primary motor impairment, set shifting and cognitive sequencing deficits predict motor sequencing performance better than simple motor performance, particularly on more complex sequencing tasks.[168]

Summary of Neuropsychological Functioning in Parkinson's Disease

PD patients demonstrate cognitive impairments in the areas of complex attentional processes, information processing speed, visuospatial orientation, procedural memory, and memory retrieval strategies. PD patients also demonstrate cognitive deficits on tests that are dependent on intact functioning of frontostriatal pathways such as tests of executive functioning, verbal fluency, working memory, and set shifting.[169] Not all cognitive domains, however, are affected by the disease process. PD patients show intact cognitive functioning in the areas of primary attention, immediate memory, recognition memory, memory storage and consolidation, and language comprehension.

PSYCHOLOGICAL FUNCTIONING IN PARKINSON'S DISEASE

Depression

Depression is the most common psychiatric manifestation of PD,[170] with approximately 40% of PD patients experiencing at least mild depression during the course of their illness.[171,172] Approximately 7% to 32% of PD patients are diagnosed with major depression according to DSM-IV diagnostic criteria.[173] Depression in PD has been linked with cognitive impairment, increased levels of disability, poorer outcomes, and caregiver burden.[172] Reported risk factors for developing depression in PD are longer duration of the disease, female sex, early-onset PD, personal history of depression, and predominantly right-sided motor symptoms.[174-177] The relationship between depression and severity of motor symptoms also has been evaluated. PD patients who predominantly have bradykinesia and gait difficulties report more depression than those PD patients who are tremor-dominant.[178] Additionally, when PD patients are in their "off" medication state, they often report more depressive symptomatology.[179]

The assessment of depression in PD patients is complicated by the overlap of the physiological symptoms of depression and the symptomatology of PD. Physiological symptoms of depression include increased fatigue, sleep difficulties, changes in appetite, and decreased libido. These symptoms also have been found in PD patients without depression. Consequently, standard depression measures that include the physiological symptoms of depression, such as the Beck Depression Inventory, may over-report the level of depression in PD patients. The Beck Depression Inventory-II (BDI-II) is a self-report questionnaire that includes 21 groups of statements measuring the cognitive, affective, and somatic/physiological symptoms of depression along a severity continuum from minimal to severe.[180] PD patients have been found to demonstrate significantly higher scores than controls on the BDI, with self-rated disability and number of recent medical problems as the greatest predictors of depressive symptoms.[181] The Geriatric Depression Inventory,[182] a self-report questionnaire with 30 true/false items, does not rely as heavily on the physiological symptoms of depression as the BDI-II; however, it is not utilized often in the research literature. The Hamilton Depression Inventory,[183] which is a self-report measure of depression frequently used in clinical studies, allows for identification and evaluation of specific symptoms of Major Depression as delineated by the DSM-IV.

The relationship between depression and cognitive functioning in PD has not been established definitively. Several studies have found more severe cognitive impairments in PD patients with depression than those without, particularly in executive functioning and memory performance.[184-191] Additionally, a longitudinal study found that PD patients with major depression demonstrate significantly greater cognitive declines over a 12-month period than PD patients with either minor depression or no depression.[192] Further research is needed to define more clearly the relationship between neuropsychological deficits and depressive symptoms in PD.

Anxiety

Approximately 40% of PD patients meet DSM-IV criteria for anxiety disorders and many more have anxiety symptoms that are insufficient to meet formal criteria.[193,194] Anxiety disorders are more prevalent in PD patients than age-matched controls;[195,196] however, anxiety often is undetected and may be underdiagnosed in this population.[197] Anxiety symptoms frequently emerge before the onset of parkinsonism,[198-202] they contribute substantially to morbidity and caregiver burden,[193] they usually co-occur with depressive symptomatology,[199,203,204] and they often worsen in patients who develop erratic motor fluctuations during "off" periods.[205-208]

Anxiety also has been related to cognitive impairment in patients with PD. Measures of anxiety on the State-Trait Anxiety Inventory were significantly and negatively correlated with RBANS (a cognitive screening measure) indexes.[209] Thus, anxiety is common in PD patients and is associated with a number of poor outcomes. Treatment of anxiety in this population may include anxiolytic medication as well as non-pharmacologic approaches such as relaxation training, exercise, and psychotherapy;[193] however, these treatments have not been studied extensively in terms of their efficacy with PD patients.[194]

Psychosis

Psychosis is a common neurobehavioral symptom in PD, affecting approximately 30% to 50% of patients over the course of the disease.[210,211] Delusions and visual hallucinations are the two most common side effects of dopaminergic therapy, occurring in 10% to 25% of PD patients.[212] Potential risk factors for the development of psychosis in PD include exposure to dopaminergic medications, older age, later stage of disease progression, dementia, greater cognitive impairment, increasing severity and duration of PD, history of depression, comorbid depression and anxiety, visual impairment, sleep disturbances, and use of multiple medications.[210,213,214] The symptoms of psychosis range widely from minor and non-threatening illusions or vivid dreams to frank visual hallucinations.[215] Visual hallucinations in PD typically occur at night, during sundowning, or when a patient is first waking up.[215] They are usually non-threatening and are not overly complex.[214] Often patients report seeing insects crawling on the floor, children playing, or a family member or friend standing in the corner of a room.[215] When the hallucinations are less vivid and non-threatening, patients typically have insight that they are not part of reality. However, as the disease progresses and the hallucinations become more vivid, they can become distressing to both the patient and caregiver. Treatment of psychosis in PD involves early detection, patient and caregiver education, analysis of risk factors, potential modification of antiparkinsonian medication, and possible adjunctive psychoactive medication such as antidepressants and antipsychotics.[210]

COGNITIVE REHABILITATION

Cognitive rehabilitation refers to methods that are used to help individuals with cognitive impairments maintain their current mental status or, if successful, improve upon or delay the decline of cognitive skills. The training usually focuses on improving memory, but strategies also have been offered for attention and concentration, visuospatial functioning, and executive functioning (eg, problem solving, sequencing, judgment). The primary goal of cognitive rehabilitation is to improve upon an individual's daily social and/or occupational functioning that has been adversely affected by cognitive declines. Cognitive rehabilitation strategies have adopted the widely known adage "If you don't use it, you will lose it" to help maintain or prevent the decline of cognitive skills.

Several definitions regarding the types of cognitive rehabilitation methods have been presented. Clare and colleagues[216] proposed three definitions that we will adopt for the remainder of the discussion. *Cognitive stimulation* has been proposed as the term for activities usually provided in a group that attempt to improve general cognitive and social functioning. *Cognitive training* is a more focused approach that utilizes guided practice or retraining on a particular skill (eg, memory training through repetition of a list learning task). Cognitive rehabilitation has been used to describe more individualized approaches that focus on patients' daily activity functioning by using their strengths to compensate for their deficits.

Only two articles have been published on cognitive training in Parkinson's disease.[217,218] Sinforiani and colleagues used a 6-week computerized cognitive training program for both motor and cognitive training in 20 early stage PD patients. They reported a significant improvement in verbal fluency, logic memory, and matrix reasoning when compared to the patients' baseline evaluations. The authors posited that this instrument should be used more widely in PD populations.[217] Sammer and colleagues[219] focused exclusively on training executive functions as compared to standard treatment in PD patients. The half of the 26 patients who participated in a 10-session working memory training program performed better on two executive function tasks as compared to no improvement in the standard care group. However, the generalizability of this training into the daily activities of PD patients was not evaluated. These authors recommend short-term specific training for PD patients based on individual needs.

Due to the lack of cognitive rehabilitation studies in PD, studies of other neurological disorders with cognitive impairments, such as AD, must be examined for their potential efficacy in PD. Several studies have investigated cognitive rehabilitation programs for episodic, prospective, and implicit memory; orientation; and visuomotor processing in AD. One such cognitive rehabilitation program with mildly impaired AD patients utilized 24 sessions of cognitive training compared to 24 sessions of computerized mental stimulation and found that the patients who participated in the cognitive rehabilitation showed improved performance on specific cognitive tasks similar to those used in the training.[220] Another study demonstrated improvements in activities of daily living (ADLs) but not memory with weekly stimulation of memory and training of ADLs.[221] Several studies have begun to investigate the role of errorless learning in the rehabilitation of memory in AD and other neurologically impaired populations with positive results.[222-226] However, we are not aware of any studies of errorless learning in PD patients. In a meta-analysis of six trials of cognitive training in AD, it was concluded that there was no empirical evidence that memory training was beneficial for improving cognitive performance in early AD.[227] It is clear that additional cognitive rehabilitation programs need to be designed and validated to support the empirical efficacy of rehabilitation in dementing illnesses. Furthermore, these programs need to be developed and evaluated specifically for PD patients who demonstrate cognitive declines that are inherently different than those of AD patients.

Memory Strategies

Cognitive rehabilitation of memory impairments can be subdivided into internal and external memory strategies (Sidebar 4-4). Internal memory strategies include cognitive activities that, if practiced and mastered, make encoding or retrieving information easier. Internal strategies include mnemonics, visual guidance, repetition, and chunking. *Mnemonics* are devices, such as rhymes or anagrams, which can aid retrieval of information. For example, a mnemonic commonly taught in grade school is "I before E except after C." The use of acronyms, or using the first letter from a group of words to create a new word, is another technique that can be useful in memorizing a list, particularly in a specified order. However, individuals with dementia are often not able to create or retrieve acronyms without assistance. Visual guidance attempts to incorporate a visual modality to aid in retrieval of verbal information. An example of a visual guidance strategy is the Method of Loci. This method requires you to visualize a familiar path (eg, through your house, or your drive to work) and then mentally associate the to-be-remembered information with landmarks on your path (eg, visualizing the items on a grocery list in atypical locations around one's house). In doing this, a connection is being made between an overlearned visual scene (one's house) and the grocery list. When you are

> ## SIDEBAR 4-4: COGNITIVE REHABILITATION STRATEGIES
>
> **Internal**
> 1. Mnemonics
> 2. Acronyms
> 3. Visual guidance-Method of Loci
> 4. Repetition
> 5. Chunking
> 6. Virtual reality
>
> **External**
> 1. Memory notebooks
> 2. Personal reminders
> 3. To-do lists
> 4. Electronic paging systems
> 5. Sticky notes
> 6. Medication timers

then at the grocery store, taking a visual tour of your house will provide you with cues to the grocery list (eg, bananas on the bed).

All of these internal memory strategies require repetition and practice to master. They must be used on a regular basis so that they become overlearned. Repetition is another internal strategy that provides additional opportunities for information to be encoded and transferred into memory stores. Most individuals have a memory limitation of five to nine pieces of information that they can hold in working memory.[95] However, chunking allows an individual to encode information more efficiently by grouping related pieces of information together to form one new piece of information. Chunking allows an individual to group between one and four pieces of information into a single chunk, thus expanding one's ability to recall large pieces of information more efficiently. For example, the number string "17762006" may be difficult to recall if you try to recall the individual numbers; however, if you chunk the items into more meaningful number arrays (eg, 1776 and 2006), then you are likely to be more successful in recalling the number series. Although several observational studies have suggested that individuals who participate in activities that require cognitive stimulation such as reading, crossword puzzles, board games, and playing musical instruments have a lower risk of developing dementia,[228,229] these cognitive stimulation exercises have not been rigorously and quantitatively evaluated in neurologically impaired populations.

Virtual reality (VR) training relies on the ability to learn automatic motor routines and implicit memory to retrain recall. VR training requires intact procedural memory, which often is left intact until later stages of many neurological diseases.[38,230-233] Researchers have suggested that VR could be used as an external stimulus to create mental images to explore motor plans. For example, a patient in a VR environment may be able to practice mental rotation in everyday life situations, such as automobile driving, or it could be used to help PD patients facilitate their gait movements or motor sequences. In a small study using VR in daily living situations (eg, eating or using the bathroom), two PD patients demonstrated mild difficulties on tasks measuring object pointing, incidental memory, and orientation in the VR environment. The PD patients were also significantly slower during all the trials, particularly in narrow virtual spaces, when compared to 10 non-neurologically compared controls.[234] With further development and evaluation, VR training programs may offer new methods to aid PD patients with both cognitive and motor rehabilitation.

External memory strategies include using compensatory devices to try to circumvent memory impairments. These compensatory devices include memory notebooks/personal reminders, to-do lists, electronic paging systems, sticky notes, and medication timers. These external aids can help improve a particular cognitive function or compensate for a specific deficit. These techniques rely on intact functioning in at least one cognitive area (eg, language) to aid in compensating for a deficit in another cognitive domain (eg, memory). Compensatory devices need to be practiced to become overlearned and a routine part of a patient's daily life. Quittre and colleagues[235] evaluated the effectiveness of using a memory book for ADL and a digital clock for time orientation in one patient with AD. They reported that this patient was able to use an agenda effectively and independently following the treatment. Furthermore, in a longitudinal study utilizing external cognitive rehabilitation strategies, Abrisqueta-Gomez and colleagues[236] reported that five AD patients showed cognitive improvements 1 year following the treatment, but that these improvements were not maintained into the second year. It is clear that more rigorous investigations incorporating much larger sample sizes in a variety of neurologically impaired populations, including PD, are needed to determine the efficacy of cognitive rehabilitation.

Emotional Strategies

A review of the literature on emotional processing in PD found that PD patients have deficits in emotional expression, which could result in interpersonal communication problems.[237] Several studies have offered suggestions on emotional rehabilitative treatments for PD patients with deficits in emotional expression, including social skills training[238,239] and the use of different means of communication to compensate for specific areas of dysfunction.[240,241]

Case Study

Mr. K is a 71-year-old, right-handed man who was diagnosed with idiopathic PD when he was 65 years old. He has been married for 48 years, and has three adult children. He completed college and earned a bachelor of science degree in mechanical engineering. He worked as an engineer for 30 years prior to retiring at the age of 67. His Hoehn and Yahr stage is a 3 while "on" medication and a 3.5 when "off" medication, placing him in the moderate stage of disease progression. His primary PD motor complaints are bradykinesia, bilateral tremor in his hands, and disabling dyskinesias when "on" his medication. His medical history is significant for high blood pressure controlled with diet and medication and prostate cancer treated with surgery. He reported recent declines in his short-term memory over the past year. He and his wife agreed that his mood has declined slightly over the past couple of years, with increased irritability and anhedonia.

A baseline neuropsychological evaluation was conducted to assess his current level of cognitive and psychological functioning. On baseline testing, his intellectual functioning was estimated to be in the high average range premorbidly, which was consistent with his educational and occupational attainment. Mr. K's scores on short-term verbal and nonverbal learning fell within the low average to average range. He was able to encode the information presented to him, and although his learning curve over several trials was somewhat flat, he was able to recall 9/12 words and 4/6 pictures by the final trial. His performance on immediate and delayed free recall was mildly impaired. However, his recognition memory for the verbal and nonverbal material was average. Mr. K's information processing speed was moderately slowed, demonstrating his difficulties with bradyphrenia. He showed some difficulties in switching between two tasks. However, Mr. K did not demonstrate orientation, attention, naming, visuospatial, language fluency or comprehension, or executive functioning deficits. He denied anxiety and any hallucinations. His score on a depression inventory revealed mild depressive symptoms.

Following the baseline evaluation, Mr. K was referred for cognitive rehabilitation to aid his memory abilities. Cognitive rehabilitation during early stages of memory impairment has its greatest impact because patients are able to learn, problem solve, practice, and visualize, which are necessary skills for utilization of internal and external memory strategies. Mr. K, who was accustomed to working with visual plans in his occupation, was able to learn the Method of Loci strategy for recalling grocery lists and his "to-do" lists. Mr. K used his house as his overlearned route, and he used his sense of humor to place objects in each of the rooms (eg, bananas in the bathtub). Mr. K also began to use a medication timer with an alarm to aid in his ability to take his medication at prescribed times. Although somewhat resistant at first, Mr. K also began to carry a memory notebook with him with a list of his medications and his schedule, his physicians' names and telephone numbers, and his family's names and telephone numbers. Mr. K's initial resistance was due to his self-report that he always had been able to remember this information without help and he did not want to be "tied" to his memory book all the time. However, Mr. K was encouraged to use the memory book for 2 weeks as a trial period.

Due to Mr. K's report of increased depression and mood changes, he was referred for an evaluation with a psychiatrist to determine whether there was a need for antidepressant medication and/or psychotherapy. Mr. K agreed to see the psychiatrist and he was prescribed an antidepressant. He refused psychotherapy; however, he agreed to contact the local PD support group. The support group was discussed thoroughly with Mr. K. It was explained to Mr. K and his family that there would be other individuals at the group who would not be as healthy or cognitively intact as he was, but that the support group provided useful information regarding progression of PD and local resources.

Mr. K was not referred for physical or occupational therapy at this time. However, Mr. K likely would have benefited from several sessions of therapy to learn new skills and strategies that he could practice. The practice would have allowed these strategies to become overlearned so that he would be able to call on them later if (or when) his memory declines. The use of assistive devices and exercises could have been practiced with him and written instructions provided to his family for home practice.

Mr. K underwent a follow-up neuropsychological evaluation 2 years following his baseline testing. Mr. K's motor disabilities had become more pronounced over the 2-year period. He had suffered several falls and his dyskinesias were more severe and present more often during the day. Mr. K's family reported that they had noticed a decline in his verbal short-term memory. He was having difficulty remembering conversations, and he was losing belongings in his house. They also remarked that they had noticed word-finding difficulties in everyday conversations.

Mr. K's neuropsychological evaluation revealed that his memory had declined from the average range to the mildly impaired range for verbal material. His learning curve remained flat over the learning trials, and he was able to recall only 6/12 words on the last trial. His immediate and delayed recall for this material also was mildly impaired. Recognition memory for the list of words was low average. His memory for nonverbal material remained relatively consistent with his previous testing. His language fluency declined to the mildly impaired range, and his information processing speed was significantly slower than his previous evaluation. Mr. K also demonstrated declines in his executive functioning, including mildly impaired performances on set shifting and problem solving. Mr. K did not demonstrate any difficulties in his visuospatial abilities, language comprehension, attention, or naming. Mr. K reported some improvements in his emotional functioning. His wife agreed that he was less irritable after he started taking an antidepressant.

Mr. K had attended several cognitive rehabilitation sessions during the 2-year period. However, he was no longer using the Method of Loci internal memory strategy on a routine basis. He stated that he found it more helpful to use the memory notebook that he carried around with him in his shirt pocket. He continued to carry his medication list and his contact information, but he also had his wife write a list of things for him to do, and he kept this task list in his memory notebook. He and his family were encouraged to structure his home environment to aid his memory. Suggested changes included keeping his medications, wallet, and keys in predetermined and highly visible areas; planning activities for outside of the home; using sticky notes on the refrigerator or a board in the kitchen to remind him of appointments or upcoming events; and providing a limited number of choices for him to choose from for activities or dinner options. Mr. K reported that he initially had attended several support group meetings, but he had not gone to a meeting in several months. He was encouraged to attend meetings more regularly to increase social interactions. His wife also was encouraged to allow their sons and daughter to take care of Mr. K at least several times a month so that she was able to attend activities that she enjoys and to reduce her caregiver stress.

Mr. K was referred to occupational therapy to help him and his family learn how to use assistive devices around the house so that he could reduce his falls. Due to his increasing memory difficulties, Mr. K would require more repetitions of task instructions, and more practice outside of the office visits for the skills to become overlearned. His family also would need to be provided with written instructions so that they would be able to practice the instructions with him on a regular basis at home.

References

1. Bassett SS. Cognitive impairment in Parkinson's disease. *Primary Psychiatry*. 2005; 12(7):50-55.
2. Stocchi F, Brusa L. Cognition and emotion in different stages and subtypes of Parkinson's disease. *J Neurol*. 2000;247 Suppl 2:II114-II121.
3. Weintraub D, Stern MB. Psychiatric complications in Parkinson disease. *Am J Geriatr Psychiatry*. 2005;13(10):844-851.
4. Locascio JJ, Corkin S, Growdon JH. Relation between clinical characteristics of Parkinson's disease and cognitive decline. *J Clin Exp Neuropsychol*. 2003;25(1):94-109.
5. Rajput AH. Prevalence of dementia in Parkinson's disease. In: Huber SJ, Cummings JL, eds. *Parkinson's Disease: Neurobehavioral Aspects*. New York: Oxford University Press; 1992:119-131.
6. Knopman DS, Boeve BF, Petersen RC. Essentials of the proper diagnoses of mild cognitive impairment, dementia, and major subtypes of dementia. *Mayo Clin Proc*. 2003; 78(10):1290-1308.
7. American Psychiatric Association. *Diagnostic and Statistical Manual of Mental Disorders*. 4th ed. Washington, DC: American Psychiatric Association, 1994.
8. Cummings JL, Benson DR. *Dementia: A Clinical Approach*. Stoneham, MA: Butterworth Publishers, Inc., 1983.
9. Emre M, Aarsland D, Brown R, et al. Clinical diagnostic criteria for dementia associated with Parkinson's disease. *Mov Disord*. 2007;22:1689-1707.
10. Ross GW, Mahler ME, Cummings JL. The dementia syndromes of Parkinson's disease: cortical and subcortical features. In: Huber SJ, Cummings JL, eds. *Parkinson's Disease: Neurobehavioral Aspects*. New York: Oxford University Press; 1992:132-148.
11. Cummings JL. Subcortical dementia. Neuropsychology, neuropsychiatry, and pathophysiology. *Br J Psychiatry*. 1986;149:682-697.
12. Alexander GE, DeLong MR, Strick PL. Parallel organization of functionally segregated circuits linking basal ganglia and cortex. *Annu Rev Neurosci*. 1986;9:357-381.
13. Lang AE, Lozano AM. Parkinson's disease: First of two parts. *N Engl J Med*. 1998;339:1044-1053.
14. Lang AE, Lozano AM. Parkinson's disease: Second of two parts. *N Engl J Med*. 1998;339:1130-1143.

15. Reitan RM, Wolfson D. *The Halstead-Reitan Neuropsychological Test Battery: Theory and Clinical Interpretation.* Tucson, AZ: Neuropsychology Press, 1993.
16. Folstein MF, Folstein SE, McHugh PR. "Mini-mental state". A practical method for grading the cognitive state of patients for the clinician. *J Psychiatr Res.* 1975;12(3):189-198.
17. Tombaugh TN, McIntyre NJ. The mini-mental state examination: a comprehensive review. *J Am Geriatr Soc.* 1992;40(9):922-935.
18. Bayles KA, Tomoeda CK, Wood JA, Montgomery EB, Jr., Cruz RF, Azuma T et al. Change in cognitive function in idiopathic Parkinson disease. *Arch Neurol.* 1996; 53(11):1140-1146.
19. Azuma T, Cruz RF, Bayles KA, Tomoeda CK, Montgomery EB, Jr. A longitudinal study of neuropsychological change in individuals with Parkinson's disease. *Int J Geriatr Psychiatry.* 2003;18(12):1115-1120.
20. Jefferson AL, Cosentino SA, Ball SK, Bogdanoff B, Leopold N, Kaplan E et al. Errors produced on the mini-mental state examination and neuropsychological test performance in Alzheimer's disease, ischemic vascular dementia, and Parkinson's disease. *J Neuropsychiatry Clin Neurosci.* 2002;14(3):311-320.
21. Huber SJ, Shuttleworth EC, Christy JA, Rice RR. A brief scale for the dementia of Parkinson's disease. *J Neuropsychiatry Clin Neurosci.* 1990;(22):183-188.
22. Muslimovic D, Post B, Speelman JD, Schmand B. Cognitive profile of patients with newly diagnosed Parkinson disease. *Neurology.* 2005;65(8):1239-1245.
23. Huber SJ, Bornstein RA. Neuropsychological evaluation of Parkinson's disease. In: Huber SJ, Cummings JL, eds. *Parkinson's Disease: Neurobehavioral Aspects.* New York: Oxford University Press; 1992:32-45.
24. Jurica PJ, Leitten CL, Mattis S. *Dementia Rating Scale-2 Professional Manual.* Lutz, FL: Psychological Assessment Resources, Inc., 2001.
25. Kiernan RJ, Mueller J, Langston W. *Cognistat.* Fairfax, CA: The Northern California Neurobehavioral Group, Inc., 1995.
26. Camicioli R, Fisher N. Progress in clinical neurosciences: Parkinson's disease with dementia and dementia with Lewy bodies. *Can J Neurol Sci.* 2004;31(1):7-21.
27. Brown GG, Rahill AA, Gorell JM, McDonald C, Brown SJ, Sillanpaa M et al. Validity of the Dementia Rating Scale in assessing cognitive function in Parkinson's disease. *J Geriatr Psychiatry Neurol.* 1999;12(4):180-188.
28. Randolph C. *Repeatable Battery for the Assessment of Neuropsychological Status.* San Antonio, TX: The Psychological Corporation, 1999.
29. Beatty WW, Ryder KA, Gontkovsky ST, Scott JG, McSwan KL, Bharucha KJ. Analyzing the subcortical dementia syndrome of Parkinson's disease using the RBANS. *Arch Clin Neuropsychol.* 2003;18(5):509-520.
30. Randolph C, Tierney MC, Mohr E, Chase TN. The Repeatable Battery for the Assessment of Neuropsychological Status (RBANS): preliminary clinical validity. *J Clin Exp Neuropsychol.* 1998;20(3):310-319.
31. Beatty WW, Ryder KA, Gontkovsky ST, Scott JG, McSwan KL, Bharucha KJ. Analyzing the subcortical dementia syndrome of Parkinson's disease using the RBANS. *Arch Clin Neuropsychol.* 2003;18(5):509-520.
32. Wechsler D. *WAIS-III Administration and Scoring Manual.* New York: The Psychological Corporation, 1997.
33. Dunn LM. *Peabody Picture Vocabulary Test (Revised Manual).* Circle Pines, MN: American Guidance Press, 1981.
34. Leiter RG. *General Instructions for the Leiter International Performance Scale.* Chicago: Stoelting, 1969.
35. Raven JC. *Guide to the Standard Progressive Matrices.* New York: The Psychological Corporation, 1973.
36. Wechsler D. *Wechsler Abbreviated Scale of Intelligence.* New York: The Psychological Corporation, 1999.
37. Loranger AW, Goodell H, McDowell FH, Lee JE, Sweet RD. Intellectual impairment in Parkinson's syndrome. *Brain.* 1972;95(2):405-412.
38. Zakzanis KK, Freedman M. A neuropsychological comparison of demented and nondemented patients with Parkinson's disease. *Appl Neuropsychol.* 1999;6(3):129-146.
39. Baldo JV, Shimamura AP, Delis DC, Kramer J, Kaplan E. Verbal and design fluency in patients with frontal lobe lesions. *J Int Neuropsychol Soc.* 2001;7(5):586-596.
40. Burgess PW, Alderman N, Evans J, Emslie H, Wilson BA. The ecological validity of tests of executive function. *J Int Neuropsychol Soc.* 1998;4(6):547-558.
41. Miyake A, Friedman NP, Emerson MJ, Witzki AH, Howerter A, Wager TD. The unity and diversity of executive functions and their contributions to complex "Frontal Lobe" tasks: a latent variable analysis. *Cognit Psychol.* 2000;41(1):49-100.
42. Sergeant JA, Geurts H, Oosterlaan J. How specific is a deficit of executive functioning for attention-deficit/hyperactivity disorder? *Behav Brain Res.* 2002;130(1-2):3-28.
43. Troyer AK, Moscovitch M, Winocur G, Alexander MP, Stuss D. Clustering and switching on verbal fluency: the effects of focal frontal- and temporal-lobe lesions. *Neuropsychologia.* 1998;36(6):499-504.
44. Barcelo F, Knight RT. Both random and perseverative errors underlie WCST deficits in prefrontal patients. *Neuropsychologia.* 2002;40(3):349-356.
45. Barcelo F, Rubia FJ. Non-frontal P3b-like activity evoked by the Wisconsin Card Sorting Test. *Neuroreport.* 1998;9(4):747-751.

46. Sergeant JA, Geurts H, Oosterlaan J. How specific is a deficit of executive functioning for attention-deficit/hyperactivity disorder? *Behav Brain Res*. 2002;130(1-2):3-28.

47. Stuss DT, Alexander MP, Hamer L, Palumbo C, Dempster R, Binns M et al. The effects of focal anterior and posterior brain lesions on verbal fluency. *J Int Neuropsychol Soc*. 1998;4(3):265-278.

48. Stuss DT, Floden D, Alexander MP, Levine B, Katz D. Stroop performance in focal lesion patients: dissociation of processes and frontal lobe lesion location. *Neuropsychologia*. 2001;39(8):771-786.

49. Zelazo P, Carter A, Reznick J, Frye D. Early development of executive function: a problem-solving framework. *Rev Gen Psychology*. 1997;1:198-226.

50. Barcelo F. Does the Wisconsin Card Sorting Test measure prefrontal function? *Span J Psychol*. 2001;4(1):79-100.

51. Manly T, Robertson I. Sustained attention and the frontal lobes. In: Rabbitt P, ed. *Methodology of Frontal and Executive Function*. Hove, UK: Psychology Press; 1997:135-153.

52. Stuss DT, Alexander MP, Hamer L, Palumbo C, Dempster R, Binns M et al. The effects of focal anterior and posterior brain lesions on verbal fluency. *J Int Neuropsychol Soc*. 1998;4(3):265-278.

53. Cummings JL. Frontal-subcortical circuits and human behavior. *Arch Neurol*. 1993; 50(8):873-880.

54. Duke LM, Kaszniak AW. Executive control functions in degenerative dementias: a comparative review. *Neuropsychol Rev*. 2000;10(2):75-99.

55. Grafman J, Litvan I. Importance of deficits in executive functions. *Lancet*. 1999; 354(9194):1921-1923.

56. Jonides J, Smith EE, Koeppe RA, Awh E, Minoshima S, Mintun MA. Spatial working memory in humans as revealed by PET. *Nature*. 1993;363(6430):623-625.

57. Malloy PF, Richardson ED. Assessment of frontal lobe functions. In: Salloway SP, Malloy PF, Duffy JD, eds. *The Frontal Lobes and Neuropsychiatric Illness*. Washington, DC: American Psychiatric Publishing, Inc.; 2001:125-137.

58. Milner B. Interhemispheric differences in the localization of psychological processes in man. *Br Med Bull*. 1971;27(3):272-277.

59. Stuss DT, Levine B, Alexander MP, Hong J, Palumbo C, Hamer L et al. Wisconsin Card Sorting Test performance in patients with focal frontal and posterior brain damage: effects of lesion location and test structure on separable cognitive processes. *Neuropsychologia*. 2000;38(4):388-402.

60. Bouquet CA, Bonnaud V, Gil R. Investigation of supervisory attentional system functions in patients with Parkinson's disease using the Hayling task. *J Clin Exp Neuropsychol*. 2003; 25(6):751-760.

61. Culbertson WC, Moberg PJ, Duda JE, Stern MB, Weintraub D. Assessing the executive function deficits of patients with Parkinson's disease: utility of the Tower of London-Drexel. *Assessment*. 2004;11(1):27-39.

62. Downes JJ, Roberts AC, Sahakian BJ, Evenden JL, Morris RG, Robbins TW. Impaired extra-dimensional shift performance in medicated and unmedicated Parkinson's disease: evidence for a specific attentional dysfunction. *Neuropsychologia*. 1989; 27(11-12):1329-1343.

63. Farina E, Gattellaro G, Pomati S, Magni E, Perretti A, Cannata AP et al. Researching a differential impairment of frontal functions and explicit memory in early Parkinson's disease. *Eur J Neurol*. 2000; 7(3):259-267.

64. Ferraro FR, Balota DA, Connor LT. Implicit memory and the formation of new associations in nondemented Parkinson's disease individuals and individuals with senile dementia of the Alzheimer type: a serial reaction time (SRT) investigation. *Brain Cogn*. 1993;21(2):163-180.

65. Knowlton BJ, Mangels JA, Squire LR. A neostriatal habit learning system in humans. *Science*. 1996;273(5280):1399-1402.

66. Milner B. Interhemispheric differences in the localization of psychological processes in man. *Br Med Bull*. 1971;27(3):272-277.

67. Morris RG, Downes JJ, Sahakian BJ, Evenden JL, Heald A, Robbins TW. Planning and spatial working memory in Parkinson's disease. *J Neurol Neurosurg Psychiatry*. 1988; 51(6):757-766.

68. Owen AM. Cognitive dysfunction in Parkinson's disease: the role of frontostriatal circuitry. *Neuroscientist*. 2004;10(6):525-537.

69. Owen AM, Roberts AC, Hodges JR, Summers BA, Polkey CE, Robbins TW. Contrasting mechanisms of impaired attentional set-shifting in patients with frontal lobe damage or Parkinson's disease. *Brain*. 1993;116(Pt 5):1159-1175.

70. Pollux PM, Robertson C. Reduced task-set inertia in Parkinson's disease. *J Clin Exp Neuropsychol*. 2002;24(8):1046-1056.

71. Taylor AE, Saint-Cyr JA. Executive function. In: Huber SJ, Cummings JL, eds. *Parkinson's Disease: Neurobehavioral Aspects*. New York: Oxford University Press, 1992: 74-85.

72. Heaton RK, Chelune GJ, Talley JL, Kay GG, Curtiss G. *Wisconsin Card Sorting Test Manual: Revised and expanded*. Odessa, FL: Psychological Assessment Resources, 1993.

73. Berg EA. A simple objective test for measuring flexibility in thinking. *J Gen Psychol*. 1948;39:15.

74. Butler M, Retzlaff P, Vanderploeg R. Neuropsychological test usage. *Professional Psychology: Research and Practice*. 1991;22:510-512.

75. Grant, DA, Berg, E. A behavioral analysis of degree of reinforcement and ease of shifting to new responses in a Weigl-type card-sorting problem. *J Exper Psychology.* 1948; 38:404-411.
76. Reitan RM, Wolfson D. A selective and critical review of neuropsychological deficits and the frontal lobes. *Neuropsychol Rev.* 1994;4(3):161-198.
77. Spreen O, Strauss E. *A Compendium of Neuropsychological Tests: Administration, Norms, and Commentary.* 2nd ed. New York: Oxford University Press, 1998.
78. Stuss DT, Levine B. Adult clinical neuropsychology: lessons from studies of the frontal lobes. *Annu Rev Psychol.* 2002;53:401-433.
79. Farina E, Gattellaro G, Pomati S, Magni E, Perretti A, Cannata AP et al. Researching a differential impairment of frontal functions and explicit memory in early Parkinson's disease. *Eur J Neurol.* 2000;7(3):259-267.
80. Green J, McDonald WM, Vitek JL, Evatt M, Freeman A, Haber M et al. Cognitive impairments in advanced PD without dementia. *Neurology.* 2002;59(9):1320-1324.
81. Muslimovic D, Post B, Speelman JD, Schmand B. Cognitive profile of patients with newly diagnosed Parkinson disease. *Neurology.* 2005;65(8):1239-1245.
82. Vingerhoets G, Verleden S, Santens P, Miatton M, De Reuck J. Predictors of cognitive impairment in advanced Parkinson's disease. *J Neurol Neurosurg Psychiatry.* 2003; 74(6):793-796.
83. Taylor AE, Saint-Cyr JA, Lang AE. Subcognitive processing in the frontocaudate "complex loop": the role of the striatum. *Alzheimer Dis Assoc Disord.* 1990;4(3):150-160.
84. Gaudino EA, Geisler MW, Squires NK. Construct validity in the Trail Making Test: what makes Part B harder? *J Clin Exp Neuropsychol.* 1995;17(4):529-535.
85. Carter CS, Mintun M, Cohen JD. Interference and facilitation effects during selective attention: an H215O PET study of Stroop task performance. *Neuroimage.* 1995; 2(4):264-272.
86. Goodglass H, Kaplan E. Assessment of cognitive deficit in the brain-injured patient. In: Gazzaniga MS, ed. *Handbook of Behavioral Neurology.* New York: Plenum Press; 1979: 3-22.
87. MacLeod CM. Half a century of research on the Stroop effect: an integrative review. *Psychol Bull.* 1991;109(2):163-203.
88. Stroop J. Studies of interference in serial verbal reactions. *J Exper Psychology.* 1935; 18:643-662.
89. Bublak P, Muller U, Gron G, Reuter M, von Cramon DY. Manipulation of working memory information is impaired in Parkinson's disease and related to working memory capacity. *Neuropsychology.* 2002;16(4):577-590.
90. Fournet N, Moreaud O, Roulin JL, Naegele B, Pellat J. Working memory functioning in medicated Parkinson's disease patients and the effect of withdrawal of dopaminergic medication. *Neuropsychology.* 2000;14(2):247-253.
91. Gilbert B, Belleville S, Bherer L, Chouinard S. Study of verbal working memory in patients with Parkinson's disease. *Neuropsychology.* 2005;19(1):106-114.
92. Kensinger EA, Shearer DK, Locascio JJ, Growdon JH, Corkin S. Working memory in mild Alzheimer's disease and early Parkinson's disease. *Neuropsychology.* 2003; 17(2):230-239.
93. O'Connor MG, Lafleche G. Amnesic syndromes. In: Snyder PJ, Nussbaum PD, Robins DL, eds. *Clinical Neuropsychology: A Pocket Handbook for Assessment.* Washington, DC: American Psychological Association; 2006:463-488.
94. Fama R, Sullivan EV, Shear PK, Stein M, Yesavage JA, Tinklenberg JR et al. Extent, pattern, and correlates of remote memory impairment in Alzheimer's disease and Parkinson's disease. *Neuropsychology.* 2000;14(2):265-276.
95. Lezak MD. *Neuropsychological Assessment.* 2nd ed. New York: Oxford University Press, 1995.
96. Bondi MW, Kaszniak AW. Implicit and explicit memory in Alzheimer's disease and Parkinson's disease. *J Clin Exp Neuropsychol.* 1991;13(2):339-358.
97. Harrington DL, Haaland KY, Yeo RA, Marder E. Procedural memory in Parkinson's disease: impaired motor but not visuoperceptual learning. *J Clin Exp Neuropsychol.* 1990; 12(2):323-339.
98. Heindel WC, Salmon DP, Shults CW, Walicke PA, Butters N. Neuropsychological evidence for multiple implicit memory systems: a comparison of Alzheimer's, Huntington's, and Parkinson's disease patients. *J Neurosci.* 1989;9(2):582-587.
98. Saint-Cyr JA, Taylor AE, Lang AE. Procedural learning and neostriatal dysfunction in man. *Brain.* 1988;111(Pt 4):941-959.
100. Warrington EK. *Recognition Memory Test.* Odessa, FL: Psychological Assessment Resources, 1984.
101. Beatty WW. Memory disturbances in Parkinson's disease. In: Huber SJ, Cummings JL, eds. *Parkinson's Disease: Neurobehavioral Aspects.* New York: Oxford University Press; 1992:49-58.
102. Green J, McDonald WM, Vitek JL, Evatt M, Freeman A, Haber M et al. Cognitive impairments in advanced PD without dementia. *Neurology.* 2002;59(9):1320-1324.
103. Muslimovic D, Post B, Speelman JD, Schmand B. Cognitive profile of patients with newly diagnosed Parkinson disease. *Neurology.* 2005;65(8):1239-1245.

104. Tierney MC, Nores A, Snow WG, Fisher RH, Zorzitto ML, Reid DW. Use of the Rey Auditory Verbal Learning Test in differentiating normal aging from Alzheimer's and Parkinson's dementia. *Psychological Assessment.* 1994;6(2):129-134.

105. Zgaljardic DJ, Borod JC, Foldi NS, Mattis P. A review of the cognitive and behavioral sequelae of Parkinson's disease: relationship to frontostriatal circuitry. *Cogn Behav Neurol.* 2003; 16(4):193-210.

106. Whittington CJ, Podd J, Kan MM. Recognition memory impairment in Parkinson's disease: power and meta-analyses. *Neuropsychology.* 2000;14(2):233-246.

107. Camicioli R, Fisher N. Progress in clinical neurosciences: Parkinson's disease with dementia and dementia with Lewy bodies. *Can J Neurol Sci.* 2004;31(1):7-21.

108. Wechsler D. *Wechsler Memory Scale-Revised Manual.* San Antonio, TX: The Psychological Corporation, 1987.

109. Wechsler D. *Wechsler Memory Scale-III Manual.* San Antonio, TX: The Psychological Corporation, 1997.

110. Downes JJ, Priestley NM, Doran M, Ferran J, Ghadiali E, Cooper P. Intellectual, mnemonic, and frontal functions in dementia with Lewy bodies: a comparison with early and advanced Parkinson's disease. *Behav Neurol.* 1998;11(3):173-183.

111. Fama R, Sullivan EV, Shear PK, Stein M, Yesavage JA, Tinklenberg JR et al. Extent, pattern, and correlates of remote memory impairment in Alzheimer's disease and Parkinson's disease. *Neuropsychology.* 2000;14(2):265-276.

112. Hannay HJ, Levin HS. Selective reminding test: an examination of the equivalence of four forms. *J Clinical Exper Neuropsychology.* 1985;7(3):251-263.

113. Rey A. *L'examen clinique en psychologie.* Paris: Presses Universitaires de France, 1964.

114. Delis DC, Kramer JH, Kaplan E et al. *The California Verbal Learning Test-II.* New York: The Psychological Corporation; 2000.

115. Shapiro AM, Benedict RH, Schretlen D et al. Construct and concurrent validity of the Hopkins Verbal Learning Test-revised. *Clin Neuropsychol.* 1999;13:348.

116. Green J, McDonald WM, Vitek JL, Evatt M, Freeman A, Haber M et al. Cognitive impairments in advanced PD without dementia. *Neurology.* 2002;59(9):1320-1324.

117. Muslimovic D, Post B, Speelman JD, Schmand B. Cognitive profile of patients with newly diagnosed Parkinson disease. *Neurology.* 2005;65(8):1239-1245.

118. Vingerhoets G, Verleden S, Santens P, Miatton M, De Reuck J. Predictors of cognitive impairment in advanced Parkinson's disease. *J Neurol Neurosurg Psychiatry.* 2003; 74(6):793-796.

119. Meyers JE, Meyers KR. *Rey Complex Figure Test and Recognition Trial.* San Antonio, TX: The Psychological Corporation, 1995.

120. Benedict RHB. *Brief Visiual Memory Test-Revised.* Lutz, FL: Psychological Assessment Resources, Inc., 1997.

121. Benton AL, Sivan AB, Hamsher K et al. *Contributions to Neuropsychological Assessment.* 2nd ed. New York: Oxford University Press, 1994.

122. Sahakian BJ, Morris RG, Evenden JL, Heald A, Levy R, Philpot M et al. A comparative study of visuospatial memory and learning in Alzheimer-type dementia and Parkinson's disease. *Brain.* 1988;111(Pt 3):695-718.

123. Sullivan EV, Sagar HJ. Nonverbal recognition and recency discrimination deficits in Parkinson's disease and Alzheimer's disease. *Brain.* 1989;112(Pt 6):1503-1517.

124. Taylor AE, Saint-Cyr JA, Lang AE. Frontal lobe dysfunction in Parkinson's disease. The cortical focus of neostriatal outflow. *Brain.* 1986;109(Pt 5):845-883.

125. Vingerhoets G, Verleden S, Santens P, Miatton M, De Reuck J. Predictors of cognitive impairment in advanced Parkinson's disease. *J Neurol Neurosurg Psychiatry.* 2003; 74(6):793-796.

126. Gronwall DMA. Paced Auditory Serial-Addition Task: A measure of recovery from concussion. *Perceptual and Motor Skills.* 1977;44:367-373.

127. Folstein MF, Folstein SE, McHugh PR. "Mini-mental state". A practical method for grading the cognitive state of patients for the clinician. *J Psychiatr Res.* 1975;12(3):189-198.

128. Posner MI, Raichle ME. *Images of Mind.* New York: Scientific American Library/Scientific American Books, 1994.

129. Conners CK, MHS staff. *Conners' Continuous Performance Test (CPT II): Computer Program for Windows Technical Guide and Software Manual.* North Tonawanda, NY: Multi-Health Systems Inc, 2000.

130. Zgaljardic DJ, Borod JC, Foldi NS, Mattis P. A review of the cognitive and behavioral sequelae of Parkinson's disease: relationship to frontostriatal circuitry. *Cogn Behav Neurol.* 2003; 16(4):193-210.

131. Rafal RD, Posner MI, Walker JA, Friedrich FJ. Cognition and the basal ganglia. Separating mental and motor components of performance in Parkinson's disease. *Brain.* 1984;107(Pt 4):1083-1094.

132. Wright MJ, Burns RJ, Geffen GM, Geffen LB. Covert orientation of visual attention in Parkinson's disease: an impairment in the maintenance of attention. *Neuropsychologia.* 1990;28(2):151-159.

133. Yamada T, Izyuuinn M, Schulzer M, Hirayama K. Covert orienting attention in Parkinson's disease. *J Neurol Neurosurg Psychiatry.* 1990;53(7):593-596.

134. Geschwind N. Language and the brain. *Sci Am.* 1972;226(4):76-83.

135. Crosson B. *Subcortical Functions in Language and Memory.* New York: Guilford Press, 1992.

136. Kaplan E, Goodglass H, Weintraub S. *The Boston Naming Test.* 2nd ed. Philadelphia, PA: Lea & Febiger, 1983.

137. Benton AL, Hamsher K. *Multilingual Aphasia Examination.* Iowa City: Department of Neurology, University of Iowa, 1983.

138. Goodglass H, Kaplan E. *Assessment of Aphasia and Related Disorders.* 2nd ed. Philadelphia: Lea & Febiger, 1983.

139. Kertesz A. *Aphasia and Associated Disorders.* New York: Grune & Stratton, 1979.

140. Jacobs DM, Marder K, Cote LJ, Sano M, Stern Y, Mayeux R. Neuropsychological characteristics of preclinical dementia in Parkinson's disease. *Neurology.* 1995; 45(9):1691-1696.

141. Azuma T, Cruz RF, Bayles KA, Tomoeda CK, Montgomery EB, Jr. A longitudinal study of neuropsychological change in individuals with Parkinson's disease. *Int J Geriatr Psychiatry.* 2003;18(12):1115-1120.

142. Beatty WW, Staton RD, Weir WS, Monson N, Whitaker HA. Cognitive disturbances in Parkinson's disease. *J Geriatr Psychiatry Neurol.* 1989;2(1):22-33.

143. Cummings JL. The dementias of Parkinson's disease: prevalence, characteristics, neurobiology, and comparison with dementia of the Alzheimer type. *Eur Neurol.* 1988; 28 Suppl 1:15-23.

144. Henry JD, Crawford JR. Verbal fluency deficits in Parkinson's disease: a meta-analysis. *J Int Neuropsychol Soc.* 2004;10(4):608-622.

145. Troyer AK, Moscovitch M, Winocur G, Leach L, Freedman M. Clustering and switching on verbal fluency tests in Alzheimer's and Parkinson's disease. *J Int Neuropsychol Soc.* 1998;4(2):137-143.

146. Benton AL, Sivan AB, Hamsher K et al. *Contributions to Neuropsychological Assessment.* 2nd ed. New York: Oxford University Press, 1994.

147. Dee HL. Visuoconstructive and visuoperceptive deficits in patients with unilateral cerebral lesions. *Neuropsychologia.* 1970;8:305.

148. Smith A. Neuropsychological testing in neurological disorders. *Adv Neurol.* 1975;7:49-110.

149. Battersby, WS, Bender MB, Pollack M, Kahn RL. Unilateral spatial agnosia (inattention) in patients with cerebral lesions. *Brain.* 1956;79(1):68-93.

150. Cummings JL, Huber SJ. Visuospatial abnormalities in Parkinson's disease. In: Huber SJ, Cummings JL, eds. *Parkinson's Disease: Neurobehavioral Aspects.* New York: Oxford University Press; 1992:59-73.

151. Freeman RQ, Giovannetti T, Lamar M, Cloud BS, Stern RA, Kaplan E et al. Visuoconstructional problems in dementia: contribution of executive systems functions. *Neuropsychology.* 2000;14(3):415-426.

152. Hovestadt A, De Jong GJ, Meerwaldt JD. Visuospatial impairment in Parkinson's disease: does it exist? *J Neurol Neurosurg Psychiatry.* 1987;50(11):1560-1561.

153. Levin BE, Tomer R, Rey GJ. Cognitive impairments in Parkinson's disease. *Neurol Clin.* 1992;10(2):471-485.

154. Montse A, Pere V, Carme J, Francesc V, Eduardo T. Visuospatial deficits in Parkinson's disease assessed by judgment of line orientation test: error analyses and practice effects. *J Clin Exp Neuropsychol.* 2001;23(5):592-598.

155. Pirozzolo FJ, Hansch EC, Mortimer JA, Webster DD, Kuskowski MA. Dementia in Parkinson disease: a neuropsychological analysis. *Brain Cogn.* 1982;1(1):71-83.

156. Cohen RA, Malloy PF, Jenkins MA, Paul RH. Disorders of attention. In: Snyder PJ, Nussbaum PD, Robins DL, eds. *Clinical Neuropsychology: A Pocket Handbook for Assessment.* Washington, DC: American Psychological Association; 2006:572-606.

157. Rogers D. Bradyphrenia in Parkinson's disease. In: Huber SJ, Cummings JL, eds. *Parkinson's Disease: Neurobehavioral Aspects.* New York: Oxford University Press; 1992:86-96.

158. Muslimovic D, Post B, Speelman JD, Schmand B. Cognitive profile of patients with newly diagnosed Parkinson disease. *Neurology.* 2005;65(8):1239-1245.

159. Pate DS, Margolin DI. Cognitive slowing in Parkinson's and Alzheimer's patients: distinguishing bradyphrenia from dementia. *Neurology.* 1994;44(4):669-674.

160. Peavy GM, Salmon D, Bear PL, Paulsen JS, Cahn DA, Hofstetter CR et al. Detection of mild cognitive deficits in Parkinson's disease patients with the WAIS-R NI. *J Int Neuropsychol Soc.* 2001;7(5):535-543.

161. Taylor AE, Saint-Cyr JA, Lang AE. Frontal lobe dysfunction in Parkinson's disease. The cortical focus of neostriatal outflow. *Brain.* 1986;109(Pt 5):845-883.

162. White RF, Au R, Durso R, Moss MB. Neuropsychological function in Parkinson's disease. In: White RF, ed. *Clinical Syndromes in Adult Neuropsychology: The Practitioners Handbook.* New York: Elsevier Science; 1992:253-286.

163. Boll TJ. The Halstead-Reitan Neuropsychology Battery. In: Filskov SB, Boll TJ, eds. *Handbook of Clinical Neuropsychology.* New York: Wiley-Interscience, 1981.

164. Vega A. Use of Purdue Pegboard and finger tapping performance as a rapid screening test for brain damage. *J Clinical Psychology.* 1969;25(3):255-258.

165. Blackburn HL, Benton AL. Simple and choice reaction time in cerebral disease. *Confinia Neurologica.* 1955;15:327-338.

166. Vingerhoets G, Verleden S, Santens P, Miatton M, De Reuck J. Predictors of cognitive impairment in advanced Parkinson's disease. *J Neurol Neurosurg Psychiatry.* 2003;74(6):793-796.

167. Tröster AI, Arnett PA. Assessment of movement and demyelinating disorders. In: Synder PJ, Nussbaum PD, Robins DL, eds. *Clinical Neuropsychology.* Washington, DC: American Psychological Association; 2006:243-293.

168. Fama R, Sullivan E, Shear P, Cahn-Weiner D. *Rate of Cognitive Decline in Alzheimer's Disease.* 2002. [Unpublished work]

169. Taylor AE, Saint-Cyr JA, Lang AE. Memory and learning in early Parkinson's disease: evidence for a "frontal lobe syndrome". *Brain Cogn.* 1990;13(2):211-232.

170. Guze BH, Barrio JC. The etiology of depression in Parkinson's disease patients. *Psychosomatics.* 1991;32(4):390-395.

171. Stocchi F, Brusa L. Cognition and emotion in different stages and subtypes of Parkinson's disease. *J Neurol.* 2000;247 Suppl 2:II114-II121.

172. Weintraub D. Depression in Parkinson's disease. *Primary Psychiatry.* 2005;12(7):45-49.

173. Veazey C, Aki SO, Cook KF, Lai EC, Kunik ME. Prevalence and treatment of depression in Parkinson's disease. *J Neuropsychiatry Clin Neurosci.* 2005;17(3):310-323.

174. Cole SA, Woodard JL, Juncos JL, Kogos JL, Youngstrom EA, Watts RL. Depression and disability in Parkinson's disease. *J Neuropsychiatry Clin Neurosci.* 1996;8(1):20-25.

175. Starkstein SE, Preziosi TJ, Bolduc PL, Robinson RG. Depression in Parkinson's disease. *J Nerv Ment Dis.* 1990;178(1):27-31.

176. Tandberg E, Larsen JP, Aarsland D, Cummings JL. The occurrence of depression in Parkinson's disease. A community-based study. *Arch Neurol.* 1996;53(2):175-179.

177. Tandberg E, Larsen JP, Aarsland D, Laake K, Cummings JL. Risk factors for depression in Parkinson disease. *Arch Neurol.* 1997;54(5):625-630.

178. Holthoff-Detto VA, Kessler J, Herholz K, Bonner H, Pietrzyk U, Wurker M et al. Functional effects of striatal dysfunction in Parkinson disease. *Arch Neurol.* 1997; 54(2):145-150.

179. Menza MA, Sage J, Marshall E, Cody R, Duvoisin R. Mood changes and "on-off" phenomena in Parkinson's disease. *Mov Disord.* 1990;5(2):148-151.

180. Beck AT. *Beck Depression Inventory-II (BDI-II).* San Antonio, TX: The Psychological Corporation, 1996.

181. Ehmann TS, Beninger RJ, Gawel MJ, Riopelle RJ. Depressive symptoms in Parkinson's disease: a comparison with disabled control subjects. *J Geriatr Psychiatry Neurol.* 1990; 3(1):3-9.

182. Yesavage JA. The use of self-rating depression scales by the elderly. In: Poon LW, ed. *Handbook for Clinical Memory Assessment of Older Adults.* Washington, DC: American Psychological Association; 1980:213-217.

183. Reynolds WM, Kobak KA. *Hamilton Depression Inventory (HDI) Professional Manual.* Lutz, FL: Psychological Assessment Resources, Inc., 1995.

184. Kuzis G, Sabe L, Tiberti C, Leiguarda R, Starkstein SE. Cognitive functions in major depression and Parkinson disease. *Arch Neurol.* 1997:54(8)):982-986. [Abstract]

185. Starkstein SE, Preziosi TJ, Berthier ML, Bolduc PL, Mayberg HS, Robinson RG. Depression and cognitive impairment in Parkinson's disease. *Brain.* 1989;112(Pt 5):1141-1153.

186. Starkstein SE, Preziosi TJ, Bolduc PL, Robinson RG. Depression in Parkinson's disease. *J Nerv Ment Dis.* 1990;178(1):27-31.

187. Starkstein SE, Rabins PV, Berthier ML, Cohen BJ, Folstein MF, Robinson RG. Dementia of depression among patients with neurological disorders and functional depression. *J Neuropsychiatry Clin Neurosci.* 1989;1(3):263-268.

188. Tandberg E, Larsen JP, Aarsland D, Cummings JL. The occurrence of depression in Parkinson's disease. A community-based study. *Arch Neurol.* 1996;53(2):175-179.

189. Troster AI, Paolo AM, Lyons KE, Glatt SL, Hubble JP, Koller WC. The influence of depression on cognition in Parkinson's disease: a pattern of impairment distinguishable from Alzheimer's disease. *Neurology.* 1995;45(4):672-676.

190. Tröster AI, Stalp LD, Paolo AM, Fields JA, Koller WC. Neuropsychological impairment in Parkinson's disease with and without depression. *Arch Neurol.* 1995;52(12):1164-1169.

191. Uekermann J, Daum I, Peters S, Wiebel B, Przuntek H, Muller T. Depressed mood and executive dysfunction in early Parkinson's disease. *Acta Neurol Scand.* 2003;107(5):341-348.

192. Starkstein SE, Mayberg HS, Leiguarda R, Preziosi TJ, Robinson RG. A prospective longitudinal study of depression, cognitive decline, and physical impairments in patients with Parkinson's disease. *J Neurol Neurosurg Psychiatry.* 1992;55(5):377-382.

193. Marsh L. Anxiety disorders in Parkinson's disease. *International Rev Psychiatry.* 2000; 12:307-318.

194. Menza M, Dobkin RD. Anxiety and Parkinson's disease. *Primary Psychiatry.* 2005; 12(7):63-68.

195. Menza MA, Robertson-Hoffman DE, Bonapace AS. Parkinson's disease and anxiety: comorbidity with depression. *Biol Psychiatry.* 1993;34(7):465-470.

196. Stein MB, Heuser IJ, Juncos JL, Uhde TW. Anxiety disorders in patients with Parkinson's disease. *Am J Psychiatry*. 1990;147(2):217-220.

197. Shulman LM, Taback RL, Rabinstein AA, Weiner WJ. Non-recognition of depression and other non-motor symptoms in Parkinson's disease. *Parkinsonism Relat Disord*. 2002; 8(3):193-197.

198. Gonera EG, van't Hof M, Berger HJ, van Weel C, Horstink MW. Symptoms and duration of the prodromal phase in Parkinson's disease. *Mov Disord*. 1997;12(6):871-876.

199. Henderson R, Kurlan R, Kersun JM, Como P. Preliminary examination of the comorbidity of anxiety and depression in Parkinson's disease. *J Neuropsychiatry Clin Neurosci*. 1992;4(3):257-264.

200. Lauterbach EC, Duvoisin RC. Anxiety disorders in familial parkinsonism. *Am J Psychiatry*. 1991;148(2):274.

201. Shiba M, Bower JH, Maraganore DM, McDonnell SK, Peterson BJ, Ahlskog JE et al. Anxiety disorders and depressive disorders preceding Parkinson's disease: a case-control study. *Mov Disord*. 2000;15(4):669-677.

202. Weisskopf MG, Chen H, Schwarzschild MA, Kawachi I, Ascherio A. Prospective study of phobic anxiety and risk of Parkinson's disease. *Mov Disord*. 2003;18(6):646-651.

203. Menza MA, Robertson-Hoffman DE, Bonapace AS. Parkinson's disease and anxiety: comorbidity with depression. *Biol Psychiatry*. 1993;34(7):465-470.

204. Schiffer RB, Kurlan R, Rubin A, Boer S. Evidence for atypical depression in Parkinson's disease. *Am J Psychiatry*. 1988;145(8):1020-1022.

205. Maricle RA, Nutt JG, Valentine RJ, Carter JH. Dose-response relationship of levodopa with mood and anxiety in fluctuating Parkinson's disease: a double-blind, placebo-controlled study. *Neurology*. 1995;45(9):1757-1760.

206. Menza MA, Sage J, Marshall E, Cody R, Duvoisin R. Mood changes and "on-off" phenomena in Parkinson's disease. *Mov Disord*. 1990;5(2):148-151.

207. Nissenbaum H, Quinn NP, Brown RG, Toone B, Gotham AM, Marsden CD. Mood swings associated with the 'on-off' phenomenon in Parkinson's disease. *Psychol Med*. 1987;17(4):899-904.

208. Siemers ER, Shekhar A, Quaid K, Dickson H. Anxiety and motor performance in Parkinson's disease. *Mov Disord*. 1993;8(4):501-506.

209. Ryder KA, Gontkovsky ST, McSwan KL, Scott JG, Bharucha KJ, Beatty WW. Cognitive function in parkinson's disease: Association with anxiety but not depression. *Aging Neuropsychology and Cognition*. 2002;9(2):77-84.

210. Marsh L. Psychosis in Parkinson's Disease. *Primary Psychiatry*. 2005;12(7):56-62.

211. Naimark D, Jackson E, Rockwell E, Jeste DV. Psychotic symptoms in Parkinson's disease patients with dementia. *J Am Geriatr Soc*. 1996;44(3):296-299.

212. Cummings JL. Neuropsychiatric complications of drug treatment of Parkinson's disease. In: Huber SJ, Cummings JL, eds. *Parkinson's Disease: Neurobehavioral Aspects*. New York: Oxford University Press;1992:313-327.

213. Sanchez-Ramos JR, Ortoll R, Paulson GW. Visual hallucinations associated with Parkinson disease. *Arch Neurol*. 1996;53(12):1265-1268.

214. Weintraub D, Stern MB. Psychiatric complications in Parkinson disease. *Am J Geriatr Psychiatry*. 2005;13(10):844-851.

215. Thanvi BR, Lo TC, Harsh DP. Psychosis in Parkinson's disease. *Postgrad Med J*. 2005;81(960):644-646.

216. Clare L, Woods RT, Moniz Cook ED, Orrell M, Spector A. Cognitive rehabilitation and cognitive training for early-stage Alzheimer's disease and vascular dementia. *The Cochrane Database of Systematic Reviews*. 2003;(4):1-12.

217. Sinforiani E, Banchieri L, Zucchella C, Pacchetti C, Sandrini G. Cognitive rehabilitation in Parkinson's disease. *Arch Gerontol Geriatr Suppl*. 2004;(9):387-391.

218. Clare L, Wilson BA, Carter G, Breen K, Gosses A, Hodges JR. Intervening with everyday memory problems in dementia of Alzheimer type: an errorless learning approach. *J Clin Exp Neuropsychol*. 2000;22(1):132-146.

219. Sammer G, Reuter I, Hullmann K, Kaps M, Vaitl D. Training of executive functions in Parkinson's disease. *J Neurol Sci*. 2006;25:248(1-2):115-119.

220. Loewenstein DA, Acevedo A, Czaja SJ, Duara R. Cognitive rehabilitation of mildly impaired Alzheimer disease patients on cholinesterase inhibitors. *Am J Geriatr Psychiatry*. 2004;12(4):395-402.

221. Avila R, Bottino CM, Carvalho IA, Santos CB, Seral C, Miotto EC. Neuropsychological rehabilitation of memory deficits and activities of daily living in patients with Alzheimer's disease: a pilot study. *Braz J Med Biol Res*. 2004;37(11):1721-1729.

222. Kixmiller JS. Evaluation of prospective memory training for individuals with mild Alzheimer's disease. *Brain Cogn*. 2002;49(2):237-241.

223. Metzler-Baddeley C, Snowden JS. Brief report: errorless versus errorful learning as a memory rehabilitation approach in Alzheimer's Disease. *J Clin Exp Neuropsychol*. 2005; 27(8):1070-1079.

224. Page M, Wilson BA, Shiel A, Carter G, Norris D. What is the locus of the errorless-learning advantage? *Neuropsychologia*. 2006;44(1):90-100.

225. Poolton JM, Masters RS, Maxwell JP. The relationship between initial errorless learning conditions and subsequent performance. *Hum Mov Sci*. 2005;24(3):362-378.

226. Sage K, Hesketh A, Ralph MA. Using errorless learning to treat letter-by-letter reading: contrasting word versus letter-based therapy. *Neuropsychol Rehabil.* 2005;15(5):619-642.

227. Clare L, Wilson BA, Carter G, Roth I, Hodges JR. Awareness in early-stage Alzheimer's disease: relationship to outcome of cognitive rehabilitation. *J Clin Exp Neuropsychol.* 2004;26(2):215-226.

228. Wilson RS, Mendes De Leon CF, Barnes LL, Schneider JA, Bienias JL, Evans DA et al. Participation in cognitively stimulating activities and risk of incident Alzheimer disease. *JAMA.* 2002;287(6):742-748.

229. Verghese J, Lipton RB, Katz MJ, Hall CB, Derby CA, Kuslansky G et al. Leisure activities and the risk of dementia in the elderly. *N Engl J Med.* 2003;348(25):2508-2516.

230. Bondi MW, Kaszniak AW. Implicit and explicit memory in Alzheimer's disease and Parkinson's disease. *J Clin Exp Neuropsychol.* 1991;13(2):339-358.

231. Harrington DL, Haaland KY, Yeo RA, Marder E. Procedural memory in Parkinson's disease: impaired motor but not visuoperceptual learning. *J Clin Exp Neuropsychol.* 1990;12(2):323-339.

232. Heindel WC, Salmon DP, Shults CW, Walicke PA, Butters N. Neuropsychological evidence for multiple implicit memory systems: a comparison of Alzheimer's, Huntington's, and Parkinson's disease patients. *J Neurosci.* 1989;9(2):582-587.

233. Saint-Cyr JA, Taylor AE, Lang AE. Procedural learning and neostriatal dysfunction in man. *Brain.* 1988;111(Pt 4):941-959.

234. Albani G, Pignatti R, Bertella L, Priano L, Semenza C, Molinari E et al. Common daily activities in the virtual environment: a preliminary study in parkinsonian patients. *Neurol Sci.* 2002;23 Suppl 2:S49-S50.

235. Quittre A, Olivier C, Salmon E. Compensating strategies for impaired episodic memory and time orientation in a patient with Alzheimer's disease. *Acta Neurol Belg.* 2005; 105(1):30-38.

236. Abrisqueta-Gomez J, Canali F, Vieira VL, Aguiar AC, Ponce CS, Brucki SM et al. A longitudinal study of a neuropsychological rehabilitation program in Alzheimer's disease. *Arq Neuropsiquiatr.* 2004;62(3B):778-783.

237. Zgaljardic DJ, Borod JC, Foldi NS, Mattis P. A review of the cognitive and behavioral sequelae of Parkinson's disease: relationship to frontostriatal circuitry. *Cogn Behav Neurol.* 2003;16(4):193-210.

238. Brozgold AZ, Borod JC, Martin CC, Pick LH, Alpert M, Welkowitz J. Social functioning and facial emotional expression in neurological and psychiatric disorders. *Appl Neuropsychol.* 1998;5(1):15-23.

239. Pitcairn TK, Clemie S, Gray JM, Pentland B. Non-verbal cues in the self-presentation of parkinsonian patients. *Br J Clin Psychol.* 1990;29(Pt 2):177-184.

240. Beatty W, Goodkin D, Weir W et al. Affective judgments by patients with parkinson's disease or chronic multiple sclerosis. *Bull Psychonom Soc.* 1989;27:361-364.

241. Raskin SA, Bloom R, Borod JC. Rehabilitation of emotional deficits in neurological populations: a multidisplinary perspective. In: Borod JC, ed. *The Neuropsychology of Emotion.* New York, NY: Oxford University Press; 2000:413-431.

Psychosocial Issues in Parkinson's Disease

Naomi D. Nelson, PhD

Introduction

Understanding Parkinson's disease (PD) as a progressive, neurodegenerative, chronic illness is not an easy task. It is a challenging task for the health care professional to learn about the complex neurological changes that patients experience, but equally important to comprehend the intricate psychosocial issues. The aim of this chapter is to help the health care professional gain competence, confidence, and compassion while learning about the psychosocial complexities of PD.

This chapter will begin with a discussion of the biopsychosocial theory, a model for understanding the interactive effects for those living with chronic illness. This theory will be followed by an introduction to the three phases PD patients experience at the onset of symptoms and/or when newly diagnosed. The chapter continues with detailed discussions of the impact of PD on the patient and family caregivers, including sections on depression and anxiety, communication, cognition, sleep, sex, and finances, concluding with guidelines for the health care professional caring for a patient with PD.

THE BIOPSYCHOSOCIAL APPROACH

Other chapters in this text discuss PD primarily using the traditional biomedical model, a model that is analytical and beneficial to science, but can easily ignore the subjective experience of the patient[1] and the psychological and social factors.[2] This section will expand on the biomedical model and begin by explaining why this model, by itself, is insufficient in describing the holistic nature of chronic illness—the blending of biological, psychological, and social dimensions.[1,3,4]

Until the late 20th century, the biomedical model was the traditional approach used by health care professionals when conceptualizing human health and illness.[5] This reductionistic model[6] emphasized infectious agents, alleviation of pain, ameliorative medications, and surgical repair, but it was limited in its understanding of the interactions among biopsychosocial factors and biological findings.[7] Eventually, health care providers had difficulty with the sole use of the biomedical approach, originally conceived as a theory based on somatic parameters. Very simply, the biological approach ignored or minimized differences in patients and between patients with chronic illness. By embracing an old world scientific view and by remaining oblivious to the sociological, psychological, and behavioral influences on health, patients received only a narrow margin of care.[8]

In 1977, a landmark article written by Dr. George L. Engel, from the University of Rochester Medical School, was published in *Science*.[4] Dr. Engel proposed that medical care required attention to psychosocial issues in addition to biological problems and suggested that respect for these data and the interview process was essential to strengthen the doctor–patient relationship and improve patient care.[9] This model closely resembled the general systems theory approach postulated by Von Bertalanffy, who argued that holistic approaches were superior to reductionistic approaches in understanding illness and behavior.[5] The systems theory scientists saw that nature is organized into a hierarchy of simple to complex units, along a continuum, which interact with and are independent from each other. This treatment of systems, whether in the biological or human laboratory, suggested that all levels of organization are linked to each other and changes in one effects change in the others. These beliefs supported the application of the biopsychosocial model to the individual care of patients and specifically to those patients living with chronic illness.[10,11]

Many health care professionals have embraced the biopsychosocial theory of care, changed some of the language, but held true to its basic assumptions for assessing the needs of patients—taking into account the interplay of biological, sociological, psychological, and environmental factors. Engel's contributions encouraged health care professionals to base their practice on the belief that patients are united, "biopsychosocial persons" rather than "biomedical persons."[3] This approach confirms what most health care professionals should be taught—that health and illness can best be understood within a holistic and multifaceted framework and that human beings are more than independent physical processes.[12]

The biopsychosocial model provides a theory that guides comprehensive medical education, patient assessment, and treatment while considering the connections between the coping resources of the patient and family, the cultural context, and the adjustments to chronic illness.[12] Additional information on the psychosocial dimensions is important because it may lead to a better understanding of the different consequences of chronic illness upon an individual.[2] This integrative psychosocial framework provides the background for addressing psychosocial issues in this chapter.

THE HEALTH CARE PROFESSIONAL AND PARKINSON'S DISEASE

Beliefs concerning the biopsychosocial meaning of illness and how illness can be controlled or managed are important for everyone involved in the clinical practice of caring for the chronically ill patient. The role of the health care practitioner is influenced by past and present personal or family experiences with chronic illness and exposure to varied and challenging roles as a professional. These experiences may result in a sensitive, competent appreciation of the interaction between the biological and psychosocial processes or an increased vulnerability and reduced objectivity in caring for these patients. Those living with a chronic illness such as PD deserve interdisciplinary communication, respect, and expertise from the health care team. Although independent practitioners may be comfortable with individual decision making, when caring for those with PD, it becomes necessary to participate in and effectively communicate with other team members.

Health care professionals first need to acknowledge the chronic, progressive nature of this neurodegenerative disorder[13] and understand that the medical therapies for patients are directed toward alleviating the cardinal symptoms: resting tremor, rigidity, bradykinesia, and postural instability.[14] Even though these physical alterations in motor functioning are visible to the patient and health care professionals, other less visible changes experienced by PD patients may cause equal or more distress. These psychosocial factors, such as well-being and quality of life, require assessment expertise and intervention formulated both by the independent health care professional and a health care team of experts knowledgeable about PD[14,15] (see Sidebar 5-1).

LIVING WITH PARKINSON'S DISEASE: IMPACT ON THE PATIENT

The Onset of Symptoms

By the time most patients are officially diagnosed with a chronic illness, they have already figured it out themselves. When compared with other chronic conditions, patients and family members may have more accurate suspicions about PD because the features are sometimes observable to those in close proximity to the patient. The visible changes that may be apparent are hand tremors or stooped posture, but more subtle cues may also be witnessed, including a weakening voice or a facial expression that does not change.[16]

Patients seeking medical care for a potentially chronic condition initially pass through various phases that can alternate between uncertainty, frustration, and confusion. For patients who begin to notice physical changes and eventually seek out the expertise of a physician, they may experience some of the emotional reactions as described in what follows.

Phase I: The Phase of Uncertainty

In this first phase, the patient and/or family member knows that the health status of the patient has changed but they are confused about what those changes may mean. This phase sometimes takes the form of secrecy because patients, friends, or family hesitate to talk about their observations in the hope that they are wrong or that the changes are transitory. Often, the patient is aware of minor neurological changes, but delays discuss-

---

Sidebar 5-1: Guidelines For The Health Care Professional

1. Learn all you can about Parkinson's disease and its influence on the patient, family, community, and health care professionals. Apply this information to your individual situation.

2. Use the "best evidence" when considering treatment interventions for your patients.

3. Become attentive to the "on-off" cycle of the medications. Attempt to schedule professional treatment and interventions during the "on" period.

4. Appreciate uncertainty, unpredictability, and ambiguity inherent in dealing with a chronic illness.

5. Encourage the patient to follow recommendations of the physician and other health care professionals, especially as related to medication, exercise, and psychological support.

6. Be alert to signs of "overwhelm" for patients and families, which manifests itself in the form of depression, isolation, and fatigue.

7. Encourage participation in a support group that provides both education and social support.

8. Encourage participation in national and community organizations for Parkinson's disease, and in their regularly scheduled exercise programs and conferences.

9. Teach the patient self-management skills and refer to a formalized class if available. Use self-efficacy tools and reinforce positive behavior as appropriate.

10. Share information about medic alert bracelets, adaptive equipment, community resources, and patient educational materials.

11. Conduct regular interdisciplinary conferences involving the physician, occupational therapist, physical therapist, speech-language pathologist, professional nurse, social worker, chaplain, and other team members.

12. Include family members or close friends in treatment sessions, especially if you suspect changes in memory.

---

ing it with others to protect them and to protect self. Both patients and families may note hand tremors, slowed thinking and movement, and changes in handwriting, but often attribute these processes to aging.[17] During this first phase, family members may become frustrated with the actions of their loved one and persuade them to seek medical attention. This frustration may cause communication difficulties later when the patient needs more assistance and even more understanding.

During the phase of uncertainty, one young woman commented to her health care provider: "I started yelling at my father when he was helping me move from my garage apartment to my new home 200 miles away. He moved so slowly going up and down the stairs and took so long to load the car. I thought he was just emotional about my leaving home, but didn't want to talk about it. He didn't laugh at my silly jokes either. After he was diagnosed with PD, I felt so guilty. I had no idea that PD would produce such changes in my relatively young father. He had become so slow."

Phase II: The Phase of Learning

During the second phase, the patient alone or with family members seeks out medical expertise and the physician confirms the PD diagnosis. At this point, patients may be reassured that there is an explanation for their problems and that treatment may be helpful. Most patients and families sense some relief when they see the physician who is able to give a diagnosis. Even though they do not like to hear the diagnosis, it explains their anxieties and observations.

What is most helpful at this phase is the willingness to learn about PD, the medications, and the treatment—all at a level comfortable for the patient and family. During this phase, the patient and health care professional benefit from forming a trusted partnership—one that may exist for years. One family therapist suggests that this is the beginning of a "chronic relationship" with the health care professional—an essential relationship for all those living with chronic illness.[5]

It is not always an easy transition from Phase I to Phase II. One woman commented: "When I heard that I had a diagnosis of Parkinson's disease, I immediately went into 'overwhelm.' All of my usual analytical thinking went flying out the window and I just started to panic right there in the doctor's office. I hid it well, though, but what I wanted to do was toss the Parkinson's books on the floor, run from the room and tell them they had made a big mistake—I didn't have Parkinson's disease. Why did I have to be pinned down to a routine of medications where there was no flexibility? On my limited budget, how was I going to afford the cost of medications not only for months ahead, but for the indeterminate future? I didn't want to learn about the complicated medication regime, how agonists work, the side effects of the medications, and the benefits of a weekly pill box. It was just too much information. I thought Parkinson's disease happened to people the age of my parents. It just didn't seem fair to be happening to me at 47, and I wasn't prepared."

Phase III: The Phase of Assimilation

In Phase III, the patient and family begin to assimilate the chronic illness into their lives, but need to be wary that the illness does not define who they are or become the focus of all their interactions and communications. They start to acknowledge that their lives are changed forever, but trust that their inner strength and external support will be stable enough to help them through the years ahead. One couple stated it this way: "Don't get us wrong, we're not happy that Bill has Parkinson's disease, but we will get through this. We've encountered other challenges in life before this and so, in a way, we've had practice for the tougher times ahead. We will be compliant with the doctor's recommendations, but we will not let Parkinson's disease rule our lives, and we won't talk about it all the time. We will find a place for this illness, just as we've found a place for other struggles like grief and loss, financial difficulties, and moving away from family."

These three phases experienced by many at the onset of PD symptoms set the stage for a more detailed discussion of the psychosocial dimensions affecting patients and family caregivers as the illness progresses.

Figure 5-1. Remaining active by engaging in stimulating leisure activities enhances quality of life for patients with Parkinson's disease.

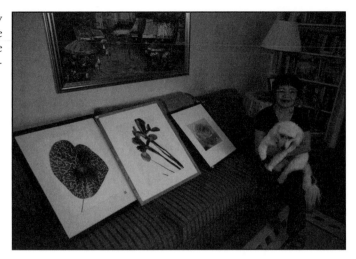

Living With Parkinson's Disease: Selected Challenges

What does PD mean to the patient? Just as there are many variants of PD, so there are many differences in the meaning and experience of the illness. As health care professionals, we must learn how the disease affects patients as individuals because there is no singular experience of living with PD.[18,19] The experience of PD supports the idiosyncratic nature of the illness, and patients state almost uniformly that it does negatively influence the quality of their lives.[20] Although "life goes on" for most patients, the assimilation of the illness into their lives is not without complexity and confusion. Astute health care professionals assess and observe the patient's positive and negative personality styles, the handling of previous crises, the influence of family dynamics, and the application of coping styles as predictors of how the patient will adapt to the diagnosis, the progression, and the treatment.[21]

There are few studies that focus on the patient's perspective on living with PD.[20,22,23] Researchers do acknowledge, however, that PD impacts both the emotional and social lives of the patient and family and contributes to stress and a sense of loss.[17,21] Whereas most environmental factors contribute to the patient's perspectives of living with PD, the rate of progression of the disease appears to be a major determinant of psychosocial stress, and the presence of dyskinesias and motor fluctuations influences quality of life.[24] One Japanese study determined that a longer duration of illness and advanced stages of the disease contributed to the perception of a more negative quality of life.[25] A larger study with veterans in the United States also supported the findings that those living with PD reported a more negative quality of life than veterans with other chronic illnesses.[26]

Illness severity by itself does not always suggest a more negative quality of life for patients with PD and those with other neurodegenerative diseases. In several studies, other domains such as meaning in life, personality, and social factors contributed significantly to the perception of quality of life as much, if not more, than illness severity (Figure 5-1).[27,28]

The patient's response to a diagnosis of PD may involve a prolonged and uncertain grieving process as well as differences in the perception of quality of life.[17] Those with younger-onset PD have reported a much more disrupted quality of life when compared with the older-onset patient.[28] Patients and caregivers may also differ in their perception of quality of life and physical progression of the illness. Several research studies suggest that the caregiver perceives the quality of life for the patient as being more negative than the patient reports. The caregiver may also perceive the severity of the illness to be greater than that experienced by the patient.[29-31]

Patients living with a chronic disease find it demanding, but facing a degenerative illness like PD is even more difficult and stressful.[21] Challenges that occur on a regular basis for patients with PD include dealing with fatigue,[32] unpredictability, changing social roles within the family, losing or adapting a new sense of identity, and living with changes in relationships.[22] Experiences with depression and psychosis, disability, postural instability, sleep disorders, lack of independence, and cognitive impairment are other significant features that impact the quality of life for those living with PD.[33-35] One qualitative study examined eight women living with PD in Sweden and identified four themes: 1) the wish for a stable body image (feeling less physically competent), 2) the wish to keep traditional female competence (not being able to do typical female duties such as household tasks, 3) the need to be accepted for the person she is (lack of understanding for "on and off" periods), and 4) the perceived stigmatization (feeling a sense of shame).[20] The responses to living with PD are not limited to these women, but they do convey an array of psychosocial reactions that tend to be negative and affect everyday activities and interactions.

A study conducted in Israel found similar perceptions when 39 patients with PD (without apparent dementia) were asked about motor, mental, and psychosocial symptoms. Over one-half of those subjects reported problems with mental changes (recall and mental clarity), motor difficulty or activity loss (tremor, writing, gait, fatigue), psychosocial difficulties (anxiety and depression), and nonspecific symptoms (constipation and insomnia). Major motor symptoms and problems with sexual functioning were reported much less frequently.[23]

Given the complexity of these psychosocial responses to living with PD, what are some ways we can help patients adapt to their illness? To begin with, studies of persons with other chronic illnesses describe the importance of social support received from others as being beneficial, especially as the illness progresses.[35] Others have noted that an optimistic attitude for both patients and caregivers may help patients deal with the basic functional disabilities they experience.[35,36] Researchers have also described that a sense of perceived control over the disease progression appeared to be associated with improved patient well-being and subsequent caregiver outcomes.[37]

Patients may be helped to assimilate PD into their lives by expressing their emotions of anger and frustration, trying to normalize each day as much as possible, avoiding social isolation, participating in exercise and support groups, grieving over their many losses, and creating a life separate from chronic illness.[5]

Depression and Anxiety

Although Dr. Parkinson's famous essay was published in 1917, the psychiatric and emotional changes were not mentioned until later,[38] and the mechanisms are still not thoroughly understood.[39] Psychological processes, like depression and anxiety, can be either important consequences of chronic disease or contributing causes.[2,40] The tendency is to assume that emotional factors and physical changes in chronic illness are unilateral and independent of each other, but relying on the biopsychosocial model as a framework for practice requires that the health care professional use an integrated approach for piecing together these complexities.

Depression is perhaps the most common psychosocial concern in PD, occurring in 40% of patients as reported in 26 studies,[40] and while the cause is still unknown, experts believe that the dopamine system plays a significant role. Both norepinephrine and serotonin, two neurotransmitters related to dopamine regulation, are critical for mood regulation but are deficient in PD.[41] This reduction in neurotransmitters may contribute to a major mood disorder that is characterized by decreased energy and motivation; feelings of helplessness, hopelessness; changes in weight, sleep, and appetite; and irritability.[42] These depressive symptoms may predate the development of motor symptoms, may fluctuate over time, and may alternate between a normal affect and a depressive state. The episodes occur more frequently when the patient is "off" the medications, and they may sometimes improve when the motor symptoms are better controlled. Treating the patient with conventional antidepressants aimed at alleviating apathy or sleeplessness may be helpful.[43]

Another form of depression is less responsive to antidepressants and may begin when the diagnosis of PD is confirmed and when the progression of motor symptoms interferes with daily functioning. This type of depression is called *reactive depression* and may be experienced by those newly diagnosed and others with more advanced disease who are losing independence and control.[42] Some older patients with depressive symptoms may be responding to a variety of life stressors—changes in financial situation, serious health problems, grieving over past losses, and negative interactions with family members or friends.[44]

Depression in PD may also co-exist with subtle cognitive symptoms such as forgetfulness, attention deficits, and problems in tracking the conversations of several individuals simultaneously. It may be difficult for the health care professional to sort out what is depression and what is cognitive decline; therefore, close communication and accurate education about PD with the patient and family members are essential. Increased emotional stress can also intensify depression, memory decline, and motor symptoms. The emergence of increased stressors enhances the critical need for a balance in all spheres of the patient's life—relationships with friends and family, work, health practices, and volunteer activities.[45-47]

Regardless of the form of depression, mood changes can profoundly affect the quality of life for those with PD,[46] those with whom they live, and their compliance with medications and the treatment plan.[47] Sometimes a health care professional may be the first to notice depression, notably when contact with the patient is more infrequent, when irritability is present, or when carelessness is observed with medications, personal appearance, and safety measures. Health care professionals may also observe the patient and misinterpret the flat affect and masked facial expression, both common in PD, to be symptoms of depression.

Occasionally, the health care professional may also recommend or reinforce the need for nonpharmacological methods for treating depression. This may include, but is not limited to, exercise (walking, tai chi, yoga, and water therapy), community education/support groups, and behavioral/cognitive counseling for individuals or families. The team approach used by health care professionals and others who provide support, encouragement, and expert clinical skills can be very therapeutic for the person who is experiencing depression.

Research on anxiety and PD is more limited than that of depression[21,48,49] and both frequently occur together.[49] In a small sample (n = 24), 38% of Parkinson's patients met the criteria for an anxiety disorder. Other larger studies (n = 205)[49] have found anxiety or nervousness to be a relatively common problem,[50,51] estimated to be between 20%[47] and

40%.[42] Motor changes, especially balance and gait problems, freezing episodes, and the potential for falls also contribute to anxiety.[51] Other manifestations may include somatic complaints such as restlessness, irritability, and muscle tension[49] and the reporting of a lower quality of life.[46]

One study that examined young- versus older-onset patients with PD reported that anxiety scores were equally present for the young- versus older-onset patients, but depression occurred more frequently in the young-onset group.[28] From these findings and anecdotal reports from patients, it is clear that anxiety as a psychosocial disturbance in PD needs more study.

Other challenges for the patient and family include communication difficulties, cognitive changes, sleep disturbances, driving concerns, sexual dysfunction, and financial stressors. These are discussed below.

Communication Difficulties

The ability to communicate is an essential component of healthy relationships, but can be impaired as PD advances. For patients with PD, communication difficulties take the form of diminished speaking volume, mumbled or fast speech, loss of facial expressions, and swallowing difficulties.[52] Many patients experience social isolation, preferring to stay at home rather than bear the humiliation of participating in discussions and activities. Patients with PD may also be self-conscious about using the telephone for fear of being misunderstood or labeled as having memory problems. For more effective communication with PD patients, see Sidebar 5-2.

SIDEBAR 5-2: TIPS FOR MORE EFFECTIVE COMMUNICATION

- Establish the habit of looking at one another while having a conversation.
- Eliminate background noise by turning off the radio or television and closing doors to noisy areas.
- Be aware that facial masking is a feature of Parkinson's disease and that emotions may be felt but not shown because of rigid facial muscles.
- Ask questions that can be answered in short sentences.
- Be patient; don't rush or force conversational responses.

Cognition Changes

The presence of memory problems in PD requires the patience and understanding of everyone because slowing of the thinking process may occur even if the memory problems are not severe. The percentage of cognitive problems for those with PD is estimated to be about 33%, especially for those with older onset.[21] It is helpful for health care professionals to reduce the anxiety for the person who has difficulty with memory and thinking functions. This involves giving the person plenty of time to think over the question rather than immediately providing the answer or hurrying the deliberation. Reading information, rather than listening to information, may also help cognition (Figure 5-2). For safety reasons, health care professionals need to be concerned about whether memory changes impair the patient's ability to organize and accurately administer medications.

Figure 5-2. Research suggests that reading is an activity that might help preserve cognitive function as we age. This patient sits in a chair that provides additional support for the neck and arms.

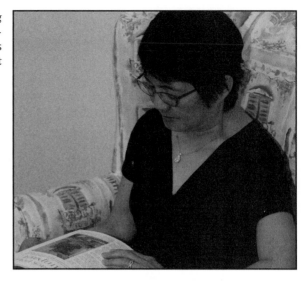

The frustration surrounding memory problems for those with PD also affects their spouses and other significant persons with whom they interact.[46] Family and friends may feel helpless when their loved one begins to experience even mild memory changes for activities that are familiar, such as the sequence of steps when putting gas in the car and performing yard work or housekeeping chores. Vigilance is necessary for observing other potentially hazardous tasks such as driving and operating dangerous equipment or machinery.

Communication between all parties is essential when a person with PD has mild memory problems. It is important to discuss how much prompting and assistance the patient desires at times of forgetfulness. For example, many frustrations occur in the car when the person with PD is driving and/or the significant other gives specific instructions about the schedule for the day or the completion of household tasks. Sometimes the person with PD will want family members to assist at the time of memory lapse; others prefer to ask for help or clarification before being corrected. Occasionally, patients with changes in memory may become agitated when reminded about their memory changes. Ask your loved one: "How and when do you want me to comment or correct you when I know you're mistaken? I don't want to be critical, but we need to work this out together."

An angry response to a reminder needs to be handled with reassurance and kindness and followed by a sensitive discussion when the stress is reduced. Communication about memory and thinking functions needs to take place at appropriate intervals because preferences and abilities may change. These communication interactions should be relaxed, private between the two persons, and should be avoided during potentially dangerous activities.

Sleep Disturbances

There are multiple factors that disrupt sleep for patients with PD.[53] Patients frequently have their sleep interrupted because of insomnia caused by PD medications (such as sedating antidepressants or anxiolytics), vivid dreams, or too much daytime napping. They may also experience daytime sleepiness due to disrupted sleep during the night or from going to bed too early in the evening.[42]

Patients should be encouraged to establish a regular bedtime and awakening time; to limit daytime napping; to avoid caffeine, food, alcohol, and excessive fluid intake prior to bedtime; and to initiate an appropriate exercise routine.[42] Health care professionals should give more attention to sleep disturbances, depression, and other non-motor aspects of PD.[54]

Driving Concerns

Throughout our lives, driving is one of the most important activities in which we engage because it represents freedom, independence, and control. Teenagers and older adults are particularly targeted for driving safety since a proportionately larger number of motor vehicle accidents occur within these two age groups.[55]

Discussions about driving concerns need to begin fairly early after the patient is diagnosed with PD. These discussions should initiate with the patient, family member, or physician and be reinforced by other health care professionals involved with patient care. Unfortunately, the "driving safety" discussion is frequently ignored or postponed because of fears of intrusion or abdication of responsibility.

Patients may be hesitant to initiate the discussion because of misperceptions that their driving habits are completely safe. Family members are reluctant to approach the patient and physician because they want to protect their loved one's independence and not upset their own routines by assuming more of the driving tasks. Physicians may be inhibited about approaching the driving issue for many reasons, among them the fear that it destroys the trusting doctor–patient relationship. All these concerns need to be acknowledged and respected, but none should be an excuse for failing to discuss this important safety issue.

There is never an ideal time for driving discussions to take place. The patient and family caregivers must be prepared to have these conversations at regular intervals because of the progressive nature of PD and changes in motor control and cognition. The short-term memory problems, tremors, dyskinesias, lack of sleep, visual problems, and effects of medications on alertness and movement cause safety hazards.[56] Chapters 9 and 14 address other driving issues.

Another significant concern is that the patient may not have an accurate assessment of his or her driving skills when compared with that of family members or the assessment of a driving examiner.[57] An occupational therapist certified in driving rehabilitation needs to evaluate driving safety for the aforementioned reasons plus other factors such as deficits in visuo-spatial skills, planning, and sequencing of steps.[57]

For purposes of discussion, let's presume that a 76-year-old husband has advanced PD and his wife is worried about his driving safety but is reluctant to start the deliberations. The wife has noticed that her husband requests that she accompany him to his appointments and errands—this is new for both of them. She believes it gives her husband more security because he asks her to be on the alert for street signs and turn signals. She also is aware that he drives more slowly and tentatively, almost to the point of it being dangerous. Prior to beginning any discussions, the wife should have completed some homework. For example, she should ride with her husband, noting his driving safety and driving hazards. She may suggest that an adult child ride with him as a passenger and that an adult child or trusted friend inconspicuously follow the patient in another car. She should also have investigated alternate plans for transportation such as taxi service, city buses, handicapped transportation, friends, the Red Cross, the faith communities and senior service agencies for possible volunteers, and local PD associations. Once other transportation has been researched, her husband may benefit from these suggestions:

1. When initiating conversations about driving, select a time of low stress and without distractions. It is not wise to discuss driving concerns of any kind while the

patient or family member is driving the car or riding as a passenger. The discussions should be rather short and reinforced later.

2. Make the driving discussions as positive as possible. Most of us will react defensively when our driving habits are questioned. "I think we should talk about some of the changes I've noticed with your Parkinson's disease. You seem to be having more problems with movement—your dyskinesias appear worse. I wonder if you are worried about how this might affect your driving safety."

3. Attempt to enlist the patient in describing any anxieties he or she has about driving. Sometimes patients will describe environmental problems rather than physical ones, but they are important clues that need attention. These concerns may include driving at night, driving in inclement weather such as ice or rain, driving on the freeways, driving to unfamiliar places, and vision changes.

4. Consider sharing concerns about your own driving. "I'm not as young anymore either. I'm worried about my vision at night, the speed of my reflexes, and driving in the city. Maybe we can work on this together, and be open to each other's suggestions."

5. If the spouse is capable of driving, he or she could drive more frequently. Some spouses, without a word, just proceed to the driver's side when they are going somewhere. The less discussion about this, the better.

6. Patients sometimes listen to the physician's recommendations more than the spouse. Make an appointment with the neurologist if necessary. If the patient doesn't initiate the driving issue, the spouse should assume that responsibility.

7. If the spouse insists on driving and has physician approval to continue, some guidelines are: minimize distractions (turn off the radio), avoid "emotionally charged" discussions, travel on familiar streets (preferably not freeways), and drive during daylight hours only.

8. If the patient still insists on driving and ignores the advice of his physician and family members, the spouse could arrange for a driver evaluation by calling the Association of Driver Rehabilitation Specialists at 1-800-290-2344, by arranging for a driver's safety course offered through the American Association of Retired Persons (AARP), or by contacting the State Department of Transportation to have a driving test retaken. In most states, issues about an individual's driving safety can be reported anonymously to the State Department of Transportation by the physician, family member, or concerned citizen. (For more information on driving, see Chapters 9 and 14.)

Sexual Dysfunction

PD has a profound effect on relationships and intimacy with others, but sexual functioning in this group of patients has been only minimally examined,[23,58,59] and the severity of the problem has not been published.[23] Few studies look at sexual functioning and neurological problems in general, but if the health care professional has concerns about these issues and the quality of the couple's relationship, a qualified clinician should be consulted.[28,51,60]

Several factors may be responsible for the scarcity of sexuality research in PD. Researchers may believe that because PD occurs primarily in older adults, the patients and their partners may no longer be interested in sex. Possible physiological changes resulting in sexual dysfunction for patients with PD have not been supported in the literature and may not be a standard component of the assessment interview.[59]

Although the documented reasons for sexual dysfunction in PD are scarce, multifaceted,[59] and complex,[51] most appear to be related to the age of the patient,[28] to dopaminergic pathways, and to Parkinson's medications.[61] Some authors consider sexual dysfunction to be rather common in PD and cite impotence, hypersexuality, and decreased libido to be the most commonly reported problems.[43]

In a recent study of sexual functioning after Deep Brain Stimulation (DBS), researchers found a small but significant change in men following surgery, but not women. In this small sample of patients, depression, anxiety, duration of illness, and improvement in severity of illness showed no relationship to changes in sexual functioning. The researchers suggest that the quality of the marital relationship may be the primary factor, but caution that more studies need to be completed to validate these findings.[62] In a study comparing younger PD patients with healthy controls, the patients were more dissatisfied with their present sexual functioning and the quality of their relationship, but sexual functioning itself was not affected. Factors included depression and unemployment.[51,63] Erectile problems, ejaculation failure, and psychological factors may account for 20% to 60% of sexual dysfunction in PD.[64]

Sexual functioning in PD may also be related to impulsive behaviors or unwelcome intrusive thoughts.[43] Three to five percent of patients may actually experience hypersexuality,[65] or unreasonable sexual demands.[43] This impulsive increased sexual drive often leads to secrecy and difficult problems for the patient and family; the situation requires openness and the expertise of a qualified health care professional.

The following clinical example illustrates the sexual functioning concerns for one patient.

Case Study

Mrs. Johnson, age 55, has been married for 20 years and was diagnosed with PD 10 years ago at the age of 45. Medications include carbidopa/levodopa (Sinemet, pramipexole [Mirapex]), and most recently apomorphine injections, a rescue drug to help with freezing episodes. She has been on antidepressants for some time—fluoxetine (Prozac)—but she is somewhat inconsistent in taking them. Although Mrs. Johnson acknowledges a positive relationship with her husband, she has been concerned for the past 2 years over her gradual disinterest in having sex. She now finds excuses for not having sex with her husband and rebuffs his attempts at physical affection. During her regular session with the occupational therapist, she casually mentions her concerns. What are some things the therapist needs to consider when patients choose to discuss sexual issues?

Prior to professional practice in occupational therapy, the therapist should have explored personal attitudes about sexuality in general, sexuality among middle-aged and older-aged adults, and sexuality for those with chronic illnesses, and should have consulted with other professionals if biases were apparent. The therapist needs to be an effective listener and reassure Mrs. Johnson of the confidentiality of their conversations and seek written approval for revealing any of the details when consultation and referral are required. The therapist discusses the impact of multiple chronic illness stressors on intimate relationships with spouses or sexual partners and everyday stressors that occur in all relationships.

The therapist should be knowledgeable about PD and understand that changes in libido may occur in some, although not in all patients and that reoccurring depression may account for disinterest in sex.[43] Additionally, the therapist should be familiar with alternate forms of physical and psychological intimacy that may be fulfilling to patients and their partners.

Mrs. Johnson begins to express vague fears that she may become excessively sleepy, feel faint or lightheaded, and that her motor problems may intensify during the sex act. She also acknowledges that over the long haul, her 20-year marriage may be in jeopardy if she continues to refuse to have sex with her husband. After a thorough assessment of the patient's concerns, the therapist should refer her to one or several appropriate health care professionals who can accurately address the possible side effects of her medications and their potential impact on libido and sexual functioning. Professionals with expertise in neurodegenerative chronic illnesses, intimacy, and sexuality are also potential referral sources.

Financial Stressors

Although the exact financial cost for patients and families living with PD is unknown, it appears to be related to illness severity, resulting in loss of employment by both the patient and the caregiver, and lack of community and government support.[66] A large study, based on 1997 figures, estimated that the annual cost burden for persons with PD was $8738 per prevalent case per year.[67] Another study conducted independently for the National Parkinson Foundation in 1997 by John Robbins Associates, and cited by Wilson, estimated that the direct per-person costs were almost identical to those of the first study—$8872.[67] One study followed 70 Parkinson's patients for 3 years and estimated that those who described their health as "poor" reported three times the total cost/capita than those rating their health as "good." By year 3, total expenditures had nearly doubled for the "poor" health groups and increased over 25% for the "good health" group. Compensated costs decreased for both groups. These figures indicate that the annual cost burden for PD is quite high at $6.6 billion in the United States, especially when considering the relatively low prevalence of the disease.[68]

LIVING WITH PARKINSON'S DISEASE: IMPACT ON FAMILY CAREGIVERS

Most of the research that describes the informal (nonpaid) care of patients with PD focuses on family members, also known as family caregivers. Although friends and neighbors sometimes fulfill this role, this section will discuss the needs and challenges of those who have the most intimate relationship with the patient, who live in close proximity, and who assume primary responsibility for the patient's day-to-day physical and emotional support. This family caregiver is usually a spouse or lifelong partner, an adult child, or other family member.

Caregiving Statistics

Family and other informal caregivers provide the backbone for the long-term supportive services system in the United States. A comprehensive study of caregiving in the United States was conducted in 1997 by the National Alliance for Caregiving and the AARP. In this randomized sample of over 1500 subjects, they defined the caregiving role as caring for persons over the age of 50 for the past 12 months, with the care defined as assistance with ADL, bathing and eating, and instrumental ADL such as paying bills and taking medication. Although this care is unpaid, its value has been estimated at $257 billion annually by the National Alliance for Caregiving and the AARP.[69]

Caregiving in Parkinson's Disease

The study of caregivers for persons with PD is not as prevalent as other illnesses, such as Alzheimer's disease (AD), and has been described as scarce.[70,71] Most studies refer to the care provided by informal caregivers as contrasted to paid (formal) caregivers. Only about 1% of published papers about PD refer to caregivers issues[72] and these studies primarily highlight tiredness or sleep disturbances,[73] fatigue,[74] stage of illness,[75] depression, and hallucinations.[47,70,72] Caregivers of patients with another neurological problem, such as cerebral vascular accidents, report three kinds of losses—loss of shared activities, loss of relationships, and loss of one's own independence.[76] The health care professional can presume that over a prolonged period of time, caregivers of patients with PD also experience these losses.

Due to the progressive nature of PD and the older age at time of diagnosis, family caregivers will ultimately be involved in the care and/or supervision of a person with PD,[77,78] and many of these caregivers will also be elderly.[78] The age of the family caregiver is a factor leading to stress, but psychological features present in patients also correlate with the emotional and social distress of the caregiver.[47,50,79]

Researchers who studied 25 couples living with PD concluded that patients and their caregivers had two similar needs: better knowledge of the disease (as related to their individual situation) and a recognition and confirmation of their reciprocal roles.[72] Caregivers also need information about PD, reduction in physical and psychological burden, a good night's sleep, and knowledge of and access to benefits and respite care.[17,18]

Caring for a person with PD was a determinant in a worsening of the caregiver's chronic illness and psychological and physical well-being when compared with elderly controls who were caregivers of partners without PD.[70,79] Caregiver suffering was found to be inversely related to the sense of control exhibited by the person with PD.[37] The health care professional is challenged to provide unrelenting support not only to the patient but also the caregiver and other family members.

A seminal project involving North American caregivers of patients with PD was initially conducted in 1992, repeated 1 year later, and again in 10 years.[80] Of the 266 eligible caregivers in 2002, 156 completed a questionnaire that asked about the impact of long-term caregiving for a loved one with PD. Results indicated that 26% of the subjects had died, 67% were being cared for by their spouse in their home, and 11% were living in a care facility. Other findings revealed that this group of caregivers were at increased risk for health problems and increased strain and that if these risks were present early in the caregiving process, 10 years later they experienced a worsening of health and poorer quality of life. Caregiver pessimism that was present early in the caregiving role was found to be a warning sign for future health problems, including depression.[80,81] Depression was present in over 20% of the caregivers and occurred at a higher rate when their spouse was in a nursing home than among those who were widowed after the beginning of the study.

Two caregiving constructs, social support and caregiver burden, are critical for understanding the complexity of underlying variables commonly experienced when caring for those with chronic illnesses. The next section will discuss these constructs more thoroughly.

Social Support

Social support for patients with PD and their caregivers is not well understood.[76] Social support usually refers to the resources or functions that are provided by a person's contacts including family members, friends, coworkers, and others.[82] Social support resources are sometimes described as serving as a stress buffer to those with chronic illness (Figure 5-3).

Figure 5-3. By taking up photography and joining a photo club, Mrs. W. found a new outlet for her creative energy and made new friends.

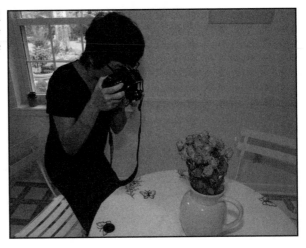

Several research studies support this view. To illustrate, when the patient's illness was more severe, spouses with a greater social support network experienced fewer depressive symptoms.[83] Other studies have compared the perception of social support usage and resources between spouses of two illness groups, PD and AD. The spouses caring for a loved one with dementia were older, had fewer children, less financial resources, and had lived with the illness a shorter period of time. The quality of the marital relationship changed for both groups, especially for women.[84]

Researchers recently examined the construct of social support in PD by comparing self-reported social support and quality of life domains between patients and caregiver-proxies.[76] The caregivers reported a lack of social support to be more problematic than the patients, and they presented a more negative view of quality of life than did the patient. Interestingly, speech and motor problems experienced by the patients were perceived to be more troublesome than that reported by the caregivers.[76] Other researchers also discuss the impact of a degenerative illness on quality of life[27,29,30] where quality of life was reported by the proxy caregivers to be more negative than that reported by the patients themselves. Others have examined perceptions of social support when motor and psychological difficulties resulting from PD were less prominent. They concluded that the patients' perceptions of chronic social support were greater when their illness symptoms were less advanced.[28]

Caregiver Burden

Caregiver burden is a term commonly used when discussing caregivers of patients with chronic illness. The definition and measurement of caregiver burden is complex and controversial.[85] It has been defined as the physical, psychological, and financial impact of caring for another person who is ill, disabled, or otherwise functionally impaired. The term is usually used in reference to informal caregivers who act in an unpaid, non-professional caregiving role as compared to formal caregivers who are usually paid to provide services to patients.[85]

Caregiver burden should be assessed at intervals during the caregiving process.[86] Several studies have investigated the factors that define caregiver burden in PD by comparing caregivers of loved ones with PD to those caring for other degenerative illnesses like AD.[87] In their study of both caregivers and patients, researchers learned that the most important variables in assessing caregiver burden were depressive symptoms in caregivers, coherence in caregivers, and functional status of patients.[34,70] To ease the burden of caregivers, health care professionals should be alert to the patient's decline in functional status, an increase in depressive symptoms, and the presence of psychiatric symptoms and refer to supportive services as soon as possible.[88]

Due to the complexity of factors, the experience of caregiver burden may differ among individuals. In one study, the strongest components of family burden were the hardships resulting from the lost income of the informal caregivers, especially those under 65 years of age.[89] These hidden costs begin early in the process of PD. Parkinson's disease specialists suggest comprehensive care from the outset and making early referrals to services such as home health agencies, social workers, and psychological counseling is critical.

Depression is common among caregivers, especially for those caring for patients with PD and AD.[90] Spouses cope with PD by maintaining their lives, encouraging the partner to remain active and involved, and by viewing their caregiving challenges secondary to other challenges.[87] Another study found that the patient's sleep disturbances and the subsequent care and supervision that resulted from lack of sleep influenced caregiver burden. Personality factors of the patient also account for caregiver burden and the emotional health of caregivers.[91] In a study comparing PD caregivers with AD caregivers, personality factors exerted significant and indirect effects on mental health and significant indirect effects on physical health. AD caregivers experienced worse emotional health than PD caregivers, but better physical health. These studies did not include various domains of personality.[91]

The quality and perseverance of caregivers is heavily influenced by the patient's advancing illness, depression, the quality of the couple's relationship,[88] the caregivers' fatigue,[74] and health problems.[92] In a study of 380 spouses caring for those with PD, as the disease progressed and the tasks of caregivers multiplied, negative changes in lifestyles, depression, and caregiver strain increased.[81] In a nonrandom convenience sample of 30 spousal caregivers of PD patients, as the physical health of the patient declined, the caregivers' health also declined, due to the decrease in their own physical functioning. The caregiver's age, years of marriage, and educational level influenced social support, psychological well-being, and financial security.[75]

In 2002, the National Parkinson Foundation initiated a new task force for caregivers.[93] Caregivers of persons with PD make up part of the estimated 52 million caregivers in the United States. Researchers are increasing their knowledge about depression, strain, and the compilation of multiple stresses that influence caregivers' lives. The experience of caregiving is sometimes positive and may lead to changes in careers and community service leadership.[94]

CONCLUSION

This chapter has reviewed the complexity of psychosocial factors for patients living with PD and their family caregivers. It becomes apparent that the comprehensive care of patients requires an integrated approach that connects all aspects of the patient's biopsychosocial needs. The care of patients with PD and their caregivers will be improved when research findings and clinical practice merge together and provide the evidence that health care professionals need for competent and compassionate care.

REFERENCES

1. Borrell-Carrio F, Suchman AL, Epstein RM. The biopsychosocial model 25 years later: principles, practice, and scientific inquiry. *Ann Fam Med.* 2004; 2(6):576-582.
2. Smith TW, Nicassio PM. Psychological practice: Clinical application of the biopsychosocial model. In: Nicassio PM, Smith TW, eds. *Managing Chronic Illness: A Biopsychosocial Perspective.* Washington, DC: American Psychological Association;1995:1-31.

3. Dowling AS. Images in Psychiatry. George Engel, M.D. (1913-1999). *Am J Psychiatry*. 2005;162:2039.
4. Engel GL. The need for a new medical model: a challenge for biomedicine. *Science*. 1977;196(4286):129-136.
5. McDaniel SH, Hepworth J, Doherty WJ. *Medical Family Therapy: A Biopsychosocial Approach to Famlies with Health Problems*. New York: Basic Books;1992:13-15, 86, 184.
6. Greenberg WM. Book Forum: Models of Psychiatry. In: Frankel RM, Quill TE, McDaniel SH, eds. *The Biopsychosocial Approach: Past, Present, Future*. Rochester, NY: University of Rochester Press; 2005.
7. Bandura A. *Self-Efficacy: The Exercise of Control*. New York, NY: W. H. Freeman & Co.; 1997:259-266.
8. Engel GL. How much longer must medicine's science be bound by a seventeenth century world view? *Psychother Psychosom*. 1992;57(1-2):3-16.
9. Engel GL. From biomedical to biopsychosocial. Being scientific in the human domain. *Psychosomatics*. 1997;38(6):521-528.
10. Nicassio PM, Smith TW. Introduction. In: Nicassio M, Smith TW, eds. *Managing Chronic Illness: A Biopsychosocial Perspective*. Washington, DC: American Psychological Association;1995:xi-xxi.
11. Yager J. Book forum: Biopsychosocial psychiatry. Dilts SL, ed. Models of the Mind: A Framework for Biopsychosocial Psychiatry. *Am J Psychiatry*. 2002;159[2001], 1612-1613. New York, NY: Brunner-Routledge.
12. Novack DH. Realizing Engel's vision: psychosomatic medicine and the education of physician-healers. *Psychosom Med*. 2003;65(6):925-930.
13. Marinus J, Visser M, Martinez-Martin P, van Hilten JJ, Stiggelbout AM. A short psychosocial questionnaire for patients with Parkinson's disease: the SCOPA-PS. *J Clin Epidemiol*. 2003;56(1):61-67.
14. Duvoisin RC, Sage J. *Parkinson's Disease: A Guide for Patient and Family*. Philadelphia: Lippincott, Williams & Wilkins;2001:23-32.
15. Marinus J, Visser M, Stiggelbout AM, Rabey JM, Martinez-Martin P, Bonuccelli U, et al. A short scale for the assessment of motor impairments and disabilities in Parkinson's disease: the SPES/SCOPA. *J Neurol Neurosurg Psychiatry*. 2004;75(3):388-395.
16. Riley DE, Lang AE. Movement disorders. In: Bradley, WG, Daroff RB, Fenichel GM, Marsden CD, eds. *Neurology in Clinical Practice Vol. II*. Boston: Butterworth-Heinemann; 1996:1731-1742.
17. Playfer JR. The therapeutic challenges in the older Parkinson's disease patient. *Eur J Neurol*. 2002;9 Suppl 3:55-58.
18. Forsyth DR. Quality of life. In: Playfer J, Hindle J, eds. *Parkinson's Disease in the Older Patient*. New York, NY: Oxford University Press, Inc.; 2001:89-95.
19. Shifren K. Individual differences in the perception of optimism and disease severity: a study among individuals with Parkinson's disease. *J Behav Med*. 1996;19(3):241-271.
20. Caap-Ahlgren M, Lannerheim L. Older Swedish women's experiences of living with symptoms related to Parkinson's disease. *J Adv Nurs*. 2002; 39(1):87-95.
21. Jahanshahi M. The psychosocial impact of Parkinson's disease and its clinical management. In: Playford E, ed. *Neurological Rehabilitation of Parkinson's Disease*. New York, NY: Martin Dunitz; 2003:25-47.
22. Habermann B. Day-to-day demands of Parkinson's disease. *West J Nurs Res*. 1996;18(4):397-413.
23. Abudi S, Bar-Tal Y, Ziv L, Fish M. Parkinson's disease symptoms—patients' perceptions. *J Adv Nurs*. 1997;25(1):54-59.
24. Marras C, Lang A, Krahn M, Tomlinson G, Naglie G. Quality of life in early Parkinson's disease: impact of dyskinesias and motor fluctuations. *Mov Disord*. 2004;19(1):22-28.
25. Morimoto T, Shimbo T, Orav JE, Matsui K, Goto M, Takemura M, et al. Impact of social functioning and vitality on preference for life in patients with Parkinson's disease. *Mov Disord*. 2003;18(2):171-175.
26. Gage H, Hendricks A, Zhang S, Kazis L. The relative health related quality of life of veterans with Parkinson's disease. *J Neurol Neurosurg Psychiatry*. 2003;74(2):163-169.
27. Nelson ND, Trail M, Van JN, Appel SH, Lai EC. Quality of life in patients with amyotrophic lateral sclerosis: perceptions, coping resources, and illness characteristics. *J Palliat Med*. 2003;6(3):417-424.
28. Schrag A, Hovris A, Morley D, Quinn N, Jahanshahi M. Young- versus older-onset Parkinson's disease: impact of disease and psychosocial consequences. *Mov Disord*. 2003;18(11):1250-1256.
29. Fleming A, Cook KF, Nelson ND, Lai EC. Proxy reports in Parkinson's disease: caregiver and patient self-reports of quality of life and physical activity. *Mov Disord*. 2005;20(11):1462-1468.
30. Trail M, Nelson ND, Van JN, Appel SH, Lai EC. A study comparing patients with amyotrophic lateral sclerosis and their caregivers on measures of quality of life, depression, and their attitudes toward treatment options. *J Neurol Sci*. 2003;209(1-2):79-85.
31. Trail M, Nelson N, Van JN, Appel SH, Lai EC. Major stressors facing patients with amyotrophic lateral sclerosis (ALS): a survey to identify their concerns and to compare with those of their caregivers. *Amyotroph Lateral Scler Other Motor Neuron Disord*. 2004;5(1):40-45.
32. Herlofson K, Larsen JP. The influence of fatigue on health-related quality of life in patients with Parkinson's disease. *Acta Neurol Scand*. 2003;107(1):1-6.

33. Schrag A, Jahanshahi M, Quinn N. How does Parkinson's disease affect quality of life? A comparison with quality of life in the general population. *Mov Disord.* 2000;15(6):1112-1118.

34. Karlsen KH, Larsen JP, Tandberg E, Maeland JG. Influence of clinical and demographic variables on quality of life in patients with Parkinson's disease. *J Neurol Neurosurg Psychiatry.* 1999;66(4):431-435.

35. Symister P, Friend R. The influence of social support and problematic support on optimism and depression in chronic illness: a prospective study evaluating self-esteem as a mediator. *Health Psychol.* 2003;22(2):123-129.

36. Lyons KS, Stewart BJ, Archbold PG, Carter JH, Perrin NA. Pessimism and optimism as early warning signs for compromised health for caregivers of patients with Parkinson's disease. *Nurs Res.* 2004;53(6):354-362.

37. Wallhagen MI, Brod M. Perceived control and well-being in Parkinson's disease. *West J Nurs Res.* 1997;19(1):11-25.

38. Hindle J. A history of Parkinson's disease. In: Playfer JV, ed. *Parkinson's Disease in the Older Patient.* London: Arnold; 2001:3-10.

39. Schrag A, Jahanshahi M, Quinn N. What contributes to quality of life in patients with Parkinson's disease? *J Neurol Neurosurg Psychiatry.* 2001; 69(3):308-312.

40. Cummings JL. Depression and Parkinson's disease: a review. Am J Psychiatry. 1992; 149(4):443-454.

41. Dubois B, Pillon B. Cognitive deficits in Parkinson's disease. *J Neurol.* 1997; 244(1):2-8.

42. Weiner WJ, Shulman LM, Lang AE. *Parkinson's Disease: A Complete Guide for Patients & Families.* New York, NY: Oxford University Press, Inc.;2001: 39, 54-56.

43. Hindle JV. Neuropsychiatry. In: Playfer JR, Hindle JV, eds. *Parkinson's Disease in the Older Patient.* New York, NY: Oxford University Press;2001:106-133.

44. Moos RH, Schutte KK, Brennan PL, Moos BS. The interplay between life stressors and depressive symptoms among older adults. *J Gerontol B Psychol Sci Soc Sci.* 2005;60(4):199-206.

45. Waters CH. *Complications of Parkinson's Disease and Its Therapy. Diagnosis and Management of Parkinson's Disease.* West Islip, NY: Professional Communications, Inc.; 2006:135-166.

46. Cubo E, Rojo A, Ramos S, Quintana S, Gonzalez M, Kompoliti K et al. The importance of educational and psychological factors in Parkinson's disease quality of life. *Eur J Neurol.* 2002;9(6):589-593.

47. Aarsland D, Larsen JP, Lim NG, Janvin C, Karlsen K, Tandberg E et al. Range of neuropsychiatric disturbances in patients with Parkinson's disease. *J Neurol Neurosurg Psychiatry.* 1999;67(4):492-496.

48. Stein MB, Heuser IJ, Juncos JL, Uhde TW. Anxiety disorders in patients with Parkinson's disease. *Am J Psychiatry.* 1990;147(2):217-220.

49. Marinus J, Leentjens AF, Visser M, Stiggelbout AM, van Hilten JJ. Evaluation of the hospital anxiety and depression scale in patients with Parkinson's disease. *Clin Neuropharmacol.* 2002;25(6):318-324.

50. Aarsland D, Larsen JP, Karlsen K, Lim NG, Tandberg E. Mental symptoms in Parkinson's disease are important contributors to caregiver distress. *Int J Geriatr Psychiatry.* 1999;14(10):866-874. Report.

51. Fitzsimmons B, Bunting LK. Parkinson's disease. Quality of life issues. *Nurs Clin North Am.* 1993;28(4):807-818.

52. Trail M, Fox C, Ramig LO, Sapir S, Howard J, Lai EC. Speech treatment for Parkinson's disease. *NeuroRehabilitation.* 2005;20(3):205-221.

53. Young A, Home M, Churchward T, Freezer N, Holmes P, Ho M. Comparison of sleep disturbance in mild versus severe Parkinson's disease. *Sleep.* 2002; 25(5):573-577.

54. Scaravilli T, Gasparoli E, Rinaldi F, Polesello G, Bracco F. Health-related quality of life and sleep disorders in Parkinson's disease. *Neurol Sci.* 2003; 24(3):209-210.

55. Aging and Driving Successfully in Texas. Austin, TX: Texas Department of State Health Services; 1993.

56. O'Neill D. Safe Mobility. In: Playfer JR, Hindle JV, eds. *Parkinson's Disease in the Older Patient.* London: Arnold; 2001:200-212.

57. Schrag A. Driving in Parkinson's disease. *J Neurol Neurosurg Psychiatry.* 2005; 76(2):159.

58. Lambert D, Waters CH. Sexual dysfunction in Parkinson's disease. *Clin Neurosci.* 1998;5(2):73-77.

59. Brown RG, Jahanshahi M, Quinn N, Marsden CD. Sexual function in patients with Parkinson's disease and their partners. *J Neurol Neurosurg Psychiatry.* 1990;53(6):480-486.

60. Chandler BJ, Brown S. Sex and relationship dysfunction in neurological disability. *J Neurol Neurosurg Psychiatry.* 1998;65(6):877-880.

61. Aarsland D, Alves G, Larsen JP. Disorders of motivation, sexual conduct, and sleep in Parkinson's disease. *Adv Neurol.* 2005;96:56-64.

62. Castelli L, Perozzo P, Genesia ML, Torre E, Pesare M, Cinquepalmi A et al. Sexual well being in parkinsonian patients after deep brain stimulation of the subthalamic nucleus. *J Neurol Neurosurg Psychiatry.* 2004; 75(9):1260-1264.

63. Jacobs H, Vieregge A, Vieregge P. Sexuality in young patients with Parkinson's disease: a population based comparison with healthy controls. *J Neurol Neurosurg Psychiatry.* 2000;69(4):550-552.

64. Kenny RA, Allcock L. Autonomic problems. In: Playfer JR, Hindle JV, eds. *Parkinson's Disease in the Older Adult.* New York, NY: Oxford University Press; 2001:171.

65. Marsh L, Callahan P. Gambling, Sex, and...Parkinson's Disease? *News & Review*, 4-5. 2006. New York, NY, Parkinson's Disease Foundation.

66. Clarke CE, Zobkiw RM, Gullaksen E. Quality of life and care in Parkinson's disease. *Br J Clin Pract*. 1995;49(6):288-293.

67. Wilson L, Huang J, Doshi D. Health care burden, prevalence, and costs of Parkinson disease. *Drug Benefit Trends*. 2002;22-40.

68. Schenkman M, Wei ZC, Cutson TM, Whetten-Goldstein K. Longitudinal evaluation of economic and physical impact of Parkinson's disease. *Parkinsonism Relat Disord*. 2001;8(1):41-50.

69. Benton W. Family caregiving in the U.S. Survey AOA-IM-97-15. Information Memorandum. 7-3-1997. Electronic citation.

70. Caap-Ahlgren M, Dehlin O. Factors of importance to the caregiver burden experienced by family caregivers of Parkinson's disease patients. *Aging Clin Exp Res*. 2002;14(5):371-377.

71. Martinez-Martin P, Benito-Leon J, Alonso F, Catalan MJ, Pondal M, Zamarbide I et al. Quality of life of caregivers in Parkinson's disease. *Qual Life Res*. 2005;14(2):463-472.

72. Pasetti C, Rossi FS, Fornara R, Picco D, Foglia C, Galli J. Caregiving and Parkinson's disease. *Neurol Sci*. 2003;24(3):203-204.

73. Happe S, Berger K. The association between caregiver burden and sleep disturbances in partners of patients with Parkinson's disease. *Age Ageing*. 2002;31(5):349-354.

74. Teel CS, Press AN. Fatigue among elders in caregiving and noncaregiving roles. *West J Nurs Res*. 1999;21(4):498-514.

75. Berry RA, Murphy JF. Well-being of caregivers of spouses with Parkinson's disease. *Clin Nurs Res*. 1995;4(4):373-386.

76. McComb MN, Tickle-Degnen L. Developing the Construct of Social Support in Parkinson's Disease. *Physical & Occup Ther Ger: Curr Trends Ger Rehab*. 2006; 24(1).

77. Bhatia S, Gupta A. Impairments in activities of daily living in Parkinson's disease: implications for management. *NeuroRehabilitation*. 2003;18(3):209-214.

78. Cram DL. *Patient Services: Caring for Caregivers, Coping with Stress*. Parkinson Report, 16-17. 2006. Miami, Florida, National Parkinson Foundation.

79. O'Reilly F, Finnan F, Allwright S, Smith GD, Ben Shlomo Y. The effects of caring for a spouse with Parkinson's disease on social, psychological and physical well-being. *Br J Gen Pract*. 1996;46(410):507-512.

80. Carter JH, Stewart BJ, Archbold PG, Inoue I, Jaglin J, Lannon M et al. Living with a person who has Parkinson's disease: the spouse's perspective by stage of disease. Parkinson's Study Group. *Mov Disord*. 1998;13(1):20-28.

81. Carter JH. *A Long-Term Follow-Up of Spouses Who Are Caring for a Partner with Parkinson Disease*. Parkinson Report. 2004. Miami, FL, National Parkinson Foundation. Pamphlet.

82. Veterans' Administration Measurement Excellence and Training Resource Information Center (METRIC). Construct Overview of Social Support: Background. U.S. Government. 11-1-2005. Electronic citation.

83. Revenson TA, Majerovitz SD. The effects of chronic illness on the spouse. Social resources as stress buffers. *Arthritis Care Res*. 1991;4(2):63-72.

84. Hooker K, Manoogian-O'Dell M, Monahan DJ, Frazier LD, Shifren K. Does type of disease matter? Gender differences among Alzheimer's and Parkinson's disease spouse caregivers. *Gerontologist*. 2000;40(5):568-573.

85. Kane RL, Priester RTAM. *Meeting the Challenge of Chronic Illness*. Baltimore: Johns Hopkins University Press;2005:38-40, 126-128.

86. Spliethoff-Kammings NG, Zwinderman AH, Springer MP, Roos RA. A disease-specific psychosocial questionnaire for Parkinson's disease caregivers. *J Neurol*. 2003;250(10):1162-1168.

87. Habermann B, Davis LL. Caring for family with Alzheimer's disease and Parkinson's disease: needs, challenges and satisfaction. *J Gerontol Nurs*. 2005;31(6):49-54.

88. Schrag A, Hovris A, Morley D, Quinn N, Jahanshahi M. Caregiver-burden in parkinson's disease is closely associated with psychiatric symptoms, falls, and disability. *Parkinsonism Relat Disord*. 2006;12(1):35-41.

89. Whetten-Goldstein K, Sloan F, Kulas E, Cutson T, Schenkman M. The burden of Parkinson's disease on society, family, and the individual. *J Am Geriatr Soc*. 1997;45(7):844-849.

90. Dura JR, Haywood-Niler E, Kiecolt-Glaser JK. Spousal caregivers of persons with Alzheimer's and Parkinson's disease dementia: a preliminary comparison. *Gerontologist*. 1990;30(3):332-336.

91. Hooker K, Monahan DJ, Bowman SR, Frazier LD, Shifren K. Personality counts for a lot: predictors of mental and physical health of spouse caregivers in two disease groups. *J Gerontol B Psychol Sci Soc Sci*. 1998;53(2):73-85.

92. Parrish M, Giunta N, Adams S. Parkinson's disease caregiving: implications for care management. *Care Manag J*. 2003;4(1):53-60.

93. Kittle G. Research reports: New task force addresses needs of Parkinson family caregivers. Parkinson Report Fall 2002, 17. Miami, Florida, National Parkinson Foundation.

94. Oblas B. *Patient's viewpoint: Parkinson's disease and families.* Parkinson Report Fall 2002, 25-28. Miami, Florida, National Parkinson Foundation.

Physical Therapy Treatment and Home Programming for Patients With Parkinson's Disease

Rhonda K. Stanley, PT, PhD; Elizabeth J. Protas, PT, PhD, FACSM

Introduction

Individuals with Parkinson's disease (PD) have difficulties with functional movement. Associated problems that impact functional movement include tremor, bradykinesia/akinesia, rigidity, and impaired postural reflexes. The overall physical effect of PD is a decrease in easy and efficient movement, as well as an increased risk for falls. A suggested key to promoting and maintaining function in patients with PD is an active lifestyle that should include regular exercise.[1] This exercise program should emphasize safe and functional movements and ideally include strengthening, flexibility, endurance, and balance activities. Numerous research studies have shown that physical therapy/exercise interventions positively impact movement problems experienced by PD patients.[2-12] What is lacking in the research literature are studies conducted to evaluate long-term carry over following a short intervention phase. The definition of "long term" is anywhere from a few weeks to a few months,[5,8,9,11-14] with the shortest being 6 weeks and the longest 6 months. Most of the studies indicate that the positive gains experienced by participants during the short-term intervention phase either decline significantly or the participants return to their baseline scores. Those participants who continue with the short-term intervention(s) on their own, following cessation of the study, are more likely to maintain the positive outcomes.

As research suggests, regular physical activity/exercise can have an impact on various problems experienced by those with PD and help maintain outcomes gained through short-term physical therapy intervention. One way to provide continued activity/exercise is for the physical therapist to provide a home program.

This chapter will review results from various research studies that looked at physical therapy and exercise interventions during a short-term phase in addition to those studies that included a long-term follow-up. We will also discuss those physical therapy interventions that appear to have the most evidence for impacting the physical problems experienced by PD patients and then provide suggestions for what activities/exercises should be included in a home program while considering safety issues. Chapter 7 covers treatment of gait abnormalities.

THE RESEARCH EVIDENCE

Before discussing the available evidence, there are several issues that need to be addressed regarding the PD physical therapy and exercise research. Although the amount of research has increased over the past 10 years, there is still a lack of published evidence as to which physical therapy interventions and exercises are the most effective.[15,16] In addition, although the quality of the research methods has also improved, there is still a shortage of randomized controlled trials. Most studies lack control of the research environment, resulting in poor internal validity (cause and effect), and use a small sample size that makes it more difficult to generalize to the entire population of patients with PD (external validity). It should also be pointed out that most research in the area has been conducted with those individuals having idiopathic PD, which is of unknown etiology and the most prevalent type of parkinsonism, making up about 75% of the cases diagnosed. Patients with idiopathic PD tend to have problems with resting tremor, bradykinesia, rigidity, postural instability, and gait difficulties. The presence and severity of each will vary from individual to individual. Prognosis for any one patient is difficult to determine when initially diagnosed because disease progression can also vary significantly between individuals. Because of this, most physical therapy interventions planned in the clinical setting are individualized based on the problem(s) the patient is experiencing. This individualized approach creates a methodological dilemma for researchers trying to decide which intervention is best for conducting a study. This, in part, contributes to our being unable to compare across research studies to determine the "best" evidence.

Two systematic Cochrane reviews have been conducted to determine "best practice" in physical therapy for those with PD.[15,16] One review looked at the efficacy of physical therapy compared to placebo and the second compared "novel" types of physical therapy interventions to "standard" interventions. These reviews encompassed eighteen studies of randomized or quasi-randomized controlled trials dating from 1981 through 2000. Study limitations included absence of randomized controlled trials, the use of small sample sizes, lack of long-term follow-up, potential publication bias, and the wide variety of interventions used. Thus, we could not combine results from various studies. The reviewers concluded that: 1) there is not enough evidence to "prove or disprove" the benefit of physical therapy for those with PD, and 2) there is not enough evidence to say which intervention(s) are the most effective. These conclusions, however, do not mean that physical therapy is ineffective for patients with Parkinson's disease but that we must establish a consensus as to what is "best practice" in physical therapy for those with this diagnosis.

CURRENT EVIDENCE

As stated earlier, physical therapy can be effective for those with idiopathic PD. Interventions that have been studied include range of motion (ROM), stretching/flexibility, strengthening, aerobic and/or graded exercises; aquatic exercises; passive, active, and segmental mobilization techniques; balance training; gait training; functional training; postural control techniques; trunk stabilization techniques; breathing exercises; proprioceptive neuromuscular facilitation (PNF); rhythmic and verbal cues; and relaxation techniques. These approaches have been studied either individually or in some combination, within individual or group sessions, with or without supervision, in a laboratory, clinic, or home environment. Physical therapy interventions for PD patients are numerous and diverse.

So what is the "best" approach? After many years of personal experience working with PD patients as a clinician and researcher, this author could argue that most of the above approaches will prove beneficial when treatment is individualized to address the patient's deficits, ie, balance training for balance problems, gait training for gait problems, verbal and cueing techniques for start initiation problems. One might ask "what do you mean when you refer to any of the aforementioned approaches?" Here again the research is limited in that there is often no clear explanation as to what specific interventions were used, making it difficult for the clinician to determine how to design the "best" treatment method.

There is also the dilemma of maintaining the benefits of any treatment once the patient is discharged from physical therapy. Herein lies the need for prescribing an appropriate home program that the individual can easily perform in an attempt to maintain any benefits that were previously achieved.

Finally, the functional and quality of life impacts for some studies are difficult to determine. Some studies tend to use impairment level outcomes rather than functional or quality of life outcomes.

CONVENTIONAL TREATMENTS

Studies that have looked at more conventional or traditional treatments used over the years for PD patients have included active and passive mobility for the extremities and spine, postural control techniques incorporating perturbations while standing on noncompliant and compliant surfaces, balance training techniques, again varying the conditions by altering the visual environment and the standing surface, graded exercises during standing and sitting, limb coordination exercises, gait exercises, and dexterity exercises.[4,5,7,8,12-14,17] Except for Schenkman's study, most incorporated a combination of the aforementioned treatment approaches. All interventions were individualized to each participant except for Villani et al and Ellis et al, who used a group intervention approach.[7,14] Those studies that included at least one outcome measure of an objective motor task and/or mobility measurement reported some improvements following the short-term intervention, although not all improvements were statistically significant. Of the previously referenced studies, six included a follow-up period after the intervention[4,5,8,12-14] ranging from 6 weeks to 6 months. All of these studies reported at least some decline at follow-up, although the amount of decline varied from study to study and between outcome measures. In none of these studies did the participants continue exercising at home between the intervention phase and the follow-up assessment.

In the Schenkman study, the intervention was specific to spinal mobility.[17] This randomized controlled trial used a series of seven graduated stages of exercises that progressed from sitting to standing. Schenkman based these exercises on the eight principles she discussed in her article. As specified, "the exercises were designed to improve mobility and coordinated movement of the spine." The primary outcome measures were functional axial rotation (FAR), functional reach (FR), and timed supine to standing. The intervention group improved on all of these measures following a 10-week program of three sessions per week. Unfortunately, no follow-up was included in the study.

The study conducted by Pellechia and colleagues incorporated water exercises for coordination of limbs and trunk control.[12] This is the only study identified that has addressed any type of aquatic therapy for PD patients. This study also incorporated PNF exercises for all limbs and exercises using Mezieres techniques (Functional Muscular Integration) for increased spinal and limb flexibility. Outcome measures included the Unified Parkinson's Disease Rating Scale (UPDRS), Self-Assessment Parkinson's Disease Disability Scale (SaPDDS), 10-meter walk, and the Zung Depression Scale. The activities of daily living (ADL) and motor sections of the UPDRS improved along with all the other measures. This study included a 3-month follow-up that indicated significant loss in the UPDRS motor score, but maintenance of the benefits found by the other measures.

The major limitations to these studies are the use of small samples, no control group, and limited information about the interventions.

Resistance Exercises and Balance Training

Few studies have looked at strength training and its impact on the problems facing patients with PD. Until recently, strength was not believed to be significantly different than in age-matched controls. Studies by Pedersen et al, Corcos et al, Kakinuma et al, and Nogaki et al looked at strength variables in patients with PD, with results indicating that the previous assumption may be inaccurate.[18-21] Therefore, in recent years there have been more studies conducted investigating strength training and its impact on balance.

In a report by Toole et al, researchers administered a progressive lower extremity (LE) strengthening program coupled with a balance training program to four individuals with PD.[22] The control group of three did not receive treatment but maintained normal activities during the 10-week study period. Strengthening exercises consisted of four resistance exercises for knee flexion and extension and ankle inversion. Knee exercises were performed on a machine using elastic exercise bands for ankle exercises. Each individual performed three sets of 10 repetitions for each exercise three times per week. Strengthening exercises were preceded by a 10-minute warm-up period of LE and trunk stretches, calisthenics, and 5 minutes on a stationary bicycle. Balance training consisted of 10 activities that varied the visual and support surface environments to challenge the participants' limits of stability. Exercises included retropulsion (posterior pull activity on fixed and foam surfaces), randomly induced anterior-posterior and lateral perturbations with feet together and feet apart, and targeted sway activities (on fixed and foam surfaces). Outcomes were based on LE strength and balance measures. Results indicated that LE strength improved in the exercise group, but not significantly, and strength declined in the control group. Balance significantly improved within the treatment group, resulting in a significant difference between groups. No follow-up occurred. A small sample size limits the study.

In a second study performed by Hirsch et al, 15 individuals with PD were divided into two groups.[23] One group received balance and strength training, the second group received only balance training. Progressive resistance training again targeted the knee flexors and extensors and the plantarflexors. Investigators used Nautilus equipment

(Nautilus Inc, Vancouver, WA) for training, which lasted 15 minutes and consisted of one set of 12 repetitions of each exercise, three times per week for 10 weeks. Balance training consisted of 30 minutes of activities on compliant (foam) and noncompliant surfaces with varied visual inputs. Activities included perturbations by a therapist for limits of stability and weight shifting exercises. Outcome measures included LE strength and balance. Improvements were seen in both groups for strength and balance, but the combined group showed greater improvements in both areas. At 4 weeks follow-up, strength had decreased by only 10% and was said to be negligible for the balance measures.

These two studies indicate that it is possible to increase LE strength in PD patients, which may have a positive impact on balance. Again, small sample sizes limit the studies.

Aerobic Exercise Interventions

Prior to the mid 1990s, there were few studies conducted investigating the impact of PD on the cardiopulmonary system. Of those published, results indicate that a high percentage of PD patients have cardiovascular abnormalities such as orthostatic hypotension, cardiac arrhythmia, and less commonly, hypertension. In addition, the disease process affects the autonomic nervous system, resulting in compromised cardiovascular reflexes, typically a blunted or fixed pulse rate.[24,25] A complicating factor is that it is unclear whether these problems are directly caused by the disease process or are side effects from PD medications, since many of the antiparkinsonian drugs cause cardiovascular side effects. In addition, a higher percentage of PD patients have obstructive pulmonary dysfunction, with the upper airways most typically involved.[26-28] Many PD patients also complain of dyspnea and fatigue.[29-31]

Few studies have been conducted looking at acute responses to aerobic exercise. One of the earlier studies, Protas et al,[32] evaluated the aerobic capacity in eight males (mean age 61) with PD and a comparison group of seven males (mean age 65) without the disease. All participants performed acute bouts of graded exercise on a stationary bicycle and an arm ergometer. Results indicated there were no differences in outcome measures between the two groups. Comparison of the LE to UE exercise indicated a significant difference in peak oxygen consumption (VO_2) between the two exercises, with the arm exercise value being lower. This last result would be expected because arm exercise usually results in lower oxygen consumption than leg exercise due to the amount of muscle mass used. The researchers concluded that PD patients can exercise using standard protocols and have comparable cardiovascular and metabolic responses to those without the disease. These investigators also graphically looked at submaximal exercise heart rate (HR) and VO_2 values between the two groups and found that PD patients had higher values than controls. The authors concluded that these individuals have a lower efficiency during exercise.

In a follow-up study, these same researchers examined the response to aerobic exercise in males and females with PD compared to those who did not.[33] They performed a one-time exercise test using a stationary bicycle and a standard protocol. Outcomes were maximum oxygen consumption (VO_{2max}) and time to maximal exercise. Comparison of VO_{2max} resulted in no significant differences between those with PD and those without PD for males and females. Relative workloads were also similar for both groups. The difference came in the measurement of time to maximal exercise and the percentage of maximum reached in each stage of exercise. Results indicate that those with PD have comparable maximum oxygen consumption, but reach maximum levels in a shorter period—meaning they were unable to exercise as long as those without PD. Additionally, at each stage of exercise, PD patients had higher VO_2 values than controls. Results indicate that those with PD are less efficient during exercise and that this may be related to their higher resting metabolic rate and a mechanical inefficiency of movement, resulting in higher energy expenditure.[34,35]

Canning et al conducted a descriptive pre-test–post-test one-group study evaluating exercise capacity in 16 individuals with mild to moderate PD[36] using a one-time exercise test with a cycle ergometer. Outcome measures included respiratory function tests, 10-meter walk test, peak work rate, peak VO_2, peak ventilation, peak respiratory exchange ratio (RER), peakHR, and dyspnea rating. For the work rate and peak VO_2 there were no significant differences between actual and predicted values. The only abnormal respiratory function tests were maximum mid-inspiratory flow rate and peak inspiratory flow rate.

Aerobic exercise intervention studies have used treadmill, stationary bicycle, and pole-striding as the mode of exercise.[37-40] Outcome variables include values for oxygen consumption, HR, RER, time to maximal exercise, pulmonary function tests, movement initiation time, and/or walk tests. Results have varied. Lacking in most of the aerobic interventions studies is the potential impact regular exercise has on functional activities such as ADL and gait.

Bridgewater and Sharpe conducted a nonrandomized comparison group study consisting of 12 weeks of aerobic exercise with mild to moderate PD patients.[37] The treatment group exercised two times weekly on a treadmill. Outcome measures included cardiorespiratory fitness, severity of parkinsonian signs, mood, functional ability, and habitual activity. Following the intervention, there were significant differences between the treatment (n = 13) and control (n = 13) group for cardiorespiratory fitness and habitual activity.

In a nonrandomized comparison group study conducted by Bergen et al, a 16-week aerobic exercise program using a stationary bicycle three times weekly resulted in a significant improvement in peak VO_2 and movement initiation time.[40] The researchers concluded that aerobic exercise will improve oxygen consumption in those with mild PD and may help reduce slowing of movement commonly seen in PD patients.

SUMMARY OF THE EVIDENCE

Most intervention studies show some improvement in various deficits associated with PD. The specifics of the intervention is not always clearly defined, making it difficult to decide exactly what might be the best practice. Many of the aforementioned studies did not include outcome measures that addressed performance-based physical function, meaning the measures were often self-report or impairment measures, rather than observation measures. Also, many of the outcome measures lack strong psychometric properties such as reliability and sensitivity to change, resulting in additional limitations in the research literature.

The therapist should choose an intervention that addresses the patient's specific problems and before discharge instruct the patient in an individualized home program designed to help maintain the benefits gained from supervised therapy. The program should be one the patient can easily follow at home independently or with assistance from a family member, friend, or caregiver.

Based on the current evidence, task specific interventions appear most effective for patients with PD. ROM and flexibility exercises may be helpful for those with mild to moderate rigidity that affects segmental movements, including extremity and spinal movement and mobility. Because strength in the LEs also appears to be impacted, therapists should include exercises specific to this area. To support this approach, research shows that weakness often seen in the LEs as an individual ages can contribute to difficulties in functional activities such as transfers, balance tasks, and gait,[41] thus strengthening exercises can be beneficial.[42] In respect to the cardiorespiratory system, it appears that moderate aerobic activity can improve exercise capacity. The method most typically examined has been with the stationary bicycle. This mode of exercise could potentially help improve aerobic capacity as well as strengthen the LEs if resistance is applied. Last but not least is balance. Balance deficits in PD patients significantly increase the risk for falls. The therapist should perform a thorough evaluation to determine the specific balance deficits and their impact on the patient's fall risk so he or she can prescribe the most appropriate balance training activities.

When trying to decide which exercises are best, research conducted with older adults provides evidence. The aging research supports that muscular strength—especially LE strength, cardiovascular endurance, flexibility, and mobility, as well as balance—declines with age, most often because of inactivity and chronic disease.[41,43] Intervention studies with various aging populations clearly show that staying active throughout one's lifetime may prevent some of the above potential declines and protect against chronic diseases and the morbidity associated with them.[42,44,45] Research using exercise interventions with more deconditioned and frail elderly populations also indicates that patients may benefit even in the later years of life.[46-48] Because PD is most typically diagnosed when an individual is in the mid- to late 50s, it makes sense to prescribe a well-rounded exercise program that addresses all of the aforementioned components.

Case Study

Mrs. H has been seen as an outpatient in a rehabilitation facility three times weekly for 3 weeks and is currently being discharged home with an exercise program. She initially came to physical therapy due to increased falls and difficulty with functional activities.

Medical Diagnosis: Idiopathic Parkinson's disease

PMH: Mrs. H is a 67-year-old divorced white female with unremarkable medical history except for idiopathic PD diagnosed at age 43. She had a fall-related fracture to the right proximal humerus 5 years ago while hiking in the mountains.

Medications: Sinemet

Social History: She lives alone in a one-story house with a small dog and has a grown son and daughter living in the same metropolitan city. Mrs. H has had a successful career as a medical doctor and professor.

Problems at Time of Initial Physical Therapy Evaluation: Although Mrs. H is currently independent in all daily activities, she initially reported an increase in falls over the previous 2 months, with three falls occurring in 1 week while she was at home. No major injuries were sustained. She was also beginning to have difficulty getting dressed, getting out of bed, and getting out of the car. Mrs. H does continue to drive although she says she is having trouble staying in an upright position behind the wheel, and she tends to lean to the right.

Her specific dressing problems included fastening her bra in back, buttoning her clothes, tying her tennis shoes, and pulling clothes on over her head. She was also having trouble washing, drying, and combing her hair because of limited overhead reach.

Mrs. H also complained of slowing of all activities, problems with balance, and difficulty with functional movements (especially rising from a chair, walking, and getting out of bed). She was particularly concerned about being unable to rise from the floor after a fall.

Mrs. H ambulated without an assistive device.

Mrs. H was not participating in a regular exercise program.

Initial Evaluation

Practice Pattern and Physical Therapy Diagnosis: Neuromuscular

Pattern A: Primary Prevention/Risk Reduction for Loss of Balance and Falling
781.2 Abnormality of gait
781.3 Lack of coordination

Pattern E: Impaired Motor Function and Sensory Integrity Associated with Progressive Disorders of the Central Nervous system
781.2   Abnormality of gait
781.3   Lack of coordination
781.9   Other conditions involving nervous and musculoskeletal systems
781.92   Abnormal posture

General Impression: Bradykinesia of all movements; flexed posture; shuffling gait with festination and decreased arm swing bilaterally, decreased heel strike (right foot greater than left), and decreased stride length; masked facies.

Fall History: Over the past week, Mrs. H has had three falls at home. One occurred on a level carpeted surface, and the patient believes she caught her toe in the carpet, causing her to trip. Because her protective reflexes are slowed, she was unable to catch herself and fell to the floor, hitting her right shoulder. The other two falls occurred when she was stepping over an object lying on the floor and, unable to clear it with her foot, she tripped and fell. Again, because of impaired righting reflexes, she was unable to catch herself and fell to the right, landing on her arm. Mrs. H says she always falls to the right.

ROM: (all active)

Upper Extremities:	Right	Left
Shoulder		
Flexion	90	110
Extension	30	35
Abduction	95	100
Adduction	WFL	WFL

	Internal rotation	50	55
	External rotation	60	70
Elbow			
	Flexion/Extension	WFL	WFL
Radioulnar			
	Pronation	60	65
	Supination	WFL	WFL
Wrist			
	Flexion	70	75
	Extension	60	65
	Radial deviation	10	15
	Ulnar deviation	20	25

Lower Extremities:

Hip			
	Flexion	90	95
	Extension	10	15
	Abduction	35	40
	Adduction	25	30
	Internal rotation	30	35
	External rotation	35	40
Knee			
	Flexion	90	100
	Extension	−10	−10
Ankle			
	Plantarflexion	30	35
	Dorsiflexion	10	15
Subtalar			
	Inversion	20	25
	Eversion	10	10

Neck/Trunk:

Cervical			
	Flexion	25	
	Extension	25	
	Lateral flexion	30	30
	Rotation	30	30
Trunk			
	Flexion	50	
	Extension	10	
	Lateral flexion	10	10
	Rotation	10	10

GROSS MMT

Upper Extremities:		Right	Left
Shoulder			
	Flexors	4+	4+
	Extensors	4	4
	Abductors	4	4
	Adductors	4	4

	Internal rotators	3+	3+
	External rotators	3+	3+
Biceps		4+	4+
Triceps		4	4
Wrist			
	Flexors/Extensors	4+	4+
	Extensors	4–	4–
	Pronators/Supinators	4	4
Grasp			

Lower Extremities:

Hip			
	Flexors	3+	3+
	Extensors	3+	3+
	Abductors	3	3
	Adductors	3	3
	Internal rotators	3	3
	External rotators	3	3
Knee			
	Flexors	3+	3+
	Extensors	3+	3+
Ankle			
	Plantar flexors	3	3
	Dorsiflexors	3	3
	Invertors	3	3
	Evertors	3	3

Neck/Trunk:

Cervical			
	Flexors	4–	
	Extensors	3+	
	Lateral flexors	3+	3+
	Rotators	3+	3+
Trunk			
	Flexors	4	
	Extensors	4–	
	Lateral flexors	3+	3+
	Rotators	3+	3+

Posture

Sitting
Thoracic kyphosis with slight shift to the right. Protracted shoulders with forward head; decreased lordosis with posterior pelvic tilt. Could not maintain upright sitting posture for longer than 5 minutes.

Standing
Slight thoracic kyphosis with slight shift to the right. Shoulders were protracted and the head forward; decreased lordosis and posterior pelvic tilt. The patient had dyskinesias in the left LE while standing.

Balance

    Sitting:
            Static   Good
            Dynamic   Good
    Standing:
            Static   Increased postural sway while standing for 1 minute
            Dynamic

                           Posterior pull test: multiple steps required in order to maintain balance, no protective reactions from UEs
                           Lateral perturbations: unable to maintain balance when nudged to the right, no protective reactions from UEs, therapist had to prevent fall; required several steps to maintain balance when nudged to the left with no protective reactions from UEs.
                           Berg Balance Scale: 38/56

Coordination

    Upper and Lower Extremities
            Bradykinesia all movements

Tone

    Upper and Lower Extremities
            Cogwheel rigidity throughout ROM of all joints bilaterally

Gait: Shuffling, festinating gait with reduced stride length and arm swing bilaterally, decreased heel strike on right greater than left. Unsteady when turning

Abnormal movements: Resting tremor bilateral upper extremities; Dyskinesias left LE

Functional Activities

Timed Up and Go:
38 seconds with assistive device

Sit to Stand:
Requires four attempts to rise from sitting in straight back chair without arm rests; unable to control descent when returning to sitting from standing

Rolling side-to-side
Increased difficulty when rolling to right or left due to lack of segmental spinal movement; patient rolls as one unit

Supine to standing
Due to patient's inability to roll to side, she comes from supine to sitting by moving legs off the plinth and pulling upper body straight up, then pushes with arms to come to standing

Plan of Care

Three times weekly for 3 weeks to include standing balance training on noncompliant and compliant surfaces, LE strengthening using elastic exercise bands and cuff weights, AROM and stretching exercise for all extremities and spine, upright sitting and standing, functional and transitional activities to increase spinal muscular endurance and strength, postural visual feedback using mirrors to increase postural awareness, gait training emphasizing heel-toe gait pattern and increased stride and arm swing.

Discharge Status

(3 weeks post initial evaluation): At time of discharge, Mrs. H exhibited increased ROM throughout the spine and shoulders, increased strength in all LE musculature, and increased ability to sit upright without shifting to the right for 15 minutes. These improvements resulted in increased ability to roll segmentally from side-to-side, making transitional movements easier and more efficient, and decreased attempts to come from sitting to standing, and a better controlled descent when returning to sitting. Mrs. H also reported a decrease in the number of falls over the 3-week period and following the two falls she did have during the first week of treatment she was able to rise from the floor without assistance. Mrs. H also reported greater ease of washing and combing her hair and getting dressed. The Berg Balance Score improved from 38 to 49/56; the Timed Up and Go from 38 to 27.

PHYSICAL THERAPY APPROACH TO CASE

As indicated by the initial evaluation, Mrs. H had lost considerable AROM in the spine and upper quadrant, resulting in difficulty in performing hygiene activities and transitional movements when coming from sitting and supine. Because the disease process impacts the upper quadrant and spine early on, it is important to prescribe ROM and flexibility activities when the individual is first diagnosed. It is not uncommon for those having PD to develop adhesive capsulitis of the shoulder joint on the involved side due to rigidity and decreased activity. Because she experienced balance impairments and falls on level carpeted surfaces, it was important to perform balance activities on both noncompliant and compliant surfaces. Large exercise mats in the clinic create a compliant surface similar to carpeting. These mats are large enough to use for practicing both static and dynamic balance activities and short-distance gait activities. Depending on the circumstances surrounding the fall, the patient should also perform balance and gait activities while carrying packages, such as a bag full of groceries. In addition, when using a functional assessment tool such as the Berg Balance Scale, the therapist may include items the individual is having difficulty with to guide task-specific activities during treatment.[49-52] Likewise, using the Timed Up and Go not only as an assessment tool, but as a treatment or practice tool also incorporates the functional tasks of coming from sitting to standing, walking, turning, and returning to sitting.[53,54] These are all difficult activities for Mrs. H and using this tool in treatment allows her to practice these tasks in a functional and goal-oriented way. The therapist could also have the patient practice the Timed Up and Go on a compliant surface such as the exercise mat. For postural abnormalities, PD patients are often unaware of postural changes that occur and when sitting or standing posture starts to shift. This was the case with Mrs. H, as she was unable to maintain upright sitting posture for more than 5 minutes and had become aware of this only when she starting having difficulty when driving. Placing a mirror in front of the individual can help him or her to see the postural shifts that may be occurring and allow them to self-correct. Research has shown that visual and auditory cues can facilitate movement initiation in patients with PD.

After 3 weeks of treatment, Mrs. H showed improvements in ROM, strength, balance, transitional movements, and a decrease in falls. The goal now is to discharge her with a home program that will help her maintain the benefits of supervised physical therapy. As noted previously, we recommend that this program be a well-rounded one that includes flexibility, strengthening and aerobic exercises, along with appropriate balance activities. Depending on the patient's independence level, the program should be easy to follow and perform. Since Mrs. H lives alone, the program should be one she can perform safely and independently.

For a series of exercises that can be recommended for a home program, see Figures 6-1 through 6-35. The therapist can be prescribe these exercises for flexibility and mobility and many can be modified for strengthening by adding elastic resistance bands or cuff weights.

Figure 6-1. Cervical rotation.

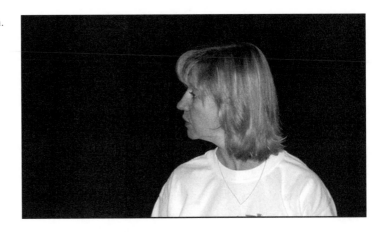

Figure 6-2. Cervical lateral flexion.

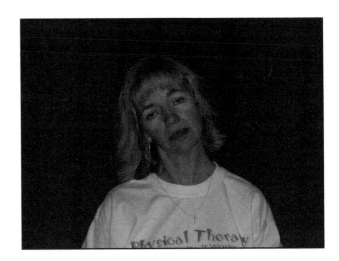

Figure 6-3. Chin tucks.

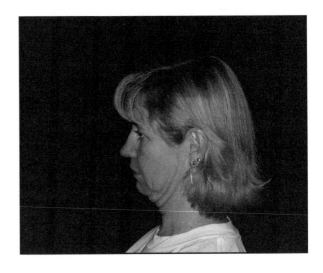

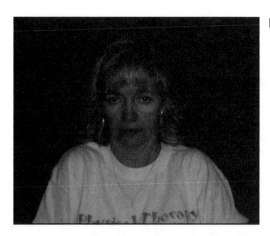

Figure 6-4. Shoulder shrugs.

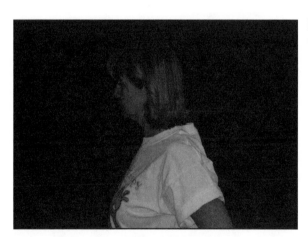

Figure 6-5. Shoulder retraction and wand exercises.

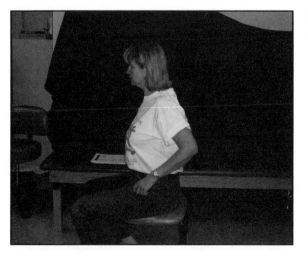

Figure 6-6. Shoulder retraction and wand exercises.

Figure 6-7. Trunk rotation.

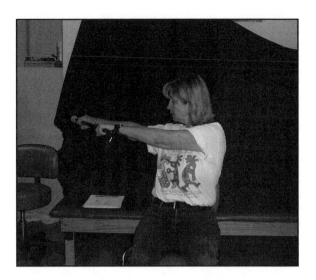

Figure 6-8. Shoulder flexion.

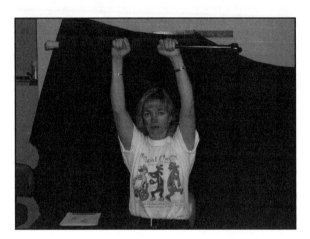

Figure 6-9. Shoulder flexion, extension, and scapular retraction.

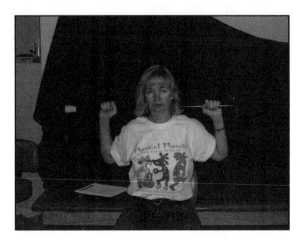

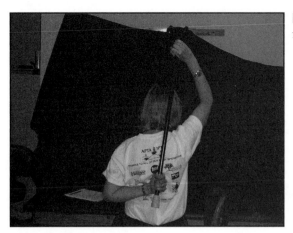

Figure 6-10. Shoulder extension, internal rotation, and adduction.

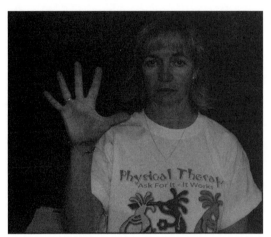

Figure 6-11. Open and close hand.

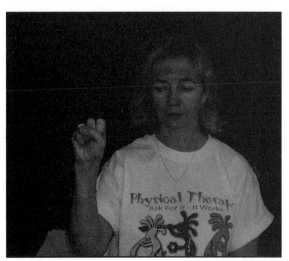

Figure 6-12. Open and close hand.

Figure 6-13. Finger opposition.

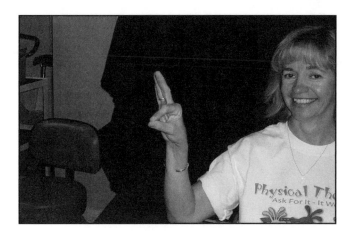

Figure 6-14. Finger opposition.

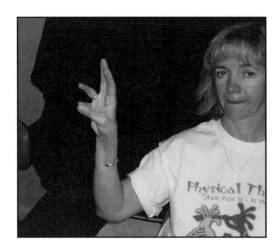

Figure 6-15. Wrist flexion and extension.

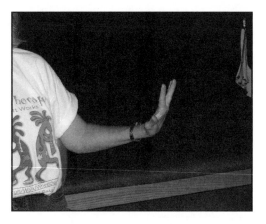

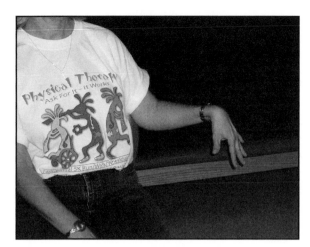

Figure 6-16. Wrist flexion and extension.

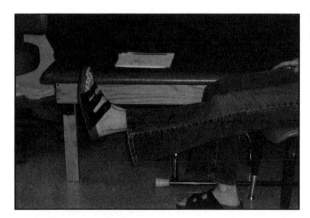

Figure 6-17. Knee and hip flexion and extension.

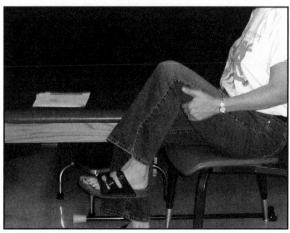

Figure 6-18. Knee and hip flexion and extension.

Figure 6-19. Hamstring stretch using a stool.

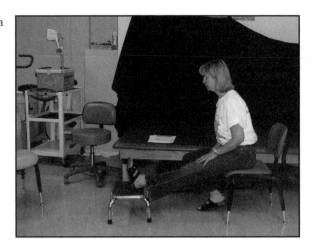

Figure 6-20. Hamstring stretch using a stool.

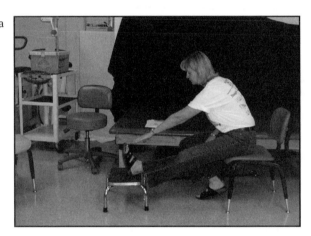

Figure 6-21. Plantarflexion and dorsiflexion.

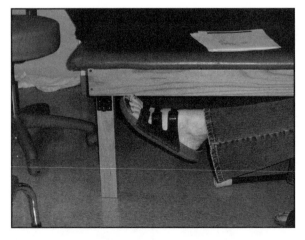

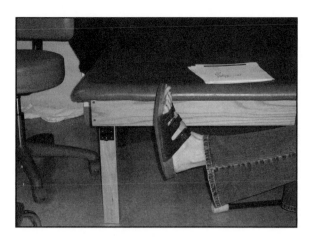

Figure 6-22. Plantarflexion and dorsiflexion.

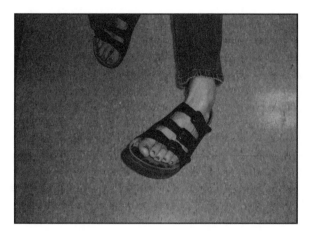

Figure 6-23. Inversion and eversion.

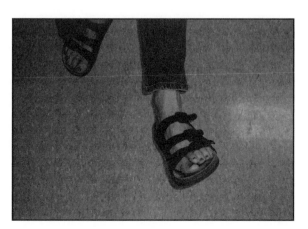

Figure 6-24. Inversion and eversion.

Figure 6-25. Bridging.

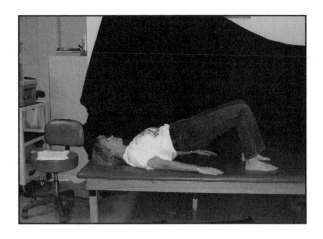

Figure 6-26. Knee rolls side to side with upper extremities abducted.

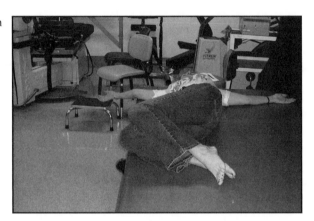

Figure 6-27. Knee rolls side to side with upper extremities abducted.

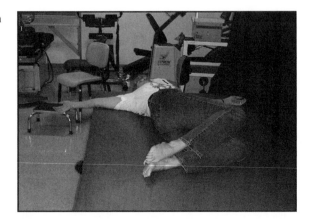

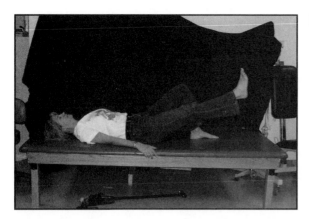

Figure 6-28. Straight leg raise.

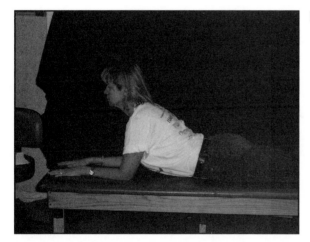

Figure 6-29. Prone on elbows.

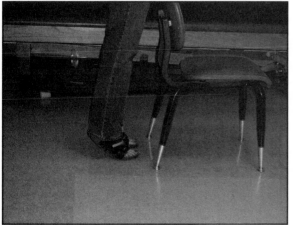

Figure 6-30. Toe raises using chair for support.

Figure 6-31. Gastrocnemius stretch using chair for support.

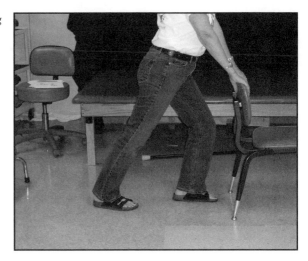

Figure 6-32. Stepping side to side using chair for support.

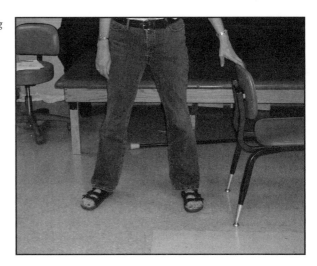

Figure 6-33. Stepping front and back using chair for support.

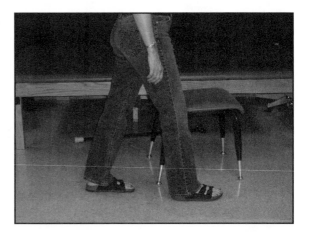

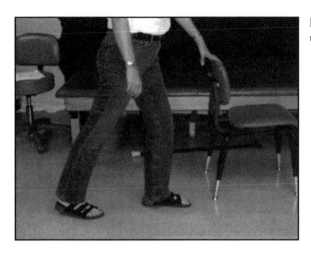

Figure 6-34. Stepping front and back using chair for support.

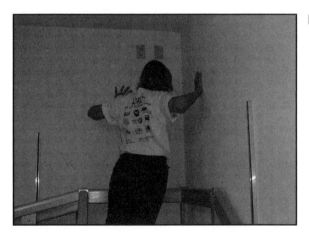

Figure 6-35. Pectoralis stretch.

REFERENCES

1. Wichman R. *Be Active!: A Suggested Exercise Program for People with Parkinson's Disease.* New York, NY: The American Parkinson Disease Association, Inc., 2000.
2. Banks MA, Caird FI. Physiotherapy benefits patients with Parkinson's disease. *Clin Rehabil.* 1989;3:11-16.
3. Comella CL, Stebbins GT, Brown-Toms N, Goetz CG. Physical therapy and Parkinson's disease: A controlled clinical trial. *Neurology.* 1994;44:376-378.
4. Dam M, Tonin P, Casson S, Bracco F, Piron L, Pizzolato G, Battistin L. Effects of conventional and sensory-enhanced physiotherapy on disability of Parkinson's disease patients. *Advances in Neurology.* 1996;69:551-555.
5. Patti F, Reggio A, Nicoletti F, Sellaroli T, Deinite G, Nicoletti Fr. Effects of rehabilitation therapy on parkinsonians' disability and functional independence. *J Neuro Rehab.* 1996;10(4):223-231.
6. Platz T, Brown G, Marsden CD. Training improves the speed of aimed movements in Parkinson's disease. *Brain.* 1998;121:505-514.
7. Villani T, Pasquetti P, Magnolfi S, Lunardelli ML, Giorgi C, Serra P, Taiti PG. Effects of physical training on straightening-up processes in patients with Parkinson's disease. *Disabil Rehab.* 1999;21(2):68-73.

8. Marchese R, Diverio M, Zucchi F, Lentino C, Abbruzzese G. The role of sensory cues in the rehabilitation of parkinsonian patients: a comparison of two physical therapy protocols. *Mov Disord.* 2000;15(5):879-883.

9. Nieuwboer A, Weerdt WD, Dom R, Truyen M, Janssens L, Kamsma Y. The effect of a home physiotherapy program for persons with Parkinson's disease. *J Rehabil Med.* 2001;33:266-272.

10. Caglar AT, Gurses HN, Mutluay FK, Kiziltan G. Effects of home exercises on motor performance in patients with Parkinson's disease. *Clin Rehabil.* 2005;19:870-877.

11. Lun V, Pullan N, Labelle N, Adams C, Suchowersky O. Comparison of the effects of a self-supervised home exercise program with a physiotherapist-supervised exercise program on the motor symptoms of Parkinson's disease. *Mov Disord.* 2005;20(8):971-975.

12. Pellecchia MT, Grasso A, Biancardi LG, Squillante M, Bonavita V, Barone P. Physical therapy in Parkinson's disease: An open long-term rehabilitation trail. *J Neurol.* 2004;251:595-598.

13. Wade DT, Gage H, Owen C, Trend P, Grossmith C, Kaye J. Multidisciplinary rehabilitation for people with Parkinson's disease: a randomized controlled study. *J Neural Neurosurg Psychiatry.* 2003;74(pt 2):158-168.

14. Ellis T, de Goede J, Feldman RG, Wolters EC, Kwakkel G, Wagenaar RC. Efficacy of a physical therapy program in patients with Parkinson's disease: a randomized controlled trial. *Arch Phys Med Rehabil.* 2005;86:626-632.

15. Deane KHO, Jones D, Playford ED, Ben-Shlomo Y, Clarke CE. Physiotherapy versus placebo or no intervention in Parkinson's disease. *The Cochrane Database of Systematic Reviews.* 2001, Issue 3.

16. Deane KHO, Jones D, Ellis-Hill C, Clarke CE, Playford ED, Ben-Shlomo Y. Physiotherapy for Parkinson's disease: a comparison of techniques (review). *The Cochrane Database of Systematic Reviews.* 2001; Issue 1.

17. Schenkman M, Cutson TM, Kuchibhatla M, Chandler J, Pieper CF, Ray L, Laub KC. Exercise to improve spinal flexibility and function for people with Parkinson's disease: a randomized, controlled trail. *J Am Geri Soc.* 1998;46:1207-1216.

18. Pedersen SH and Oberg B. Dynamic strength in Parkinson's disease. *Eur Neurol.* 1993;33:97-102.

19. Corcos DM, Chen CM, Quinn NP, McAuley J, Rothwell JC. Strength in Parkinson's disease: relationship to rate of force generation and clinical status. *Ann Neurol.* 1996;39:79-88.

20. Kakinuma S, Nogaki H, Pramanik B, Morimatsu M. Muscle weakness in Parkinson's disease: Isokinetic study of the lower limbs. *Eur Neurol.* 1998;39:218-222.

21. Nogaki H, Kakinuma S, Mormatsu M. Movement velocity dependent muscle strength in Parkinson's disease. *Acta Neurol Scand.* 1999;152-157.

22. Toole T, Hirsch MA, Forkink A, Lehman DA, Maitland CG. The effects of a balance and strength training program on equilibrium in parkinsonism: a preliminary study. *J Neuro Rehab.* 2000;14:165-174.

23. Hirsch MA, Toole T, Maitland CG, Ridger RA. The effects of balance training and high-intensity resistance training on person's with idiopathic Parkinson's disease. *Arch Phys Med Rehabil.* 2003;84:1109-1117.

24. Haapaniemi TH, Kallio MA, Korpelainen JT, Suominen K, Tolonen U, Sotaniemi KA, Myllyla VV. Levodopa, bromocriptine and selegiline modify cardiovascular responses in Parkinson's disease. *J Neurol.* 2000;415:868-874.

25. Ludin SM, Steiger MJ, Ludin HP. Autonomic disturbances and cardiovascular reflexes in idiopathic Parkinson's disease. *J Neurol.* 1987;235:10-15.

26. Neu HC, Connolly JJ, Schwertley FW et al. Obstructive respiratory dysfunction in Parkinson's patients. *Am Rev Respir Dis.* 1967;95:33-47.

27. Lilker ES, Woolf CR. Pulmonary function in Parkinson's syndrome: the effect of thalamotomy. *Can Med Assoc J.* 1968;99:752-757.

28. Sabate M, Rodriguez M, Mendez, Enriquez E, Gonzalez I. Obstructive and restrictive pulmonary dysfunction increases disability in Parkinson's disease. *Arch Phys Med Rehabil.* 1996;77(1):29-34.

29. Brown RG, Dittner A, Findley L, Wessely SC. The Parkinson fatigue scale. *Parkinsonism Relat Disord.* 2005;11:49-55.

30. Ziv I, Avraham M, Michaelov Y, et al. Enhanced fatigue during motor performance in patients with Parkinson's disease. *Neurology.* 1998;51:1583-1586.

31. Karlsen K, Larsen JP, Tandberg E, Jorgensen K. Fatigue in patients with Parkinson's disease. *Mov Disord.* 1999;14(2):237-241.

32. Protas EJ, Stanley RK, Jankovic J. Cardiovascular and metabolic responses to upper and lower extremity exercise in med with idiopathic Parkinson's disease. *Phys Ther.* 1996;76:34-40.

33. Stanley RK, Protas EJ, Jankovic J. Exercise performance in those having Parkinson's disease and healthy normals. *Med Sci Sports Exer.* 1999;31(6):761-766.

34. Levi S, Cox M, Lugon M, Hodkinson M, Tomkins A. Increased energy expenditure in Parkinson's disease. *Br Med J.* 1990;301:1256-1257.

35. Markus HS, Cox M, Tomkins AM. Raised resting energy expenditure in Parkinson's disease and its relationship to muscle rigidity. *Clin Sci.* 1992;83:199-204.

36. Canning CG, Alison JA, Allen NE, Groeller H. Parkinsons' disease: an investigation of exercise capacity, respiratory function, and gait. *Arch Phys Med Rehabil.* 1997;78:199-207.

37. Bridgewater KJ, Sharpe MH. Aerobic exercise and early Parkinson's disease. *J Neurol Rehabil.* 1996;10(4):233-241.

38. Koseoglu F, Inan L, Ozel S, et al. The effects of a pulmonary rehabilitation program on pulmonary function tests and exercise tolerance in patients with Parkinson's disease. *Funct Neurol.* 1997;12(6):319-325.

39. Baatile J, Langbein WE, Weaver F, Maloney C, Jost MB. Effect of exercise on perceived quality of life of individual with Parkinson's disease. *J Rehabil Res Dev.* 2000;37(5):529-534.

40. Bergen J, Toole T, Elliott RG III, Wallace B, Robinson K, Maitland CG. Aerobic exercise intervention improves aerobic capacity and movement initiation in Parkinson's disease patients. *NeuroRehabil.* 2002;17:161-168.

41. Spirduso WW, Francis KL, MacRae PG. *Physical Dimensions of Aging.* 2nd ed. Champaign, IL: Human Kinetics; 2005.

42. Clark DO. The effects of walking on lower body disability among older blacks and whites. *Am J Public Health.* 1996;86:57-61.

43. Hughes VA, Frontera WR, Wood M, et al. Longitudinal muscle strength changes in older adults: influence of muscle mass, physical activity, and health. *J Geront: Biol Sci.* 2001;56A:B209-B217.

44. Paffenbarger RS, Lee IM. Physical activity and fitness for health and longevity. *Res Quarterly Exer Sport.* 1996:62(Suppl):S11-S28.

45. Mazzeo RS, Tanaka H. Exercise prescription for the elderly. *Sports Med.* 2001;31:809-818.

46. Fiatarone Singh MA. Exercise comes of age: rationale and recommendations for a geriatric exercise prescription. *J Geront.* 2002;57(5):M262-M282.

47. Fiatarone MA, Marks EC, Ryan ND, Meredith C, Lipsitz LA, Evans WJ. High intensity strength training in nonagenerians. *JAMA.* 1990;263:3029-3034.

48. Fiatarone MA, O'Neill EF, Ryan ND, et al. Exercise training and nutritional supplementation for physical frailty in very elderly people. *N Engl J Med.* 1994;330(25):1769-1775.

49. Berg K, Wood-Dauphinee S, Williams JI, Gayton D. Measuring balance in the elderly: preliminary development of an instrument. *Physiother Can.* 1989;41:304-311.

50. Berg K, Maki B, Williams JI, Holiday P, Wood-Dauphinee S. A comparison of clinical and laboratory measures of postural balance in an elderly population. *Arch Phys Med Rehabil.* 1992;73:1073-82.

51. Berg K, Wood-Dauphinee S, Williams JI, Maki B. Measuring balance in the elderly: validation of an instrument. *Can J Public Health.* 1992;2:S7-11.

52. Berg K, Wood-Dauphinee S, Williams JI. The Balance Scale. Reliability assessment for elderly residents and patients with an acute stroke. *Scan J Rehabil Med.* 1995;27:27-36.

53. Podsiadlo D, Richardson S. The Timed "Up & Go": A test of basic functional mobility for frail elderly persons. *J Am Geriatr Soc.* 1991;39:142-148.

54. Morris S, Morris ME, Iansek R. Reliability of measurements obtained with the Timed "Up & Go" Test in people with Parkinson's disease. *Phys Ther.* 2001;81:810-818.

GAIT CHARACTERISTICS AND INTERVENTION STRATEGIES IN PATIENTS WITH PARKINSON'S DISEASE

Denis Brunt, EdD, PT; Elizabeth Protas, PT, PhD, FACSM; Mark Bishop, PhD, PT

GAIT IN IDIOPATHIC PARKINSON'S DISEASE

Idiopathic Parkinson's disease (PD) is a result of the progressive loss of dopamine-producing neurons of the substantia nigra in the brain stem.[1] Dopaminergic medication may increase the amount of dopomine produced by the remaining neurons, an effect that will last for approximately 5 years. As a result of this progressive disease, a number of clinical motor signs become apparent, including a gait that can be primarily characterized by hypokinesia and akinesia.[2] *Hypokinesia* refers to a slowness of gait characterized by a short step length and decreased ground clearance. The term *shuffling gait* is often used to describe how patients with PD walk. The fear of falling may also contribute to the hypokinetic characteristics of PD gait. Akinesia is manifested in the inability of PD patients to initiate gait or in "freezing" during gait. Freezing, or sudden cessation of walking,[1] usually occurs while turning or when confronted with environmental constraints such as a doorway or an approaching target.[3-5] According to Giladi et al,[3] it is unclear if freezing is a severe form of akinesia or whether it should be considered as a separate entity. Fahn[6] believes that akinesia describes hypokinesia and bradykinesia and that freezing should be considered as a separate motor disturbance. However, others consider freezing as at least a type of akinesia[4-7] or maybe an advanced stage of akinesia.[5]

TABLE 7-1

Mean Characteristics of Parkinson's Disease Gait "On" and "Off" Medication

Gait Characteristic	"Off" Medication	"On" Medication
Velocity (m/min)	50.9	69.3 (69.25)
Stride Length (m)	.94	1.24 (1.27)
Cadence (steps/min)	108	112 (109.64)
DLS (% of Gait Cycle)	33.03	30.4 (33.76)

Data from O'Sullivan et al[11] and Bond and Morris[12]

Knutsson[8] and Murray et al[9] provided early accounts of PD gait. Both described a gait that was significantly slower than healthy elderly, with a decreased stride length and increased double support time. Patients displayed limited hip and knee extension in stance and decreased plantarflexion following terminal stance. In swing, there was decreased initial knee flexion and hip flexion (and therefore reduced toe clearance) and a lack of knee extension in terminal swing. Plantarflexion was diminished or absent at loading, probably due to the lack of a heel strike. Arm swing was significantly decreased and trunk and pelvic motion were not reciprocal. These characteristics contribute to a short step length and therefore gait hypokinesia. It is interesting that cadence was thought to be similar to normal elderly gait.

Recent papers have provided detailed information on parameters of PD gait and the effect of anti-parkinsonian medication on these parameters.[10,11] Table 7-1 shows mean data reported by O'Sullivan et al[11] both on and off medication. As can be seen, significant improvements were reported for gait velocity and stride length. Although cadence increased and double limb support decreased, these changes were not statistically significant. The data in parentheses are from Bond and Morris[12] and are very much in agreement with the data of O'Sullivan et al.

Morris et al[10] showed that PD patients could in fact increase cadence and that there was a strong relationship between cadence and stride length. Their subjects walked to the beat of a metronome. Up to a certain cadence (approximately 120 steps/min) there is a linear relationship between cadence and stride length. However, stride length for the PD subjects is less than normal controls at each level of cadence. Obviously, the extent to which stride length can continue to increase depends, in part, on the individual's stature. At this point (termed break point) cadence and not step length may continue to increase to modulate gait velocity. Step length at the break point is far less for PD patients compared to controls. At a given cadence, step length is greater and the break point occurs at an increased cadence when patients are "on" versus "off" medication. Blin et al[13] also reported that distance (step length) and velocity parameters of gait improved following medication, yet timing parameters (stride duration) remained statistically unchanged. Together, these data show that with medication PD patients can increase stride length, but that the absolute stride length values are consistently less than control values. It appears, therefore, that a shorter step length contributes more to decreased velocity in PD patients than cadence.[11,14]

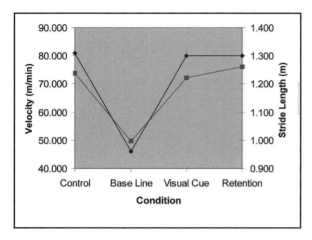

Figure 7-1. Stride length and gait velocity are shown for control subjects and Parkinson's disease subjects when 'on' medication (baseline condition). Stride length and velocity increased to control values when subjects were to step to lines on the floor (visual cue). Subjects were able to maintain this improvement following removal of the lines (retention).

EXTERNAL SENSORY CUEING TO IMPROVE GAIT IN PARKINSON'S DISEASE

Strategies have emerged that may be used in rehabilitation as an adjunct to medication. Morris et al[15,16] asked PD subjects to walk on a floor where lines were placed at distances equal to the stride length of matched controls. Baseline results are shown in Figure 7-1, where velocity and stride length for PD patients on medication (baseline) are significantly less than age matched controls. However, these values were similar to control values following the use of the visual cue. Similar patterns emerged for double support time and cadence, although the change in cadence was not so impressive. Of interest is that results were similar when PD subjects were asked to develop a mental image of the control step length and concentrate on that step length during gait.[16] It also appears that step length increases when parallel stripes simply provide an optic flow and not a target for foot strike.[17] However, it was also shown that improvement in gait variables to visual cues or attention to step length was to some extent due to the testing environment and experimenter encouragement. That is, subjects' performance decreased as they walked between experimental trials when they thought data were not being collected.[16] It is perhaps not surprising, therefore, that gait of PD patients has also been shown to improve following verbal instruction (for example, walk fast, take longer steps)[18] or by walking in time to a rhythmic auditory signal.[19]

Both Morris et al[16] and Bagley et al[20] reported that there is some retention of increased step length following the removal of the visual cues (see Figure 7-1). However, retention of performance appears to be degraded if PD patients have to perform an attentive task while walking.[16] This degradation of walking is proportional to the level of complexity of task interference. Subjects were asked to verbalize phrases of different complexity while walking. Stride length, velocity, and cadence decrease compared to percent of control values as the task becomes more complex while double support time increases. The change in cadence was again less impressive. Similar effects on gait have been shown when patients were asked to carry a tray of glasses while walking.[12] These data are shown in Figure 7-2. For healthy subjects, no differences were noted between control gait and gait

Figure 7-2. The effect of dual task interference on gait parameters in subjects with Parkinson's disease. While carrying a tray of glasses stride length and gait velocity significantly decreased in patients with Parkinson's disease yet had no effect on normal controls.

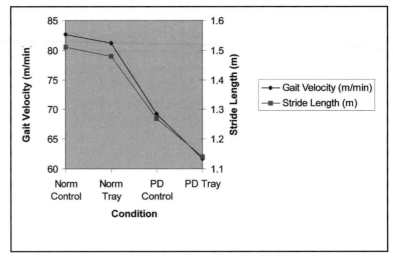

when carrying a tray of glasses for both velocity and stride length. However, a significant decrease from the control condition for both variables is apparent for PD patients. For both groups, no changes were noted for cadence or double support time.

EFFECT OF SUBTHALAMIC NUCLEUS (STN) STIMULATION ON GAIT IN PARKINSON'S DISEASE

PD is initially treated with medication. Both with time and disease progression, the use of medication becomes less effective, resulting in drug-induced fluctuation of motor behaviors and the presence of involuntary movements, or dyskinesias.[21] It has been shown that Deep Brain Stimulation (DBS) that targets the STN improves those motor behaviors that are typically responsive to levadopa therapy.[22] Recent studies have reported improvement on the gait scores of the Unified Parkinson's Disease Rating Scale (UPDRS) (item 30) following bilateral STN stimulation.[22-25] In general, it appears that the gait score improved with stimulation and off medication compared to preoperative off medication with greater improvement when on medication post-surgery.[26]

Quantitative gait analysis would appear to support the UPDRS data to the extent that increased gait velocity would result from STN stimulation.[14,27,28] To fully comprehend the effects of stimulation, researchers have observed gait with subjects off medication and stimulation, off medication and on stimulation, on medication and off stimulation, and on medication and on stimulation. In general, it appears that both medication and stimulation greatly improve gait parameters. However, gait further improves when on medication post-surgery. The data in Table 7-2 are taken from Faist et al.[28] It can be seen that gait velocity increases when either on stimulation or on medication, but velocity increases further when on both medication and stimulation. It is also apparent that the increase in velocity is due to an increase in step length as cadence varies very little between conditions. As expected, double stance time decreases and swing time increases as a percent of the gait cycle with the increase in velocity. Of further significance is that the variability of the gait decreased with this increase in velocity. Table 7-3 shows the coefficients of variation of velocity, stride length, cadence, and double support. The decrease in variability is

	No Medication		Medication	
Gait Characteristics	**No Stimulation**	**Stimulation**	**No Stimulation**	**Stimulation**
Velocity (m/s) (1.07)*	35	96	94	1.19
Stride length (m) (1.15)*	34	99	92	1.20
Cadence (steps/m) (112)*	122	118	121	119
Double stance (%) (18)	39	22	23	21
Swing (%) (42)*	33	38	39	39

TABLE 7-2

Effect of Subthalamic Nucleus Stimulation on Gait Parameters

* Control values.
% Percent of gait.

From Faist M, Xie J, Kurz D, et al. Effect of bilateral subthalamic nucleus stimulation on gait in Parkinson's disease. *Brain.* 2001;124(Pt 8):1590-1600.

apparent and the greatest increase occurred when the patients were on medication following surgery. It is also significant to note that the incidence of freezing in PD is thought to increase with variability of gait parameters.[27]

GAIT INITIATION IN PATIENTS WITH PARKINSON'S DISEASE

Hypokinesia is often used to describe the gait of PD patients where the velocity is known to be slow due primarily to short step lengths.[8-12] Gait initiation (GI) in PD patients has also been shown to be slow. In GI, the antagonist muscles at the ankle control the backward movement of the center of pressure to initiate dorsiflexion moments and a pendulum-like motion at the ankle. Prior to toe-off of the swing limb, there is a distinct increase in the anterior/posterior ground reaction under the swing limb. In our lab, we have shown a strong relationship between ground reaction forces of the swing limb and the intended velocity of GI as determined by time to swing toe-off. The swing limb hip abductors also create a lateral movement of the center of pressure toward the swing limb to propel the center of mass toward the stance limb. In addition, the coordination of stance knee flexion with the swing limb hip abductors prepare for the movement of the center of mass toward the stance limb.[29] The mechanism of this frontal plane movement is less impaired in PD patients compared to the forward acceleration of the center of mass.[29] Further explanation of the ground reaction forces and EMG activity during GI appears in Figure 7-3.

TABLE 7-3

Coefficient of Variation (%) of Gait Parameters Following Subthalamic Nucleus Stimulation

Gait Characteristics	No Medication		Medication	
	No Stimulation	Stimulation	No Stimulation	Stimulation
Velocity (7)*	22	12	12	8
Stride length (5.9)*	21.3	11.9	11.8	7.6
Cadence (2.7)*	9.8	4.1	5.7	3.9
Double stance (11.9)*	18.8	13.6	16.1	11.8

* Control values.

From Faist M, Xie J, Kurz D, et al. Effect of bilateral subthalamic nucleus stimulation on gait in Parkinson's disease. *Brain.* 2001;124(Pt 8):1590-1600.

Figure 7-3. EMG and force plate data from one patient in the fast group. First vertical line represents movement onset while the second vertical line swing limb toe-off. EMG activity approximates a normal pattern with bilateral activation of the tibialis anterior (TA) and reciprocal inhibition of the soleus (Sol). Peak propulsive forces (FX). under the swing limb is 12% body weight (see arrow). Pattern of vertical ground reaction forces (Fz) demonstrate a normal unloading of the stance limb (40% body weight) and loading of the swing limb (60% body weight). Time to swing toe-off was 630 ms..

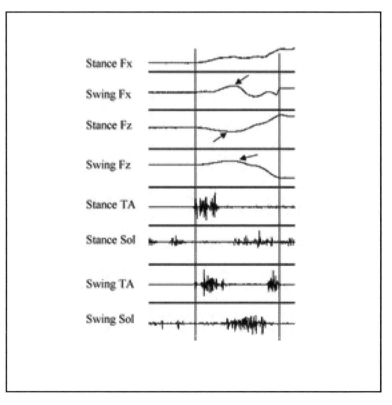

In normal GI, onset of tibialis anterior and soleus inhibition creates the backward movement of the center of pressure and an increase in the anterior ground reaction force. Motion is initiated at the ankles to destabilize upright posture and begin the process of GI. In PD patients, it appears that the burst of tibialis anterior is more variable[29] and reduced in amplitude.[29,30] In addition, the soleus may not be inhibited, resulting in a co-contraction or delayed onset of tibialis anterior. Either a reduction in tibialis anterior EMG, soleus co-contraction with the tibialis anterior, or absent tibialis anterior activity will result in a decrease in the backward movement of the center of pressure[29,30] and a decreased forward velocity of the center of mass.[30,31] Consequently, there is a prolonged time to swing limb toe-off and a short swing limb step length.

We identified two groups of PD patients based on their speed of GI as measured by the time to swing limb toe-off.[32] All patients were tested in the "on" state approximately 1.5 hours following the administration of their medication. The mean time to swing toe-off was 750 milliseconds (ms) (SD = 100 ms). Subjects whose time to toe-off was greater than 800 ms were placed in a slow PD group, whereas those whose time was less than 700 ms were placed in a fast PD group. Mean time to swing toe-off from the onset of movement was 628 ms (fast group) and 859 ms (slow group).

Analysis of different EMG patterns and ground reaction forces between the fast and slow group provides some explanation as to why patients with PD begin to walk slowly. Figure 7-3 shows data from a patient in the fast group. As illustrated in the caption, GI begins by bilateral inhibition of the soleus and activation of tibialis anterior. Consequently, there is an increase in the swing limb forward ground reaction force. The center of mass is propelled forward. In addition, there is a loading of the swing limb and unloading of the stance limb vertical ground reaction force. This is a component of the movement of the center of mass toward the stance limb. The center of mass thus moves forward and toward the stance limb. However, although the pattern of EMG and force plate activity appears relatively normal, the execution of the task was slow. In this trial, time to swing toe-off (second vertical line) was 630 ms. The peak of swing limb anterior-posterior ground reaction force (see arrow) was 12% body weight and the slope to peak 40% body weight/sec. Equivalent values for healthy elderly subjects were 500 ms, 17% body weight, and 56% body weight/sec. Eighty-six percent of the fast group (and 100% of the elderly group) showed normal timing of the tibialis anterior where onset was before or at the same time as movement onset (see Figure 7-3). This pattern of muscle activity was present in only 25% of the slow group.

Figure 7-4 shows a single trial from a subject in the slow group. In this case, there is no inhibition of the soleus and tibialis anterior activity does not begin until pre-swing. In this trial, peak swing limb anterior-posterior ground reaction force was 10% body weight, the slope to the peak 19.44% body weight/sec, and time to swing limb toe-off was 766 ms. The main burst of tibialis anterior activity for 58% of the slow group occurred just before toe-off of the swing limb. Tibialis anterior activity at this time is in preparation for swing phase and occurs as the limb is being unloaded. In this instance, it was control by the soleus that initiated a fall forward to begin walking. According to Halliday et al,[33] the center of mass in PD patients during quiet stance is in fact further forward than normal. Further trunk flexion may then be sufficient to initiate gait, a selected strategy that requires the late inhibition of soleus activity.

Muscle activity at the ankle dictates the forward velocity of gait initiation. As we have shown in Figure 7-3, and according to Gantchev et al,[30] even when the onset of tibialis anterior activity is normal in PD patients, diminished EMG amplitude is responsible for the decreased ground reaction forces. A further decrease in velocity of initiation would be expected with disease severity because an inverse trend exists between propulsive forces and the severity of the disease as determined by the Hoehn and Yahr scale.[34] A recent

Figure 7-4. EMG and force plate data from a patient from the slow group. Abreviations same as Figure 7-3. Peak swing Fx (at arrow) was 10% body weight and swing toe-off was 766 ms. Soleus activity continues until pre-swing tibialis anterior activity. The pattern of Fz loading and unloading remains symmetrical.

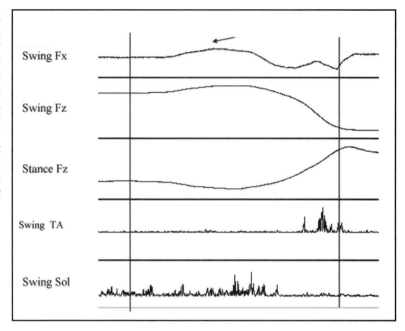

study has also demonstrated significant and positive changes in peak anterior-posterior ground reaction force and backward movement of the center of pressure following STN stimulation.[35]

GAIT TERMINATION IN PATIENTS WITH PARKINSON'S DISEASE

Gait termination occurs as the result of decelerating the forward motion of the center of mass. As such, stopping represents a transitional activity that moves us from rhythmical gait to standing still. In those with PD, a decreased ability to internally control changes in the center of mass during self-directed activities such as getting up from a chair, turning, or stopping is commonly associated with falls.[36-38] Difficulty stopping or turning is a characteristic of elderly fallers,[39] stroke survivors,[40] and those with parkinsonism (PD).[41,42] Individuals with PD are of particular concern because they are five times more likely to experience a fall-related injury than the general older population.[43]

Understanding how one stops, therefore, has implications for people who may be at risk of injuring themselves as a result of their inability to stop effectively. A number of factors must be examined when considering this topic. For example, frail elderly fallers have strength deficits in the hip and ankle musculature important during stopping. Balance, peripheral sensation, and reaction times must be considered. Another consideration is that stopping is at least one motor program.[44] Crenna et al[45] suggested that when healthy adults are rapidly terminating gait, the muscle activity generated in response to cue to stop is produced by a flexible set of motor commands in the stance limb, and by a single motor program in the swing limb. As such, difficulty activating this program or programs, for example in the context of PD, will also affect a person's ability to stop. Additionally, freezing of gait may lead to involuntary termination of gait, which is a transient phenomenon common to those patients with PD.[46]

During a planned stop, there occurs a volitional decision to stop at a certain position in space. This implies that not only is there enough time available to appropriately identify a suitable, satisfactory place to stop free of obstacles and other impediments, but also to determine how much braking force is required and how rapidly it needs to be produced to slow the body and maintain dynamic balance. Three phases of planned gait termination have been identified: preparatory brake, fast brake, and final brake.[47] The goal of preparatory braking is described as the reduction of forward velocity and adjustment of posture for ensuing phases. During fast braking, a rapid reduction in kinetic energy occurs. In the final brake phase, the remainder of the forward velocity is reduced as the center of pressure moves quickly ahead of the center of mass due to increased activity of the plantar flexors, and, finally, the center of mass is brought within the base of support. Hirokawa[48] noted a decrease in forward velocity over the last three steps during stopping. Similarly, Wearing et al[49] showed that subjects had already slowed by the second to last step.

Subjects with PD tend to slow their gait velocity even earlier than these studies in healthy adults would indicate. We have noted that those with PD slow velocity several steps earlier than healthy peers and enter the final step at only 84% of forward velocity. O'Kane et al[50] noted a similar early slowing strategy in subjects with neurological balance impairments who were performing a planned stop, which these authors speculated might be a compensatory strategy to reduce the challenges of controlling posture.

In contrast, an unplanned stop may be defined as a termination of gait that occurs without prior planning; that is, an event occurs that requires the rapid termination of forward gait. Perhaps more commonly, the occurrence has always been present (a pothole in the foot path) and it suddenly comes to our notice. Jaeger and Vanitchatchavan[51] identified predominant mechanisms to reduce forward velocity included a diminution of acceleration forces at push-off of the trailing leg and an increase in deceleration forces of the leading leg. These findings were replicated by Jian et al[47] and in our laboratory.[52] That is, there is an interaction between the stance and swing limbs that occurs. This interaction becomes more evident as the velocity of gait increases.[53,54]

Jaeger and Vanitchatchavan[51] reported critical periods during the stance phase of gait. As long as the signal stop occurred before 18% of stance time, subjects were able to stop on the next step. After this, the time to stop increased, as subjects had to take an extra step. Based on the timing of the signal, three mechanisms have been identified to stop the forward motion of the body.[55] First, the subject could increase the extension of the leading limb, thereby keeping the center of mass behind the lead foot. This was achieved predominantly by strong activation of the soleus and activation of the quadricep and gluteus maximus muscles. Second, there was a reduction in push-off from the stance limb (soon to become a swing limb). A large burst of activity from the tibialis anterior muscle reduces the effect and output from the ankle plantar flexors. In this instance, gluteus medius and hamstrings slow and limit hip flexion, in effect holding the swing leg back. This process was summarized by Crenna et al[45] as distal to proximal activation in the lead limb, and proximal to distal activation in the trailing limb. Hase and Stein[55] described a third scenario that occurs when the first two mechanisms described are ineffective in controlling the motion of the center of mass. If the signal to stop occurred after midstance, there was insufficient time for subjects to reduce push-off power and ready the swinging limb to maintain extension. In this case, subjects either rose onto their toes to convert kinetic to potential energy, or took another step.

Work in our laboratory indicates that the braking impulse generated under the stance limb is modulated differently by those with PD when compared to healthy age-matched peers without PD. Figure 7-5 contains mean data from control subjects and those with PD and demonstrates that the control subjects remain able to modify braking impulse under the stance limb with a signal to stop that occurs at peak loading during stance.[52] Subjects

Figure 7-5. Mean anterior-posterior force graphs of all unplanned stopping trials. Control subjects are shown in the top graph and trials are shown in which the signal to stop occurred at heel-strike (HS), first peak loading (Pk1), and midstance (MS). The bottom graph represents data from a group of subjects with PD (Hoehn and Yahr 1 to 3). Note that the mean graph of trials at Pk1 for the group with PD is very similar to that for the control group at MS. The vertical dashed lines indicate the approximate timing of the light signal. The vertical bar represents 40% body weight, the arrow 100ms and the direction of travel. For the HS trial, note the increase in area above the zero line. This is indicates an increase in the braking impulse.

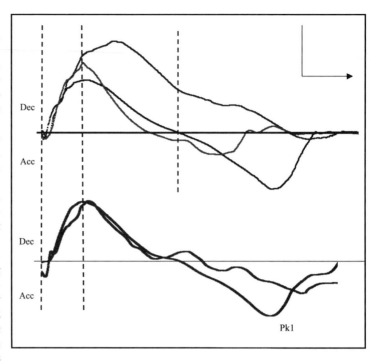

with PD, however, tended to have the same contribution from braking changes regardless of the timing of the signal to stop, while the control group was able to increase braking to a greater extent with an early signal. The changes were likewise reflected in the ability to recruit muscle activity during time-critical conditions. For example, healthy older adults appear to be able to generate both stance limb and swing limb changes during unplanned stopping, even with a signal to stop that occurs late in stance phase. Those with PD increased amplitude in key muscle groups but to a fraction (25% in tibialis anterior, for example) of that demonstrated by healthy adults.

Additionally, subjects with PD show patterns of muscle activation that differ when comparing planned and unplanned stopping when, in contrast, it appears that healthy adults use similar patterns in both. Healthy older adults used muscle activation patterns in the distal stance limb that were similar during both planned and unplanned stopping (increased tibialis anterior during push-off and decreased soleus during mid and late stance), altering the magnitude of their motor response but not the pattern. During unplanned stopping, this pattern of activation—increased gastrocnemius and tibialis anterior, decreased soleus activation—is comparable to the "push-off" reduction pattern noted by Hase and Stein.[55]

Subjects with PD, in contrast, demonstrated differing patterns of muscle activation between tasks. During planned stopping, these subjects increased distal leg muscle activity (above that of walking) of the stance limb, resulting in co-contraction at the ankle and when stopping was unplanned, subjects decreased tibialis anterior activation and increased soleus of stance limb. Also during unplanned stopping, subjects with PD increased activation of soleus activation of the swing limb to a greater extent than the control group. These subjects also tended to increase gluteus medius activity more than con-

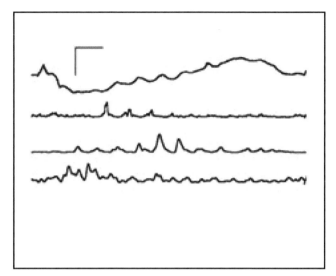

Figure 7-6. Anterior-posterior force and EMG data from one subject with PD during planned stopping. TA = tibialis anterior, SOL = soleus, GM = gluteus medius. The vertical bar represents 40% body weight and 0.08mV, the horizontal line, 100ms.

trol subjects. We speculate that this increase in activation may be similar to the "extensor muscle pattern" (gluteus maximus, quadriceps, and soleus) reported by Hase and Stein[55] and is likely required by subjects with PD to generate deceleration forces because there was less modulation of muscular activity and ground reaction forces by the stance limb.

Intriguingly, we noted that difficulty stopping was related more to functional measures (gait speed) than disease severity (Hoehn and Yahr, for example) although our data were limited to those with H&Y scores of less than three. Nonetheless, during unplanned stopping, subjects who walked slower than 1 m/s generated deceleration force at a significantly faster rate than faster-walking peers. That is, although they walked more slowly, forces were generated very rapidly, indicating an increase in limb stiffness. These subjects had been less able to modulate force under the trailing limb and were totally reliant on the leading limb to stop.

In studies in our lab, subjects with PD (as a group) tend to take more steps when stopping suddenly. For example, in a recent study, a larger number of trials in the groups of subjects with PD (35%) occurred predominantly because of several subjects with very high percentage of trials (>50%) in which these individuals used the two-step strategy. Tirosh and Sparrow[56] speculated that the increased frequency of "extra steps" observed when they compared older and younger adults performing unplanned stopping might have been needed to ensure medial lateral stability after anterior-posterior forces were controlled. So, although different than the control group, we consider the "extra step" strategy to be necessary and functional for the PD group. However, we speculate that reliance on a single strategy to stop would place individuals with PD at greater risk of failure to stop, and that an alternate strategy may be required or beneficial.

Also noteworthy are observations of alternating bursts of tibialis anterior and soleus activity in slower walkers with PD (Figure 7-6). These alternating bursts are similar to those noted by others during postural adjustments prior to activities such as initiating gait,[57] rising up onto the toes,[58] sit to stand,[59] or hip abduction. For example, a common mechanism to initiate gait is to inhibit soleus activity and pull the center of pressure behind the center of mass using tibialis anterior contraction or gravity. During gait initiation, it is hypothesized that the alternating tibialis anterior and soleus activity arises from an inability to activate or superimpose the central program to destabilize the subject's posture. Perhaps the bursting of activity, noted in our studies, reflects an inability to superimpose a stopping program or programs onto that of walking.

FREEZING DURING GAIT

Freezing of gait (FOG) is a motor symptom of PD that is different from bradykinesia, rigidity, or postural instability.[60] Approximately 50% of persons with advanced PD experience unexpected but transient interruptions to their movement, leading to the common consideration of FOG as a later onset feature of PD; however, FOG also occurs in approximately 7% to 16% of early idiopathic PD.[5,61] In early stage PD, FOG is generally of short duration and mainly seen in the form of hesitation during movement initiation or turning.[62] Schaafsma et al[62] indicated that most FOG episodes last less than 10 seconds and only a few last more than 30 seconds. As PD progresses, the episodes of FOG become more frequent and disabling, often leading to falls.[5,61] FOG is more common in the "off" medication state and if FOG occurs during the "on" medication state it often does not respond to levodopa therapy.[63] Development of FOG appears to be associated with the akinetic-rigid form of PD,[5] and with a patient having gait disturbance as the initial motor symptom, more advanced disease, cognitive decline, and depression.[61] The presence of tremor as the initial motor symptom seems to be protective for development of FOG.

FOG often occurs during turning movements and while patients attempt to start walking; however, FOG may also appear during unobstructed walking, while crossing narrow spaces, coming to a threshold such as a doorway, when reaching a target, or when trying to negotiate obstacles. FOG is more common in crowded places and in time-restricted, stressful situations. Visual inputs can, perhaps counter-intuitively, both cause and alleviate FOG. For example, FOG frequently occurs when patients attempt to cross a threshold, but marks on the floor can be used to normalize stride length during gait and overcome an episode of freezing.[10,15,16] Fortunately, given the variety of presentation and timing of FOG, Giladi et al[61] have constructed a specific questionnaire that can help clinicians screen for the presence of FOG and assess subjective severity.

Schaafsma et al[62] described three different types of FOG. The first occurs when the person is unable to start walking (start hesitation) or fails to continue to move forward (akinesia). The second occurs when a patient's legs "tremble in place." When this "tremble" of the legs during FOG is analyzed using time series analyses, the trembling is distinct from classic tremor in terms of frequency and complexity. The third type of presentation consists of shuffling forward with small steps.

Recent studies have indicated that patients with FOG walk differently from those who do not. Persons who experience FOG have an abnormal stride length and cadence during the three steps prior to freezing.[64] Another study observed that patients with FOG have increased stride-to-stride variability compared to patients without FOG while walking without apparent freezing episodes.[65] Extending work presented in 2001, Nieuwboer et al[66] compared distal muscle activity timing and magnitude during the three steps prior to an episode of FOG to both normal gait and voluntary stopping. These data suggest that FOG represents a phenomenon separate from planned or voluntary stopping given the statistical differences between the conditions. However, the pattern of increased tibialis anterior muscle activity during pre-swing on the stance limb associated with increased gastrocnemius activity of the swing limb is similar to the pattern of distal muscle activity identified during planned stopping, and dramatic increases in activity are related to unplanned stopping.[52,53]

INTERVENTIONS TO IMPROVE BALANCE IN PATIENTS WITH PARKINSON'S DISEASE

Although improving balance in individuals with PD is a common goal, few studies have reported balance outcomes after a physical intervention. Schenkman and her group[67] conducted a randomized controlled trial in 46 people with PD using an intervention to improve axial mobility. The intervention involved a series of progressively more challenging spinal flexibility exercises. The functional reach, a measure used to assess anterior standing balance, increased significantly after the intervention; however, this intervention was not specifically related to balance. Possibly, improved spinal flexibility enabled an improvement in balance. In another study, 40 individuals in stage III PD (Hoehn & Yahr scale) underwent a program consisting of exercise, cued walking, stepping, and motor function strategies for 30 days. The program resulted in improvements in static balance (timed tandem and single limb stance), as well as number of single limb steps in 15 seconds and functional reach for both individuals with PD who fell or did not fall.[68] The outcomes of this study were compared with performance by age-matched controls, but all of the 40 patients underwent the intervention. The incidence of falling was not followed after the intervention.

FALLS IN THE ELDERLY AND INTERVENTIONS TO PREVENT FALLS

There are multiple intrinsic and extrinsic factors that contribute to the increased risk of falls seen in elderly people. Intrinsic factors include conditions such as poor vision, postural hypotension, adverse cognitive effects of polypharmacy, and reduced lower extremity muscle strength contribute to falls, as do neurologically mediated gait and balance problems. Extrinsic factors include environmental hazards such as throw rugs and uneven surfaces as well as low lighting, use of an assistive device, or unstable shoes.[69,70] Considerable research has been done on interventions to prevent falls in the elderly, and these interventions significantly reduce the proportion of older people who fall at least once as well as the monthly rate of falling.[71,72] Given that the reasons for falls are multi-factorial, a multi-factorial fall risk assessment and management program should be effective; however, exercise programs are effective as well.[71,72] Shumway-Cook and colleagues[73] demonstrated that an upright balance and gait training program reduced falls in community-dwelling older adults.

FALLS IN PARKINSON'S DISEASE

In contrast to elders who fall, individuals with neurologic deficits tend to fall more frequently and experience gait and balance deficits secondary to intrinsic causes.[74] In a recent study of 548 patients with neurological diseases, 34% had fallen once or more during the previous 12 months, and falls were most frequent (62%) in patients with Parkinson's disease compared to individuals with other neurological diagnoses.[74] Disturbed gait was associated with 55% of the falls in individuals with PD.[74] Ashburn and her group[75] compared individuals with PD who were fallers and non-fallers and reported that 40% of the sample had fallen within the last 12 months. The fallers reported a median of 3 falls in 12 months. Furthermore, the fallers were more impaired and had poorer measures of mobility and balance than the non-fallers. Seventy-five percent of the fallers were either in Stage II or III of the Hoehn & Yahr impairment scale, and had higher scores on the UPDRS (28.3 for the fallers compared to 22 for non-fallers). When subjects with PD are compared to aged-matched controls, 51% of the PD subjects with moderately advanced disease fell during a 6-month period compared to only 15% in the controls.[75] Others have observed that 59% over a 3-month period and 68% over a 1-year period of those with PD fell.[36,76] Seventy percent of the falls in people with PD are due to intrinsic, patient-related factors compared to 50% in controls who fall due to extrinsic factors (due to the environment).[36] Recurrent falls in PD are more common in people taking benzodiazepines.[36] People with PD who fall tend to take more steps to complete a test of mobility, had a reduced functional reach, and greater postural sway when completing dual tasks.[75] Schaafsma and her group[77] found that stride to stride time variability was greater indicating more impairment both on and off anti-parkinsonian medications in individuals with PD who fell, and this was not correlated with symptoms of tremor, rigidity, or bradykinesia. Fear of falling is reported by 45.8% of the patients with PD, and 44.1% of the patients report reduced daily activities as a result of falling.[36] It would appear that falls are more frequent, more often due to intrinsic factors, and result in a restriction of activity compared to elders without PD who fall.

INTERVENTIONS TO IMPROVE GAIT IN PATIENTS WITH PARKINSON'S DISEASE

Few studies have tried to isolate different components of rehabilitation interventions. Several studies examined the efficacy of using motor control strategies in patients with PD. Stefaniwsky and Bilowit[78] comparing 10 patients with PD and 5 healthy subjects found that movement initiation was significantly slower in the patients with PD compared to healthy subjects. After daily in-home exercises using sensory stimuli to facilitate movement initiation for a 3-week period, the patients demonstrated comparable movement initiation speeds to the healthy individuals. In another study, standing weight shifting was compared in 34 people with stage I or II PD and 34 neurologically intact subjects.[79] Reduced ability to shift weight from one lower extremity to another was observed in both disability stages of PD when compared to the controls. All groups improved weight shifting responses after continuous video feedback when compared to end of trial feedback. Although this study evaluated the response following a single session, and did not use a training strategy over several weeks, it supports the notion that sensory stimuli can influence movement control in individuals with PD when performing complex motor tasks. In a similar fashion, visual and auditory sensory cues as well as levodopa can modify gait movements and muscle activation in some patients with PD.[80-82] Visual cues such as lines on the floor improve step length in individuals with PD, whereas auditory cues enhance gait speed.[82]

Two recent Cochrane reviews, one evaluating various physical therapy techniques for PD and another the efficacy of physical therapy compared to a placebo or no intervention control in PD, identified a relatively small number of randomized controlled trials. Only 7 trials investigating techniques of physical therapy with 142 patients were considered to be of adequate quality for review. Eleven trials with 280 patients were considered in the review investigating the value of various physical therapy programs versus placebo and no intervention. Both reviews pointed out many problems in methodology, with a minority of trials reporting a positive outcome. There was considerable variability in the treatment interventions studied. They concluded that there is insufficient evidence to support or refute the efficacy of physical therapy in PD.[83,84] A more recent randomized controlled trial investigating the long-term effect of multidisciplinary rehabilitation inter-

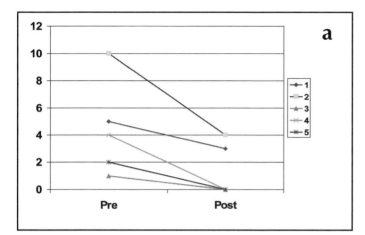

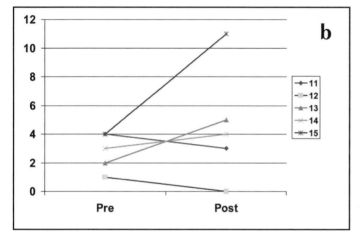

Figure 7-7a,b. Comfortable gait speed after 6 weeks of physical and medical therapy and follow-up.

vention enrolled 144 people with PD. Although there was an improvement in mobility after a 6-week intervention, there was a significant decline in mobility over 6 months.[85,86] There was also a significant loss of subjects (30%) at the 6-month assessment. The multidisciplinary intervention involved only 10 hours of individual treatment and 10 hours of group activities (such as talks with experts and relaxation) once a week for 6 weeks. It was difficult to determine how much specific gait and balance training was conducted. Another randomized controlled trial using a cross-over design randomly assigned 68 subjects with idiopathic PD to physical therapy plus medical therapy for 6 weeks, followed by 6 weeks of medical therapy alone, followed by 6 weeks of physical therapy plus medical therapy.[87] The physical therapy intervention consisted of stretching, strengthening, functional training, gait training over-ground and on the treadmill with external auditory cueing, balance training, and relaxation. The training was conducted twice a week for 1½ hours. Testing occurred at baseline and at 6-week, 12-week, and 3-month follow-up. The gait and balance training comprised 30 minutes of the total training, but no specific details of the training were described. Significant differences occurred between groups in comfortable walking speed, mobility, the activities of daily living (ADL) scale of the UPDRS, and the total UPDRS score after 6 weeks (Figure 7-7a,b). Significant differences were also found at 3 months compared to baseline on walking speed, the UPDRS ADL, and total scores. This intervention improved gait, and maintained the improvement during a 3-month follow-up.

There is some limited evidence that multidimensional rehabilitation interventions can improve gait outcomes in individuals with PD.

Gait and Step Training

Studies have been published demonstrating that humans with neurological conditions can improve gait by either training ambulation on a treadmill with no body weight support or with body weight support.[88-96] The degree of locomotor recovery has been shown to be significantly related to the type of locomotor training used in patients with neurological conditions.[89,90,97] Other studies report similar gait outcomes with task-specific gait training or body weight supported training in individuals with neurologic deficits.[98,99] Several recent reports suggest that ambulation training using body weight support for individuals with PD results in improvements in gait.[100-102] These reports were either case reports or small sample sizes, used varying training intervals, or used no balance or fall measures. Several authors reported increased gait speeds after treadmill training[101,103] or repetitive training of compensatory stepping in individuals with PD.[104] Pohl and his group reported increased gait speeds and stride length immediately after a single session of either speed-dependent treadmill training or limited progressive treadmill training compared to conventional gait training or a no-intervention waiting period.[103] Miyai et al[101] reported an increase in gait speed from .93 m/s to 1.18 m/s following gait training using body weight supported treadmill training 3 days/week for 1 month. These increases in gait speed were maintained for up to 4 months following treatment. In another study, patients with PD underwent training consisting of pull perturbations for 14 days and demonstrated an increase of gait speed from 0.64 m/s to 0.77 m/s. This increase was accompanied by an increase in cadence (0.80 steps/s to 0.87 steps/s) and step length (0.80 m to 0.87 m), but there was no control-group comparison. Similar step training in healthy elders resulted in an increase in step initiation time.[105]

A randomized, controlled pilot study of a specific gait and step training intervention in individuals with idiopathic PD was recently published.[106] Eighteen men with PD were randomly assigned to a training or control group. Subjects were called for 2 weeks prior to and after an 8-week period about any falls. Gait speed, cadence, and step length were tested on an instrumented walkway. Subjects were timed while stepping onto and back down from an 8.8 cm step for five consecutive steps. Other measures included a functional reach test, timed 360-degree turn, and a Berg Balance Scale. Gait training consisted of walking on a treadmill at a speed greater than fastest over ground walking speed while walking in four directions and while supported in a harness for safety. Step training consisted of suddenly turning the treadmill on and off while the subject stood in the safety harness facing either forward, backward, or sideways. Training occurred 1 hour per day, 3 times per week for 8 weeks. Only 10 subjects had a fall during the 2-week pre- and post-observation period. Significant reduction occurred in falls in the training group (4.4 +/- 3.5 pre and 1.6 +/- 1.8 post), but not in the control group (2.3 +/- 1.6 pre and 3.8 +/- 4.1 post) (Figure 7-8a,b). Subjects in the trained group had a reduction in falls with three exhibiting no falls during the 2 weeks after the intervention, whereas only two in the control group had a reduction (4 to 3 and 1 to 0). Gait speed increased significantly in the trained group from 1.28 m/s +/- .33 to 1.45 m/s +/- .37, but not in the control group (1.26 m/s pre and 1.27 m/s post). The cadence increased for both groups from 112.8 to 120.3 steps/min for the training group and 117.7 to 124.3 steps/min for the control. Stride lengths increased for the trained group, but not the control. The 5-step test speed increased significantly in the trained group from .40 steps/s +/- .08 to .51 steps/s +/- .12, and in the control group (.36 steps/s +/- .11 to .42 steps/s +/- .11). Functional reach and

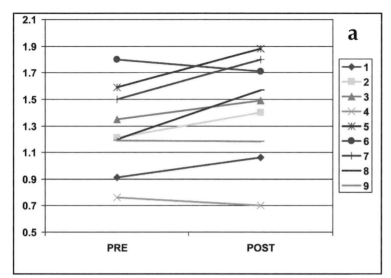

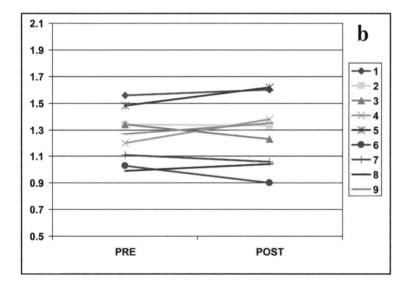

Figure 7-8a,b. Comparison of pre and post gait speed for subjects receiving training and control.

timed 360-degree turns did not differ among the groups. The Berg Balance Scale also was not different between groups. Although this is a small study, it suggests that this type of gait and step training resulted in a reduction in falls and improvements in gait speed and stride length as well as dynamic balance (5-step test) in these individuals with PD.

Limited evidence to date suggests that balance and the spatial and temporal characteristics of gait in individuals with PD can be improved in response to physical therapy intervention strategies. The interventions with the best evidence follow motor learning strategies that are task specific to gait and balance deficits and occur under progressively more demanding conditions.

Case Study

Mr. D is a 55-year-old male with a 6-year history of Parkinson's disease with postural instability gait deficit-type PD. His Hoehn & Yahr disability stage was 3.5 with loss of postural reflexes and bilateral symptoms. His medications were as follows: Sinemet 25/100 every 2 hours, Comtan every 4 hours, and Sinemet CR 25/100 once per day. He reported a Schwab and England Activities of Daily Living Scale of 75%, indicating that he was independent in 75% of his activities. Mr. D experienced severe freezing episodes during 40% to 60% of the day and he displayed dyskinesias in both the upper and lower extremities. He would fall on average 10 times per day, and he had frequent on/off phenomena that could be sudden. He required a walker to ambulate at times. He underwent DBS surgery with the placement of electrodes bilaterally in the STN. Post-surgery, his medications remained the same except that he no longer required medication at night. His gait and balance tests were as follows:

	Pre	Post
UPDRS Motor Subscale (on medications)	42	24
Gait speed (m/s)	1.18	1.43
Cadence 9 (steps/min)	98	114
Stride length (m)	1.4	1.5
Time to turn 360 degrees (sec)	5.9	2.2
5-step test (sec)	10	10.6
Functional reach (in)	6.2	10
Berg Balance Scale	55	52

There were no significant differences in limits of stability measures before or after surgery. He continued to fall approximately 10 times per day. He subjectively reported improved appetite, better sleeping, and that he was less emotionally labile. He noticed minimal change in his mobility.

Although Mr. D demonstrated improvement on his UPDRS Motor Score, increased usual gait speed and cadence, a reduction in the time to turn 360 degrees, and an increased functional reach, it should be noted that his spatial and temporal gait measures were within normal limits prior to the surgery. The faster time to turn 360 degrees could suggest fewer problems with step initiation. Likewise, the increased functional reach suggests improved forward balance. Note that the Berg Balance Scale score was within normal limits even though this individual had serious balance deficits and fell often each day.

Conclusion

Mr. D had severe fluctuation in his movement disorders as well as dyskinesias. These objective measures of gait and balance suggest that his function was not improved by the DBS.

REFERENCES

1. Morris ME, McGinley J, Huxham F, Collier J, Iansek R. Constraints on the kinetic, kinematic and spatiotemporal parameters of gait in Parkinson's disease. *Human Movement Science*. 1999;18:461-483.
2. Morris ME, Matyas TA, Iansek R, Summers JJ. Temporal stability of gait in Parkinson's disease. *Phys Ther*. 1996;76(7):763-777.

3. Giladi N, McMahon D, Przedborski S, Flaster E, Guillory S, Kostic V et al. Motor blocks in Parkinson's disease. *Neurology*. 1992;42(2):333-339.
4. Kompoliti K, Goetz CG, Leurgans S, Morrissey M, Siegel IM. "On" freezing in Parkinson's disease: resistance to visual cue walking devices. *Mov Disord*. 2000; 15(2):309-312.
5. Lamberti P, Armenise S, Castaldo V, De Mari M, Iliceto G, Tronci P et al. Freezing gait in Parkinson's disease. *Eur Neurol*. 1997;38(4):297-301.
6. Fahn S. The freezing phenomenon in parkinsonism. *Adv Neurol*. 1995;67:53-63.
7. Dietz MA, Goetz CG, Stebbins GT. Evaluation of a modified inverted walking stick as a treatment for parkinsonian freezing episodes. *Mov Disord*. 1990; 5(3):243-247.
8. Knutsson E. An analysis of Parkinsonian gait. *Brain*. 1972;95(3):475-486.
9. Murray MP, Sepic SB, Gardner GM, Downs WJ. Walking patterns of men with parkinsonism. *Am J Phys Med*. 1978;57(6):278-294.
10. Morris M, Iansek R, Matyas T, Summers J. Abnormalities in the stride length-cadence relation in parkinsonian gait. *Mov Disord*. 1998;13(1):61-69.
11. O'Sullivan JD, Said CM, Dillon LC, Hoffman M, Hughes AJ. Gait analysis in patients with Parkinson's disease and motor fluctuations: influence of levodopa and comparison with other measures of motor function. *Mov Disord*. 1998; 13(6):900-906.
12. Bond JM, Morris M. Goal-directed secondary motor tasks: their effects on gait in subjects with Parkinson disease. *Arch Phys Med Rehabil*. 2000;81(1):110-116.
13. Blin O, Ferrandez AM, Pailhous J, Serratrice G. Dopa-sensitive and dopa-resistant gait parameters in Parkinson's disease. *J Neurol Sci*. 1991;103(1):51-54.
14. MacKay-Lyons M. Variability in spatiotemporal gait characteristics over the course of the L-dopa cycle in people with advanced Parkinson disease. *Phys Ther*. 1998;78(10):1083-1094.
15. Morris ME, Iansek R, Matyas TA, Summers JJ. Ability to modulate walking cadence remains intact in Parkinson's disease. *J Neurol Neurosurg Psychiatry*. 1994;57(12):1532-1534.
16. Morris ME, Iansek R, Matyas TA, Summers JJ. Stride length regulation in Parkinson's disease. Normalization strategies and underlying mechanisms. *Brain*. 1996;119(Pt 2):551-568.
17. Azulay JP, Mesure S, Amblard B, Blin O, Sangla I, Pouget J. Visual control of locomotion in Parkinson's disease. *Brain*. 1999;122(Pt 1):111-120.
18. Behrman AL, Teitelbaum P, Cauraugh JH. Verbal instructional sets to normalise the temporal and spatial gait variables in Parkinson's disease. *J Neurol Neurosurg Psychiatry*. 1998;65(4):580-582.
19. Thaut MH, McIntosh GC, Rice RR, Miller RA, Rathbun J, Brault JM. Rhythmic auditory stimulation in gait training for Parkinson's disease patients. *Mov Disord*. 1996;11(2):193-200.
20. Bagley S, Kelly B, Tunnicliffe N, Turnbull GI, Walker J. The effect of visual cues on the gait of independently mobile Parkinson's disease patients. *Physiother*. 1991;77:415-420.
21. Lozano AM, Mahant N. Deep brain stimulation surgery for Parkinson's disease: mechanisms and consequences. *Parkinsonism Relat Disord*. 2004;10 Suppl 1:S49-S57.
22. Kumar R, Lozano AM, Kim YJ, Hutchison WD, Sime E, Halket E et al. Double-blind evaluation of subthalamic nucleus deep brain stimulation in advanced Parkinson's disease. *Neurology*. 1998;51(3):850-855.
23. Doshi PK, Chhaya NA, Bhatt MA. Bilateral subthalamic nucleus stimulation for Parkinson's disease. *Neurol India*. 2003;51(1):43-48.
24. Kumar R, Lozano AM, Sime E, Halket E, Lang AE. Comparative effects of unilateral and bilateral subthalamic nucleus deep brain stimulation. *Neurology*. 1999;53(3):561-566.
25. Limousin P, Krack P, Pollak P, Benazzouz A, Ardouin C, Hoffmann D et al. Electrical stimulation of the subthalamic nucleus in advanced Parkinson's disease. *N Engl J Med*. 1998;339(16):1105-1111.
26. Hamani C, Richter E, Schwalb JM, Lozano AM. Bilateral subthalamic nucleus stimulation for Parkinson's disease: a systematic review of the clinical literature. *Neurosurgery*. 2005;56(6):1313-1321.
27. Hausdorff JM, Cudkowicz ME, Firtion R, Wei JY, Goldberger AL. Gait variability and basal ganglia disorders: stride-to-stride variations of gait cycle timing in Parkinson's disease and Huntington's disease. *Mov Disord*. 1998; 13(3):428-437.
28. Faist M, Xie J, Kurz D, Berger W, Maurer C, Pollak P et al. Effect of bilateral subthalamic nucleus stimulation on gait in Parkinson's disease. *Brain*. 2001; 124(Pt 8):1590-1600.
29. Elble RJ, Cousins R, Leffler K, Hughes L. Gait initiation by patients with lower-half parkinsonism. *Brain*. 1996;119(Pt 5):1705-1716.
30. Gantchev N, Viallet F, Aurenty R, Massion J. Impairment of posturo-kinetic co-ordination during initiation of forward oriented stepping movements in parkinsonian patients. *Electroencephalogr Clin Neurophysiol*. 1996;101(2):110-120.
31. Martin M, Shinberg M, Kuchibhatla M, Ray L, Carollo JJ, Schenkman ML. Gait initiation in community-dwelling adults with Parkinson disease: comparison with older and younger adults without the disease. *Phys Ther*. 2002;82(6):566-577.

32. Brunt D, Bishop MD, Kim HD, Marjarma-Lyons J, Ko MS. Abnormal ankle muscle activity contributes to slowness of gait initiation in Parkinson's disease. In Review. 2006.

33. Halliday SE, Winter DA, Frank JS, Patla AE, Prince F. The initiation of gait in young, elderly, and Parkinson's disease subjects. *Gait Posture.* 1998;8(1):8-14.

34. Crenna P, Gringo C, Giovannini P, Piccolo I. The initiation of gait in Parkinson's disease. In: Beradelli A, Benecke R, Manfredi M, Marsden CD, eds. *Motor Disturbances.* London: Academic Press;1998:161-173.

35. Liu W, McIntire K, Kim SH, Zhang J, Dascalos S, Lyons KE et al. Bilateral subthalamic stimulation improves gait initiation in patients with Parkinson's disease. *Gait Posture.* 2006;23(4):492-498.

36. Bloem BR, Grimbergen YA, Cramer M, Willemsen M, Zwinderman AH. Prospective assessment of falls in Parkinson's disease. *J Neurol.* 2001; 248(11):950-958.

37. Morris M, Iansek R, Smithson F, Huxham F. Postural instability in Parkinson's disease: a comparison with and without a concurrent task. *Gait Posture.* 2000; 12(3):205-216.

38. Morris ME, Huxham FE, McGinley J, Iansek R. Gait disorders and gait rehabilitation in Parkinson's disease. *Adv Neurol.* 2001;87:347-361.

39. Tinetti ME, Williams TF, Mayewski R. Fall risk index for elderly patients based on number of chronic disabilities. *Am J Med.* 1986;80(3):429-434.

40. Kirker SG, Simpson DS, Jenner JR, Wing AM. Stepping before standing: hip muscle function in stepping and standing balance after stroke. *J Neurol Neurosurg Psychiatry.* 2000;68(4):458-464.

41. Gray P, Hildebrand K. Fall risk factors in Parkinson's disease. *J Neurosci Nurs.* 2000;32(4):222-228.

42. Morris ME, Iansek R. Gait disorders in Parkinson's disease: a framework for physical thrapy practice. *Neuro Report.* 1997;21:125-131.

43. Johnell O, Melton LJ, III, Atkinson EJ, O'Fallon WM, Kurland LT. Fracture risk in patients with parkinsonism: a population-based study in Olmsted County, Minnesota. *Age Ageing.* 1992;21(1):32-38.

44. Bai O, Nakamura M, Shibasaki H. Compensation of hand movement for patients by assistant force: relationship between human hand movement and robot arm motion. *IEEE Trans Neural Syst Rehabil Eng.* 2001;9(302):307.

45. Crenna P, Cuong DM, Breniere Y. Motor programmes for the termination of gait in humans: organisation and velocity-dependent adaptation. *J Physiol.* 2001; 537(Pt 3):1059-1072.

46. Bloem BR, Hausdorff JM, Visser JE, Giladi N. Falls and freezing of gait in Parkinson's disease: a review of two interconnected, episodic phenomena. *Mov Disord.* 2004; 19(8):871-884.

47. Jian Y, Winter DA, Ishac MG, Gilchrist L. Trajectory of the body GOG and COP during initiation and termination of gait. *Gait Posture.* 1993;17:170-179.

48. Hirokawa S. Normal gait characteristics under temporal and distance constraints. *J Biomed Eng.* 1989;11(6):449-456.

49. Wearing SC, Urry S, Smeathers JE, Battistutta D. A comparison of gait initiation and termination methods for obtaining plantar foot pressures. *Gait Posture.* 1999; 10(3):255-263.

50. O'Kane FW, McGibbon CA, Krebs DE. Kinetic analysis of planned gait termination in healthy subjects and patients with balance disorders. *Gait Posture.* 2003;17(2):170-179.

51. Jaeger RJ, Vanitchatchavan P. Ground reaction forces during termination of human gait. *J Biomech.* 1992;25(10):1233-1236.

52. Bishop MD, Brunt D, Kukulka C, Tillman MD, Pathare N. Braking impulse and muscle activation during unplanned gait termination in human subjects with parkinsonism. *Neurosci Lett.* 2003;348(2):89-92.

53. Bishop MD, Brunt D, Pathare N, Patel B. The interaction between leading and trailing limbs during stopping in humans. *Neurosci Lett.* 2002;323(1):1-4.

54. Bishop M, Brunt D, Pathare N, Patel B. The effect of velocity on the strategies used during gait termination. *Gait Posture.* 2004;20(2):134-139.

55. Hase K, Stein RB. Analysis of rapid stopping during human walking. *J Neurophysiol.* 1998;80(1):255-261.

56. Tirosh O, Sparrow WA. Gait termination in young and older adults: effects of stopping stimulus probability and stimulus delay. *Gait Posture.* 2004;19(3):243-251.

57. Burleigh-Jacobs A, Horak FB, Nutt JG, Obeso JA. Step initiation in Parkinson's disease: influence of levodopa and external sensory triggers. *Mov Disord.* 1997; 12(2):206-215.

58. Frank JS, Horak FB, Nutt J. Centrally initiated postural adjustments in parkinsonian patients on and off levodopa. *J Neurophysiol.* 2000;84(5):2440-2448.

59. Bishop M, Brunt D, Pathare N, Ko M, Marjama-Lyons J. Changes in distal muscle timing may contribute to slowness during sit to stand in Parkinsons disease. *Clin Biomech.* (Bristol, Avon) 2005;20(1):112-117.

60. Bartels AL, Balash Y, Gurevich T, Schaafsma JD, Hausdorff JM, Giladi N. Relationship between freezing of gait (FOG) and other features of Parkinson's: FOG is not correlated with bradykinesia. *J Clin Neurosci.* 2003;10(5):584-588.

61. Giladi N, McDermott MP, Fahn S, Przedborski S, Jankovic J, Stern M et al. Freezing of gait in PD: prospective assessment in the DATATOP cohort. *Neurology.* 2001;56(12):1712-1721.

62. Schaafsma JD, Balash Y, Gurevich T, Bartels AL, Hausdorff JM, Giladi N. Characterization of freezing of gait subtypes and the response of each to levodopa in Parkinson's disease. *Eur J Neurol.* 2003;10(4):391-398.
63. Panisset M. Freezing of gait in Parkinson's disease. *Neurol Clin.* 2004;22(3 Suppl):S53-S62.
64. Nieuwboer A, Dom R, De Weerdt W, Desloovere K, Fieuws S, Broens-Kaucsik E. Abnormalities of the spatio-temporal characteristics of gait at the onset of freezing in Parkinson's disease. *Mov Disord.* 2001;16(6):1066-1075.
65. Hausdorff JM, Schaafsma JD, Balash Y, Bartels AL, Gurevich T, Giladi N. Impaired regulation of stride variability in Parkinson's disease subjects with freezing of gait. *Exp Brain Res.* 2003;149(2):187-194.
66. Nieuwboer A, Dom R, De Weerdt W, Desloovere K, Janssens L, Stijn V. Electromyographic profiles of gait prior to onset of freezing episodes in patients with Parkinson's disease. *Brain.* 2004;127(Pt 7):1650-1660.
67. Schenkman M, Cutson TM, Kuchibhatla M, Chandler J, Pieper CF, Ray L et al. Exercise to improve spinal flexibility and function for people with Parkinson's disease: a randomized, controlled trial. *J Am Geriatr Soc.* 1998;46(10):1207-1216.
68. Stankovic I. The effect of physical therapy on balance of patients with Parkinson's disease. *Int J Rehabil Res.* 2004;27(1):53-57.
69. Tinetti ME. Performance-oriented assessment of mobility problems in elderly patients. *J Am Geriatr Soc.* 1986;34(2):119-126.
70. Tinetti ME, Baker DI, McAvay G, Claus EB, Garrett P, Gottschalk M et al. A multifactorial intervention to reduce the risk of falling among elderly people living in the community. *N Engl J Med.* 1994;331(13):821-827.
71. Chang JT, Morton SC, Rubenstein LZ, Mojica WA, Maglione M, Suttorp MJ et al. Interventions for the prevention of falls in older adults: systematic review and meta-analysis of randomised clinical trials. *BMJ.* 2004;328(7441):680.
72. Gillespie AR. Interventions to reduce falls in the elderly. *Cochrane Library.* 2004; 4:1-204.
73. Shumway-Cook A, Gruber W, Baldwin M, Liao S. The effect of multidimensional exercises on balance, mobility, and fall risk in community-dwelling older adults. *Phys Ther.* 1997;77(1):46-57.
74. Stolze H, Klebe S, Zechlin C, Baecker C, Friege L, Deuschl G. Falls in frequent neurological diseases—prevalence, risk factors and aetiology. *J Neurol.* 2004; 251(1):79-84.
75. Ashburn A, Stack E, Pickering RM, Ward CD. A community-dwelling sample of people with Parkinson's disease: characteristics of fallers and non-fallers. *Age Ageing.* 2001;30(1):47-52.
76. Wood BH, Bilclough JA, Bowron A, Walker RW. Incidence and prediction of falls in Parkinson's disease: a prospective multidisciplinary study. *J Neurol Neurosurg Psychiatry.* 2002;72(6):721-725.
77. Schaafsma JD, Giladi N, Balash Y, Bartels AL, Gurevich T, Hausdorff JM. Gait dynamics in Parkinson's disease: relationship to Parkinsonian features, falls and response to levodopa. *J Neurol Sci.* 2003;212(1-2):47-53.
78. Stefaniwsky L, Bilowit DS. Parkinsonism: facilitation of motion by sensory stimulation. *Arch Phys Med Rehabil.* 1973;54(2):75-77.
79. Krasilovsky G, Gianutsos J. Effect of video feedback on the performance of a weight shifting controlled tracking task in subjects with parkinsonism and neurologically intact individuals. *Exp Neurol.* 1991;113(2):192-201.
80. Morris ME. Movement disorders in people with Parkinson disease: a model for physical therapy. *Phys Ther.* 2000;80(6):578-597.
81. Richards CL, Malouin F, Bedard PJ, Cioni M. Changes induced by L-Dopa and sensory cues on the gait of parkinsonian patients. In: Wollacot M, Horak F, eds. *Posture and Gait: Control Mechanisms.* Eugene, OR: University of Oregon Books;1992:126-129.
82. Suteerawattananon M, Morris GS, Etnyre BR, Jankovic J, Protas EJ. Effects of visual and auditory cues on gait in individuals with Parkinson's disease. *J Neurol Sci.* 2004;219(1-2):63-69.
83. Deane KH, Jones D, Playford ED, Ben Shlomo Y, Clarke CE. Physiotherapy for patients with Parkinson's Disease: a comparison of techniques. *Cochrane Database Syst Rev.* 2001;(3):CD002817.
84. Deane KH, Jones D, Ellis-Hill C, Clarke CE, Playford ED, Ben Shlomo Y. A comparison of physiotherapy techniques for patients with Parkinson's disease. *Cochrane Database Syst Rev.* 2001;(1):CD002815.
85. Trend P, Kaye J, Gage H, Owen C, Wade D. Short-term effectiveness of intensive multidisciplinary rehabilitation for people with Parkinson's disease and their carers. *Clin Rehabil.* 2002;16(7):717-725.
86. Wade DT, Gage H, Owen C, Trend P, Grossmith C, Kaye J. Multidisciplinary rehabilitation for people with Parkinson's disease: a randomised controlled study. *J Neurol Neurosurg Psychiatry.* 2003;74(2):158-162.
87. Ellis T, de Goede CJ, Feldman RG, Wolters EC, Kwakkel G, Wagenaar RC. Efficacy of a physical therapy program in patients with Parkinson's disease: a randomized controlled trial. *Arch Phys Med Rehabil.* 2005;86(4):626-632.
88. da CI, Jr., Lim PA, Qureshy H, Henson H, Monga T, Protas EJ. Gait outcomes after acute stroke rehabilitation with supported treadmill ambulation training: a randomized controlled pilot study. *Arch Phys Med Rehabil.* 2002;83(9):1258-1265.

89. Visintin M, Barbeau H, Korner-Bitensky N, Mayo NE. A new approach to retrain gait in stroke patients through body weight support and treadmill stimulation. *Stroke.* 1998;29(6):1122-1128.
90. Hesse S, Bertelt C, Schaffrin A, Malezic M, Mauritz KH. Restoration of gait in nonambulatory hemiparetic patients by treadmill training with partial body-weight support. *Arch Phys Med Rehabil.* 1994;75(10):1087-1093.
91. Macko RF, DeSouza CA, Tretter LD, Silver KH, Smith GV, Anderson PA et al. Treadmill aerobic exercise training reduces the energy expenditure and cardiovascular demands of hemiparetic gait in chronic stroke patients. A preliminary report. *Stroke.* 1997;28(2):326-330.
92. Protas EJ, Holmes SA, Qureshy H, Johnson A, Lee D, Sherwood AM. Supported treadmill ambulation training after spinal cord injury: a pilot study. *Arch Phys Med Rehabil.* 2001;82(6):825-831.
93. Waagfjord J, Levangie PK, Certo CM. Effects of treadmill training on gait in a hemiparetic patient. *Phys Ther.* 1990;70(9):549-558.
94. Wernig A, Nanassy A, Muller S. Maintenance of locomotor abilities following Laufband (treadmill) therapy in para- and tetraplegic persons: follow-up studies. *Spinal Cord.* 1998;36(11):744-749.
95. Wernig A, Muller S, Nanassy A, Cagol E. Laufband therapy based on 'rules of spinal locomotion' is effective in spinal cord injured persons. *Eur J Neurosci.* 1995;7(4):823-829.
96. Wernig A, Muller S. Laufband locomotion with body weight support improved walking in persons with severe spinal cord injuries. *Paraplegia.* 1992;30(4):229-238.
97. Richards CL, Malouin F, Wood-Dauphinee S, Williams JI, Bouchard JP, Brunet D. Task-specific physical therapy for optimization of gait recovery in acute stroke patients. *Arch Phys Med Rehabil.* 1993;74(6):612-620.
98. Nilsson L, Carlsson J, Danielsson A, et al. Walking training of patients with hemiparesis at an early stage after stroke: a comparison of walking training on a treadmill with body weight support and walking training on the ground. *Clin Rehabil.* 2001;15(5):515-527.
99. Laufer Y, Dickstein R, Chefez Y, Marcovitz E. The effect of treadmill training on the ambulation of stroke survivors in the early stages of rehabilitation: a randomized study. *J Rehabil Res Dev.* 2001;38(1):69-78.
100. Jackson AJ, Porter JW, Merrell KA, Burt BT. The effects of harness supported treadmill ambulation training on the gait characteristics of a person with Parkinson's disease. *Med Sci Sports Exer.* 2000;32:S236.
101. Miyai I, Fujimoto Y, Yamamoto H, Ueda Y, Saito T, Nozaki S et al. Long-term effect of body weight-supported treadmill training in Parkinson's disease: a randomized controlled trial. *Arch Phys Med Rehabil.* 2002;83(10):1370-1373.
102. Miyai I, Fujimoto Y, Ueda Y, Yamamoto H, Nozaki S, Saito T et al. Treadmill training with body weight support: its effect on Parkinson's disease. *Arch Phys Med Rehabil.* 2000;81(7):849-852.
103. Pohl M, Rockstroh G, Ruckriem S, Mrass G, Mehrholz J. Immediate effects of speed-dependent treadmill training on gait parameters in early Parkinson's disease. *Arch Phys Med Rehabil.* 2003;84(12):1760-1766.
104. Jobges M, Heuschkel G, Pretzel C, Illhardt C, Renner C, Hummelsheim H. Repetitive training of compensatory steps: a therapeutic approach for postural instability in Parkinson's disease. *J Neurol Neurosurg Psychiatry.* 2004; 75(12):1682-1687.
105. Rogers MW, Johnson ME, Martinez KM, Mille ML, Hedman LD. Step training improves the speed of voluntary step initiation in aging. *J Gerontol A Biol Sci Med Sci.* 2003;58(1):46-51.
106. Protas EJ, Mitchell K, Williams A, Qureshy H, Caroline K, Lai EC. Gait and step training to reduce falls in Parkinson's disease. *NeuroRehabilitation.* 2005; 20(3):183-190.

8

OPTIMIZING MOVEMENT AND PREVENTING FALLS IN PARKINSON'S DISEASE: STRATEGIES FOR PATIENTS AND CAREGIVERS

Meg E. Morris, BScPT, Grad Dip (Geron), MAppSc, PhD; Frances Huxham, PhD; Hylton B. Menz, PhD; Fiona Dobson, BScPT, PhD; Pagamas Piriyaprasarth, BScPT; Pamela Fok, BScPT; Robert Iansek, PhD; Kimberly J. Miller, BScPT, MSc

INTRODUCTION

This chapter explores treatment strategies that people with idiopathic Parkinson's disease (PD) can implement to make mobility easier and safer, and to cope with fluctuations in their ability to move. Although PD is a progressive neurodegenerative condition, these strategies can be valuable in assisting individuals with PD to remain active and engaged for as long as possible in their homes and communities. Suggestions are also made about how caregivers can enable people with PD to retain their highest levels of independence and safety.

PD is prevalent, particularly among older people. It is estimated that 5 million people in the world have PD, with more than 1.5 million in the United States and a further 1.5 million in Europe. Falls are very common, with one study showing that 68% of community dwelling older people fall per year.[1] People with PD also fall frequently, and up to 25% of people report a serious fracture within the first 10 years after diagnosis.[2] PD results from a neurotransmitter imbalance in the feedback loop between the basal ganglia and motor cortex, due to unremitting and progressive death of dopamine producing neurons in the basal ganglia, deep within the brain.[3] These neurons normally secrete dopamine, which enables skilled movement sequences to run quickly and with little attention. The reason for cell death in this region is unknown, although environmental toxins or a genetic pre-disposition might possibly increase the risk.[4]

The loss of neurons in the substantia nigra and the resulting neurotransmitter imbal-ance produce characteristic movement disorders. These include hypokinesia, akinesia, freezing, dyskinesia, rigidity, tremor, balance, and postural instability.[5] *Hypokinesia* affects virtually all people with PD and refers to reduced movement speed and size.[6] Slowness in performing rapidly alternating movement sequences is known as *bradyki-nesia.*[7] *Akinesia* refers to an absence of movement associated with an inability to initiate long or complex sequences. *Freezing* is an abrupt cessation of movement midway through a long or complex locomotor sequence[5,7] and typically occurs when there is an environ-mental trigger such as a doorway or support surface change.[5,7-9] Some people with PD experience freezing when attempting to stop actions such as walking or turning around.[9] *Dyskinesias* or involuntary over-activity of muscles can present in various ways. They can be seen as random wriggling or writhing movements, or as tics.[9] Dyskinesias can also present as abnormal dystonic postures of body segments such as the wrist or foot.[10] *Rigidity* or increased resistance of muscles to passive movements can be evident, particu-larly toward the end of the levodopa dose.[9] *Resting tremor* is common in the early stages, whereas balance problems are more common as the disease progresses.[5,11] Hypokinesia, akinesia, and *balance problems* are the major contributing factors that limit mobility in people with PD.[5,7]

STRATEGIES AND EXERCISES TO ENHANCE MOVEMENT IN PATIENTS WITH PARKINSON'S DISEASE

Medication can provide considerable relief from the movement disorders that arise in PD, particularly in the early stages of the condition. Although optimal management is provided by a multidisciplinary team,[12] medication plays an important role in improv-ing overall mobility, independence, and quality of life. Most often, PD progresses slowly, and the rate of progression influences the medication adjustments that are necessary to maintain an individual at his or her optimum level of function.

Numerous strategies have been advocated to assist people to cope with movement symptoms that occur despite drug management.[5] These strategies are summarized in a recent systematic review of the literature by Morris.[13] PD affects the performance of well-learned movement sequences such as walking, running, dancing, turning, speak-ing, and driving. Allied health interventions such as physical therapy, speech therapy, and occupational therapy aim to reduce activity limitations and increase participation in societal roles, rather than simply targeting impairments. One approach that has been shown to be effective in addressing hypokinesia and akinesia is to teach people strategies to bypass the defective basal ganglia in order to move more quickly and easily.[5] This can be achieved by the use of attentional strategies, whereby the person focuses his or her thoughts on moving in a particular way in order to utilize intact frontal cortical regions of the brain to drive motor performance.[5,14] For example, the person can be trained to think about walking with long strides, to use large handwriting strokes or to speak with a loud voice. By focusing attention on a critical aspect of the movement, it can be easier to move quickly. There is also research to show that external visual cues or auditory cues can assist people to move more quickly and with large amplitude movements. Examples include using lined paper to guide the size of handwriting strokes, using markers on the floor to assist the person to commence stepping or to lengthen his or her stride, or button-ing a shirt in time to a metronome in order to dress more quickly.[10] Progressive resistance strength training programs and physical activity programs might also assist people to move more easily, although large randomized controlled clinical trials are required to measure their effectiveness. Physical therapy usually has little long-term effect on dyskinesia, dystonia, or tics—these are usually managed by adjusting the medication dose or schedule.[5]

Several recent randomized controlled clinical trials have measured the effects of movement strategy training and exercise programs. Wade and colleagues[15] evaluated the effects of a 6-week multidisciplinary rehabilitation program on mobility in 144 people with PD. Each week, a 2-hour session of individualized rehabilitation (physical therapy, speech pathology, and nursing) and another 2 hours of group activities were delivered. After the 6 weeks of intervention, the only significant improvement was seen for the timed stand-walk-sit test; all other variables showed negligible changes. At the 6-month follow-up, deterioration was evident in most variables, including disability, quality of life, and caregiver burden. Even though Wade's study used a controlled clinical trial design, the frequency of physical therapy was limited to only once per week for 6 weeks.

A randomized controlled trial by Ellis et al[16] obtained more promising results. This was conducted in 68 people with PD in the United States and the Netherlands and compared the effects of physical therapy in addition to medication with medication alone over a 6-week period. The intensity of physical therapy dosage was two 1.5-hour treatments per week, and the aim was to improve gait and balance in order to enhance mobility and the performance of activities of daily living (ADL). The improvement in mobility was greater in the physical therapy group than for the control group and improvements were retained for 3 months. One limitation of this study was difficulty in controlling the similarity of participants in the crossover design across two sites in two different countries. There were differences in baseline performance for the US group compared to the Dutch group, most notably for motor performance. In addition, 11 subjects did not have full data sets and patients did not receive a standardized physical therapy program.

Recently, some of the results of the "RESCUE" European trial on movement strategy training have been reported.[17] This study evaluated the effect of external rhythmic cues (auditory and visual) on walking performance including walking speed, step length, and step frequency. Walking was tested, both with and without a dual-motor task of carrying a tray of drinks from one room to another. This study was the first to be conducted within the participant's own home environment rather than in a laboratory setting. The results were evaluated from 18 people with idiopathic PD and 10 matched controls. It was shown that during dual-motor tasks within the home environment, people with PD walked 34% slower and had a 36% greater reduction in step length than people without PD. During dual-motor tasks, people with PD were able to effectively increase their step length when using external rhythmic cues, and they were more successful at using auditory cues (an auditory tone from an earpiece) than visual cues (an LED flash of light on a pair of clear glasses). Although there was a trend for increased walking speed when external cues were used, this was not significant for either cue. No major changes in step frequency were shown with the use of external cues. A restriction in the design of this study was that the external cueing frequency was set only to each participant's preferred walking rate. The timing of auditory cues appears to be a key determinant of walking performance and a cueing frequency set higher than the preferred walking rate might have improved the walking speed. Changes in baseline performance before and after cueing intervention were also found, indicating the possibility of a practice effect within the study. Alternatively, this effect may imply that practice is beneficial. The use of a home environment setting may provide findings that better reflect the true nature of everyday performance; however, the varied nature of each environment in this study (eg, different distances, obstacles, types of turns, and number of doorways) may have affected the outcomes.

FALL PREVENTION IN COMMUNITY-DWELLING PEOPLE

An increased risk of falling is common among people with PD, particularly in those over 2.5 on the Hoehn and Yahr (H&Y) scale.[18] While approximately one-third of the older population fall in a year,[23] in PD almost twice the incidence occurs.[1] People with PD are particularly likely to experience repeated falls.[19] One quarter of those who fell in the Bloem et al[19] study fell more than once in 6 months, increasing to one half over a year in Wood et al.[1] People with PD have a relative risk of 6.1 compared to controls for a single fall and a relative risk of 9.0 for repeated falls.[19]

Falling is more likely to result in both injuries and serious injury in people with PD than their peers. A retrospective review of hospital outpatients in the United Kingdom revealed a fracture rate of 15% in 200 patients with PD, compared to 7.5% in patients with other conditions.[20] The most common fracture in the PD group occurred at the hip, rather than in the forearm as in the other patients.[20] Many people with PD do not regain the ability to walk independently after a fracture, despite rehabilitation. There is also a higher rate of osteoporosis in this group, which further increases the fracture risk.

Balance disturbance is a symptom that develops later in the condition. In the most widely used measure of overall disease severity, the H&Y scale,[18] an abnormal response to perturbation in standing represents progression from bilateral mild-to-moderate disease (H&Y 2.5) to bilateral mild-to-moderate disease with postural instability (H&Y 3.0). The mean H&Y of those who fell in the three cited studies was only 2.0 to 2.7.[1,19,20] Bloem et al[19] argued that this apparent anomaly can be explained by the limited mobility of more severely affected patients, a suggestion supported by the greater incidence of falls when in the "on" phase of medication than in the more severe "off" phase.[19,21] Less overt balance impairment early in PD is suggested by a growing body of evidence for altered postural responses in standing. These include increased stiffness of ankles and trunk;[22] enlarged destabilizing medium latency postural responses and diminished stabilizing long latency responses;[23] inadequate and delayed control of the center of mass, especially backwards,[24] and also laterally if the base of support is narrowed and reduced; and narrowed limits of stability.[24]

The ability to predict which people with PD will fall is poor. The strongest predictor for future falls is a previous fall.[1] Unlike healthy elderly people who often fall due to a slip or trip, falls in people with PD are generally intrinsic or "person specific," such as walking and balance difficulties. Although around 70% of PD patient falls are intrinsic,[19] foot clearance is reduced in PD,[25] increasing the risk of tripping. The reduced capacity for force generation in PD[26] also makes recovery from a slip or trip more difficult. Another factor that no doubt contributes both to the incidence and the severity of falls is the abnormal pattern of protective balance reactions. Not only are these responses delayed and undersized, but they occur in abnormal directions.[22] The arms, for example, are adducted toward the body, rather than stretching out to protect the face in the event of a fall.

Falls in people with PD are particularly likely to occur during walking. Between 24%[19] and 40%[21] of falls in this condition are associated with turning, and patients who report freezing episodes are twice as likely to suffer a fall than those who do not freeze.[21] At this time, there is little known about the capacity of people with PD to adapt their walking patterns dynamically to adjust to the demands of functional activity, such as turning, avoiding or stepping over or under obstacles, traversing slopes, or carrying objects. A number of studies have demonstrated that people with PD have greater difficulty with concurrent task performance than their peers.[27,28] As this is believed to result from the withdrawal of attention from gait and balance to the concurrent task, it may be that they will experience similar difficulties when undertaking more complex adaptive gait tasks.

In the Multiple Tasks Test, performed by repeating the Timed Up and Go test in increasingly more difficult form, people with PD prioritize cognitive concurrent tasks higher than unimpaired older subjects, further reducing the amount of attention paid to the gait and balance requirements of the task.[29]

FALL PREVENTION IN HOSPITALS AND RESIDENTIAL CARE

Very little data are available on the incidence and prevalence of falls among people with PD who are hospitalized or who live in residential care. Thus at the present time it is necessary to extrapolate falls prevention strategies from existing knowledge in the aging literature. Falls among hospitalized older people are a major concern, with rates of between 13% and 32% of admitted patients reported in the literature.[30,31] The combination of physiological and/or cognitive impairments associated with acute illness and an unfamiliar environment makes the likelihood of falling while in the hospital extremely high. This situation is made even more complex by the need for health care providers to encourage older people to regain functional independence during their hospital stay.

A recent systematic review revealed that although there are a number of clearly identifiable risk factors for falls in hospitals (including the use of psychoactive medications, confusion or disorientation, gait impairment, visual impairment, and incontinence), the currently available risk assessment tools fail to classify a high percentage of fallers and therefore require further validation.[32] In the absence of an accurate assessment tool, it has been suggested that environmental safety measures be routinely adopted and modifiable risk factors targeted in all patients.[32]

Although several single-factor intervention studies have been undertaken with mixed results, two recent multifaceted randomized controlled trials have demonstrated significant reductions in falls while in the hospital. A targeted multifactorial intervention study conducted in a subacute hospital setting in Australia found that the use of a falls risk alert card, an exercise program, an education program, and provision of hip protectors reduced falls by 30%.[33] A similar risk reduction was observed in a cluster randomized trial conducted in the United Kingdom,[34] in which the intervention group received a targeted intervention addressing visual impairment, medication assessment, advice on changing position slowly to prevent orthostatic hypotension, physical therapy referral for those with mobility problems, addition of bedrails where appropriate, footwear advice, and ensuring a nurse call bell was within reach. Thus, it appears that many hospital falls can be prevented with targeted, multifactorial interventions. However, the translation of these research results to clinical practice is clearly dependent on adequate staffing and resources.[35]

Falls are also a significant problem in residential aged care facilities (ie, hostels and nursing homes), with falling rates up to three times greater than for older people living independently in the community.[36] The risk factors for falls in residential care are similar to those in the community, including muscle weakness, gait and balance disorders, visual impairment, and cognitive impairment.[37] However, incontinence and the use of antipsychotic medications are more prevalent in residential care and are of greater importance in relation to falls in this setting.[36,38,39]

As is the case with hospital settings, falls prevention programs in residential aged care facilities should ideally be multifaceted and address physical risk factors, medication assessment, environmental safety issues, and awareness-raising among staff. There have now been three multifaceted randomized controlled trials that have demonstrated reductions in falling rates in residential care. Ray et al[40] reported a 19% reduction in recurrent falls in nursing home residents who received an individualized program of environmental safety, wheelchair use, psychotropic medication use, and ambulation advice and intervention. Greater reductions in falls (approximately 40%) were reported by Jensen et al[41] and Becker et al[42] for intervention studies involving staff education, exercise programs, and medication assessment. The effectiveness of any falls prevention program in residential care, however, depends on a range of location-specific factors and the characteristics of the residential population. In particular, it has been shown that intervention programs are less successful in facilities with a higher proportion of residents with cognitive impairment.[43]

A final consideration with regard to falls in people with PD is the provision of hip protectors to prevent injury. Hip protectors are constructed of dense molded plastic and are designed to disperse the impact force applied to the hip in the event of a sideways fall. Although hip protectors may reduce the risk of fracture when worn correctly, their overall efficacy is limited by incorrect positioning and variable compliance.[44] The main barrier to compliance with hip protectors is general discomfort and the extra effort required to wear them, particularly in older people with urinary incontinence.[43,45] Thus, it would appear that hip protectors should only be considered for older people who have a high risk of falling and fracturing, and who are highly motivated to wear them.[45] Nevertheless they would appear to have particular application in people with PD, who tend to be underweight and are especially likely to fall when turning, which is more likely to result in hip fracture (odds ratio 7.9[46]).

ROLE OF THE CAREGIVER

Caregivers can play a major role in assisting people with PD to move more easily, prevent falling, and participate in a range of activities and societal roles. In clinical circles, it is argued that supportive caregivers with a positive outlook and life-long commitment to the relationship enhance patient outcomes. In addition, effective treatment of PD appears to be facilitated by educating and training both the caregiver and the person with the disease.[5] Caregivers are most often husbands and wives, although sons and daughters, other relatives, close friends, or occasionally employed staff may perform this role. The characteristic feature of their role is the provision of physical, psychological, and social support to varying degrees over the course of disease progression. Because PD always affects the motor system, there can be a significant caregiver role in helping patients manage their medication regimen, move more easily, and prevent falls, particularly in H&Y stages III and IV of disease progression. Furthermore, changes in cognitive function are common, necessitating assistance with higher order executive function, such as planning, sequencing of activities, and three-dimensional construction tasks.

Most people who enter a caregiver role have little prior experience of chronic disease management, disability, or how to oversee the types of complex medication regimens that typically occur in PD. Over the course of the disease, caregiver burden can become a significant issue.[47-50] At the time of diagnosis, many caregivers express a need for quick access to user-friendly information about the causes, typical disease progression, types of treatment available, and likely outcomes in the short- and long-term. Although medical information is most often sought, counseling services can be beneficial in allowing individuals or couples to adjust to the diagnosis and reset their short-term goals. Often the diagnosis is made around the time of retirement, sometimes requiring travel or relocation plans to be reconsidered or adjusted. For those aged 75 or older, the spouse may be experiencing his or her own age-related difficulties or chronic diseases, adding complexity to the caregiving role. Few are initially aware that PD is a chronic degenerative condition that relentlessly progresses over time and that no cure currently exists. Because only symptomatic treatment is available and movement disorders and postural instability gradually worsen, families need to make progressive adjustments and adaptations over time. They need to learn the most effective methods for enabling their loved ones to move more easily, prevent falls, and participate as fully as possible in family, work, leisure, and societal roles.

There are many practical strategies that caregivers can use to enhance quality of life. Having a partner who understands and can help to de-brief about the disease, its progression, and the way that it leads to variable motor performance, can be a tremendous support. On a more practical level, caregivers can tactfully provide reminders about when the medication is due, which tablets to take, and when to contact the medical practitioner if the response to medication has become unsatisfactory. Use of a medication dosette box, in which tablets are placed into compartments labeled with the time to be taken, can be an excellent method for ensuring that medication has actually been taken and avoids duplication. Likewise, wrist watches can now be purchased with multiple alarms that can be set to ring at the times throughout the day and night when medication is scheduled to be taken. Reminders can also be provided by portable alarm clocks placed in a bag or pocket. Because some patients' medication regimens are very complex, it can be useful to have another person monitoring them. Missed doses may result in marked hypokinesia, akinesia, and freezing, whereas doses taken too close together can result in dyskinesia. Some patients are prescribed liquid levodopa preparations that the person drinks as needed. Although this form of administration tends to be used for people who are fully cognitively intact or those with young-onset PD, it can still be useful for a person in a caregiving role to keep an eye on their use and outcomes.

Caregivers can provide very helpful assistance by reinforcing the movement strategies in a tactful way. Subtle phrases from the caregiver such as "long steps" may be helpful if steps start to shuffle. Similarly, "forward and up" or "nose over knees" may assist rising from a chair, or "arc turn" may be useful when turning around becomes problematic.[12] Likewise, an auditory cue such as a clap may help to overcome a freezing episode.[51] Understanding of the environmental impact on movement disorders can also provide great assistance. Minimizing clutter around the home, maintaining clear pathways, or planning visits to shops during less chaotic periods of the day can all be simple but effective ways of maximizing the use of movement strategies. In some situations when movement becomes more restricted, the caregiver may provide physical assistance to guide movements such as turning the head and facilitating the legs over the bed to help with getting out of bed.[12]

CONCLUSION

Due to the complexity of motor and non-motor complications of PD as well as the steady yet slow progression of the condition, a multidisciplinary team approach to care appears to be optimal, particularly when significant emphasis is placed on the caregiver as well as the person with the disease. The major goal of movement rehabilitation and medical management is to assist the person and his or her caregiver to maintain the highest possible quality of life, to maintain well-being, and to minimize distress. This is enhanced by educating them about the likely course and consequences of the disease, as well as by teaching strategies to enhance movement, manage medications, maintain physical activity, and reduce falls.

References

1. Wood BH, Bilclough JA, Bowron A, Walker RW. Incidence and prediction of falls in Parkinson's disease: a prospective multidisciplinary study. *J Neurol Neurosurg Psychiatry.* 2002;72(6):721-725.

2. Johnell O, Melton LJ, III, Atkinson EJ, O'Fallon WM, Kurland LT. Fracture risk in patients with parkinsonism: a population-based study in Olmsted County, Minnesota. *Age Ageing.* 1992;21(1):32-38.

3. Alexander GE, Crutcher MD. Functional architecture of basal ganglia circuits: neural substrates of parallel processing. *Trends Neurosci.* 1990;13(7):266-271.

4. Tanner CM, Aston DA. Epidemiology of Parkinson's disease and akinetic syndromes. *Curr Opin Neurol.* 2000;13(4):427-430.

5. Morris ME. Movement disorders in people with Parkinson disease: a model for physical therapy. *Phys Ther.* 2000;80(6):578-597.

6. Morris ME, Iansek R, Matyas TA, Summers JJ. Stride length regulation in Parkinson's disease. Normalization strategies and underlying mechanisms. *Brain.* 1996;119(Pt 2):551-568.

7. Morris ME, Huxham FE, McGinley J, Iansek R. Gait disorders and gait rehabilitation in Parkinson's disease. *Adv Neurol.* 2001;87:347-361.

8. Morris ME, Huxham F, McGinley J, Dodd K, Iansek R. The biomechanics and motor control of gait in Parkinson disease. *Clin Biomech.* (Bristol, Avon) 2001;16(6):459-470.

9. Morris ME, Iansek R. Gait disorders in Parkinson's disease: a framework for physical therapy practice. *Neuro Report.* 1997;21:125-131.

10. Bilney BE, Morris ME, Denisenko S. Physical therapy for people with movement disorders arising from basal ganglia dysfunction. *New Zealand Journal of Physical Therapy.* 2003; 32(2):94-100.

11. Smithson F, Morris ME, Iansek R. Performance on clinical tests of balance in Parkinson's disease. *Phys Ther.* 1998;78(6):577-592.

12. Morris M, Iansek R. An interprofessional team approach to rehabilitation in Parkinson's disease. *Europ J Phys Med Rehabil.* 1997;7(6):166-170.

13. Morris ME. Impairments, activity limitations and participation restrictions in Parkinson's disease. In: Refshauge K, Ada L, Ellis E, eds. *Science-Based Rehabilitation: Theories into Practice.* London: Butterworth Heinemann, 2005.

14. Landers M et al. An external focus of attention attenuates balance impairments in patients with Parkinson's disease who have a fall history. *Phys Ther.* 2005; 91:152-158.

15. Wade DT, Gage H, Owen C, Trend P, Grossmith C, Kaye J. Multidisciplinary rehabilitation for people with Parkinson's disease: a randomised controlled study. *J Neurol Neurosurg Psychiatry.* 2003;74(2):158-162.

16. Ellis T, de Goede CJ, Feldman RG, Wolters EC, Kwakkel G, Wagenaar RC. Efficacy of a physical therapy program in patients with Parkinson's disease: a randomized controlled trial. *Arch Phys Med Rehabil.* 2005;86(4):626-632.

17. Rochester L, Hetherington V, Jones D, et al. The effect of external rhythmic cues (auditory and visual) on walking during a functional task in homes of people with Parkinson's disease. *Arch Phys Med Rehabil.* 2005;86(5):999-1006.

18. Hoehn MM, Yahr MD. Parkinsonism: onset, progression and mortality. *Neurology.* 1967;17(5):427-442.

19. Bloem BR, Grimbergen YA, Cramer M, Willemsen M, Zwinderman AH. Prospective assessment of falls in Parkinson's disease. *J Neurol.* 2001;248(11):950-958.

20. Genever RW, Downes TW, Medcalf P. Fracture rates in Parkinson's disease compared with age- and gender-matched controls: a retrospective cohort study. *Age Ageing.* 2005;34(1):21-24.

21. Gray P, Hildebrand K. Fall risk factors in Parkinson's disease. *J Neurosci Nurs.* 2000; 32(4):222-228.

22. Carpenter MG, Allum JH, Honegger F, Adkin AL, Bloem BR. Postural abnormalities to multidirectional stance perturbations in Parkinson's disease. *J Neurol Neurosurg Psychiatry.* 2004;75(9):1245-1254.

23. Bloem BR, Beckley DJ, van Hilten BJ, Roos RA. Clinimetrics of postural instability in Parkinson's disease. *J Neurol.* 1998;245(10):669-673.

24. Horak FB, Dimitrova D, Nutt JG. Direction-specific postural instability in subjects with Parkinson's disease. *Exp Neurol.* 2005;193(2):504-521.

25. Murray MP, Sepic SB, Gardner GM, Downs WJ. Walking patterns of men with parkinsonism. *Am J Phys Med.* 1978;57(6):278-294.

26. Corcos DM, Chen CM, Quinn NP, McAuley J, Rothwell JC. Strength in Parkinson's disease: relationship to rate of force generation and clinical status. *Ann Neurol.* 1996; 39(1):79-88.

27. O'Shea S, Morris ME, Iansek R. Dual task interference during gait in people with Parkinson disease: effects of motor versus cognitive secondary tasks. *Phys Ther.* 2002;82(9):888-897.

28. Rochester L, Hetherington V, Jones D, Nieuwboer A, Willems AM, Kwakkel G et al. Attending to the task: interference effects of functional tasks on walking in Parkinson's disease and the roles of cognition, depression, fatigue, and balance. *Arch Phys Med Rehabil.* 2004;85(10):1578-1585.

29. Bloem BR, Valkenburg VV, Slabbekoorn M, Willemsen MD. The Multiple Tasks Test: development and normal strategies. *Gait Posture.* 2001;14(3):191-202.

30. Mion LC, Gregor S, Buettner M, Chwirchak D, Lee O, Paras W. Falls in the rehabilitation setting: incidence and characteristics. *Rehabil Nurs.* 1989;14(1):17-22.

31. Vlahov D, Myers AH, al Ibrahim MS. Epidemiology of falls among patients in a rehabilitation hospital. *Arch Phys Med Rehabil.* 1990;71(1):8-12.

32. Oliver D, Daly F, Martin FC, McMurdo ME. Risk factors and risk assessment tools for falls in hospital in-patients: a systematic review. *Age Ageing.* 2004;33(2):122-130.

33. Haines TP, Bennell KL, Osborne RH, Hill KD. Effectiveness of targeted falls prevention programme in subacute hospital setting: randomised controlled trial. *BMJ.* 2004;328(7441):676.

34. Healey F, Monro A, Cockram A, Adams V, Heseltine D. Using targeted risk factor reduction to prevent falls in older in-patients: a randomised controlled trial. *Age Ageing.* 2004;33(4):390-395.

35. Oliver D. Prevention of falls in hospital inpatients: agendas for research and practice. *Age Ageing.* 2004;33(4):328-330.

36. Rubenstein LZ, Josephson KR, Osterweil D. Falls and fall prevention in the nursing home. *Clin Geriatr Med.* 1996;12(4):881-902.

37. Clinical practice guidelines for the assessment and prevention of falls in older people. 2004. National Institute for Clinical Excellence. Pamphlet.

38. Lipsitz LA, Jonsson PV, Kelley MM, Koestner JS. Causes and correlates of recurrent falls in ambulatory frail elderly. *J Gerontol.* 1991;46(4):M114-M122.

39. Luukinen H, Koski K, Laippala P, Kivela SL. Risk factors for recurrent falls in the elderly in long-term institutional care. *Public Health.* 1995;109(1):57-65.

40. Ray WA, Taylor JA, Meador KG, Thapa PB, Brown AK, Kajihara HK et al. A randomized trial of a consultation service to reduce falls in nursing homes. *JAMA.* 1997;278(7):557-562.

41. Jensen J, Lundin-Olsson L, Nyberg L, Gustafson Y. Fall and injury prevention in older people living in residential care facilities. A cluster randomized trial. *Ann Intern Med.* 2002;136(10):733-741.

42. Becker C, Kron M, Lindemann U, Sturm E, Eichner B, Walter-Jung B et al. Effectiveness of a multifaceted intervention on falls in nursing home residents. *J Am Geriatr Soc.* 2003;51(3):306-313.

43. Jensen J, Nyberg L, Gustafson Y, Lundin-Olsson L. Fall and injury prevention in residential care—effects in residents with higher and lower levels of cognition. *J Am Geriatr Soc.* 2003;51(5):627-635.

44. Parker MJ, Gillespie WJ, Gillespie LD. Hip protectors for preventing hip fractures in older people. *Cochrane Database Syst Rev.* 2005;(3):CD001255.

45. Patel S, Ogunremi L, Chinappen U. Acceptability and compliance with hip protectors in community-dwelling women at high risk of hip fracture. *Rheumatology* (Oxford). 2003;42(6):769-772.

46. Cumming RG, Klineberg RJ. Fall frequency and characteristics and the risk of hip fractures. *J Am Geriatr Soc.* 1994;42(7):774-778.

47. Carter JH, Stewart BJ, Archbold PG, Inoue I, Jaglin J, Lannon M et al. Living with a person who has Parkinson's disease: the spouse's perspective by stage of disease. Parkinson's Study Group. *Mov Disord.* 1998;13(1):20-28.

48. McRae C, Sherry P, Roper K. Stress and family functioning among caregivers of persons with Parkinson's disease. *Parkinsonism and Related Disorders.* 1999;5:69-75.

49. Fernandez HH, Tabamo RE, David RR, Friedman JH. Predictors of depressive symptoms among spouse caregivers in Parkinson's disease. *Mov Disord.* 2001; 16(6):1123-1125.

50. Trend P, Kaye J, Gage H, Owen C, Wade D. Short-term effectiveness of intensive multidisciplinary rehabilitation for people with Parkinson's disease and their carers. *Clin Rehabil.* 2002;16(7):717-725.

51. Morris ME, Iansek R. Characteristics of motor disturbance in parkinson's disease and strategies for movement rehabiitation. *J Human Movement Sci.* 1996;15:649-669.

AN OCCUPATIONAL THERAPY MODEL OF TREATMENT FOR PARKINSON'S DISEASE

Marilyn Trail, MOT, OTR

INTRODUCTION

Few could argue that as occupational therapists we have a responsibility to provide our patients with the most current and effective forms of treatment. Evidence-based practice arose from a concern that patients were receiving interventions unsupported by scientific inquiry. Practicing evidence-based treatment—a form of quality assurance—means we must be accountable to our patients, other heath care providers, insurance companies, the community, and to ourselves as health care professionals.

Perhaps now is the time to forever rid our occupational therapy clinics of pegboards, ring arcs, clothes pin trees, and other equipment and rote activities that have been shown to be ineffective as well as demeaning and inappropriate for adults. Substantiation from the literature, research studies, and good clinical practice can supply us with more effectual treatment interventions as occupational therapy moves into the 21st century. This does not mean that we throw away our clinical judgment and experience, but rather acknowledge that in some cases, treatment techniques we have used in the past may not be the best. The aim of this chapter is to describe the impairments caused by Parkinson's disease that impede the patient's ability to engage in occupations and review the best evidence to describe treatment interventions and solutions that occupational therapists can draw on when working with this challenging group of patients.

A Review of the Literature

Although there is general agreement in the literature that occupational therapy is an important adjunctive treatment for persons with PD, there is limited evidence supporting its value.[1] Reviewers investigating the efficacy of occupational therapy for the treatment of PD [1-3] found some studies to be of questionable merit, others undertaken by physical therapists and nurses, some classified as rehabilitation and others as exercise, and only a few studies involved specific occupational therapy therapeutic interventions. In a 2001 Cochrane review, Deane and colleagues[2] found two randomized controlled trials on occupational therapy intervention for PD, both of which they deemed to be methodologically flawed.

A 2003 Delphi survey of best practice occupational therapy for PD in the United Kingdom found that although there was no consensus on what constituted best practice, current practice emphasizes functional goals, mobility, and self care with little emphasis on social and psychological aspects of occupation.[4] Furthermore, many of the occupational therapists surveyed reported that they lacked adequate training to treat this group of patients.

Tse and Spalding[5] reviewed the implications of motor control and motor learning theory for occupational therapy treatment of patients with PD and inferred that "motor learning knowledge provides techniques that may enhance learning skills of PD patients."

Functional environmentally specific tasks and active rather than passive patient participation are inherent to the practice of occupational therapy,[6] rendering the tenets of motor learning theory especially suitable for occupational therapists to apply when working with this patient population.

Treatment Models from Other Disciplines

Schenkman and Butler developed a comprehensive model of care for patients with PD for physical therapy practice.[7] They differentiated between impairments that occur as direct effects of central nervous system (CNS) pathology (which will not be improved by physical therapy or occupational therapy), those that occur indirectly because of musculoskeletal alterations, and those that result from a composite of CNS and non-CNS impairment. They drew on treatment techniques based on Bobath (neurodevelopment treatment), Feldenkrais, and Knott and Voss (proprioceptive neuromuscular facilitation), proposing that musculoskeletal impairments contribute to patients' total disability, restrict their ability to perform activities of daily living, and impede normal movement patterns. Schenkman endorsed the importance of exercises for spinal flexibility, suggesting that tightness may contribute to poor balance, falls, functional limitations, and bradykinesia. She also emphasized techniques to decrease rigidity, including relaxation, and pointed out that decreased chest expansion might play a role in terminal pneumonia.

Rogers[8] emphasized the need to teach patients with PD the biomechanical features of an action and the use of cognitive strategies to help alter ineffective movement patterns. The musculo-skeletal-biomechanical factors include the structure and properties of muscles, joints, and soft tissues and the physical laws governing movement.[8]

Carr and Shepherd[9] and Morris[10] based their models of PD treatment on motor control and motor learning theory. They postulated that slowness of movement and difficulties initiating movement rather than rigidity are the major deficits underlying the poverty of motor performance experienced by PD patients. Musculoskeletal changes (eg, forward head, flexed posture) also contribute to reduced speed and difficulty in initiating gait. Carr and Shepherd[9] cited lack of evidence in the motor learning literature that passive or therapist-controlled movement or active nonspecific exercise will carry over to improve performance on specific tasks. They emphasized that tasks should always be practiced in the environment where they take place and recommend teaching the biomechanical features of an action.

Carr and Shepherd[9] pointed out that the presence of depression, dementia (more significant in older clients with advanced disease), memory impairment, and visual perceptual motor deficits should be considered when planning a therapeutic intervention.

Morris[10] based her protocol on the pathogenesis of PD and an evaluation of the evidence for therapeutic intervention. Her model emphasized that normal movement can be obtained by teaching clients to compensate for the basal ganglion pathology with frontal cortical control mechanisms. External cues (ie, visual, auditory, proprioceptive) can assist clients with cognitive deficits. Morris,[10] like Carr and Shepherd,[9] and Rogers[8] advocated task-specific training regimes.

All of the aforementioned theorists agree that patients with PD benefit from physical activity and home exercise programs, and that therapy should begin early in the disease course to help preserve musculoskeletal flexibility, prevent inactivity and deconditioning, minimize mental decline, and help patients find solutions to functional problems.

A Theoretical Approach to the Occupational Therapy Management of the Patient with PD

The occupational therapist can perhaps best approach the treatment of the PD patients using elements of motor learning theory (which was developed in response to new ideas in the motor learning literature and the limitations of the neurodevelopment theory),[11] the task oriented approach (which organizes movement around a behavioral goal),[12] Schmidt's[13] principles of skill acquisition (conceptual model of human performance), and Morris's,[10] Carr and Shepherd's,[9] and Schenkman and Butler's[7] treatment models for PD.

Mathiowetz and Haugen[11] described a task-oriented approach for treatment of patients with CNS dysfunction based on a systems model of motor control. The literature on motor learning supports "a functional approach to treatment in which movement patterns and components of tasks should be practiced in relation to functional tasks." Poole[14] applied principles of motor learning to occupational therapy treatment and emphasized the importance for therapists to gain knowledge of the teaching-learning process and how we acquire skills. She, like Mathiowetz, advocated a functional approach to treatment based upon motor learning theory.

Shumway-Cook and Woollacott[12] describe three goals of the task-oriented approach: 1) Resolve, reduce, or prevent impairment; 2) Develop effective task-specific strategies; and 3) Adapt functional goal-orientated strategies to changing task and environmental conditions. These goals should be applied simultaneously during the same therapy session.

Opinions as to whether to focus on recovering normal or previous strategies to perform a task such as dressing or to teach the patient compensatory strategies are mixed. Whereas Tse and Spaulding[5] indicated that training the patient in alternative strategies to perform tasks might be the more realistic goal, others recommended focusing on recovery of function.[15] Morris[10] suggested that for PD patients, learning novel movements may not be as important as relearning functional tasks such as dressing and writing. Schenkman and Butler[7] recommended that specific impairments such as decreased range of motion (ROM) should be treated if they interfere with physical performance or if they will lead to injury of loss of function.

All of the aforementioned are important considerations, but treatment decisions should also be made on a case-by-case basis depending on the patient's cognitive status and capacity to learn, stage of disease and degree of impairment, the difficulty of the task itself, the environment where the task will be performed, and the patient's changing needs. As the disease advances and the ongoing loss of motor skills results in his or her increased inability to perform ADL, teaching compensatory strategies, and adapting the environment is a more appropriate mode of therapeutic intervention. Impairments resulting from PD are typically individualized, and thus therapy needs to be customized to each patient's specific goals and needs.

INCORPORATING LEARNING THEORY INTO OCCUPATIONAL THERAPY TREATMENT OF PATIENTS WITH PARKINSON'S DISEASE

Schmidt's work on motor learning and motor performance[13,16] provides useful concepts on how we learn and methods to instill learning that are helpful to occupational therapy practice. He defined motor learning as "a set of processes associated with practice or experience leading to relatively permanent changes in the capacity for responding." He distinguished between motor performance (which is seen in a practice session) and motor learning (a permanent change seen after the session). Learning thus involves a permanent change in behavior. Variables that affect motor learning are 1) practice, 2) feedback, 3) stages of learning, and 4) type of task.[16] Another important learning concept influencing outcome of occupational therapy treatment is the ability to transfer what was learned from one activity to another. For instance, to apply the skills learned for handwriting to other graphic tasks.

Actual physical practice is essential to acquiring a skill. Schmidt suggested that long practice periods can become tedious and detrimental to learning.[13] He distinguished between blocked practice whereby all of the trials of a given task (like donning shoes) are practiced during a single treatment session before moving to another activity (like donning a shirt) during another, separate session. He theorized that whereas blocked practice leads to better practice performance, random practice (ie, practice donning shoes, shirt, and trousers within the same occupational therapy treatment session), promotes learning.

Morris[10] recommended that performance can be improved for individuals with PD by training them to break down long or complex sequences into parts and then to practice each part separately. Schmidt[13] suggested breaking serial tasks of very long duration into components for part practice and later switching to whole; however, if the task has parts that are closely connected or that require rapid action, they should be practiced together. Ma and Trombly[17] found that part practice depended on the organization and complexity of the task whereas whole task performance resulted in more forceful and smoother movement. The author believes that if part practice is used, it should be early in training. As soon as possible, the practice should move toward whole task performance. Carr and Shepard[9] also recommended practice of whole action tasks while pointing out that given the deficits exhibited by patients undergoing rehabilitation, it is sometimes necessary to have patients practice one part of an action critical to the whole performance.

In the occupational therapy clinic, drill is sometimes used to enhance a patient's skill on a particular task. This type of practice, however, does not simulate reality. In actuality, people do not engage in daily activities such as buttoning or donning socks by performing them repetitiously. Although blocked practice might appear to be effective after an hour-long treatment session, it does not contribute to lasting learning as does random practice, or varying the activities.[13]

Another important element in learning is feedback, given either verbally or through demonstration.[9] There are perhaps few occupational therapists who have not, at some time in their careers, found themselves saying "good job" or "that was good" when the performance is only fair or poor. We say this because we want to be positive, we want to keep the patient engaged and motivated, and we want to provide reinforcement. Although we want to encourage our patients, the feedback given should always reflect the true performance. Schmidt[13] pointed out that because feedback is important to performance and learning, some types are more helpful that others, and we should be aware of the message we are conveying when responding to a patient's execution of a task.

If practice is to result in learning, our patients need to know when their endeavors are successful (the button goes through the hole) and when they are making errors (the button went through the wrong hole). This knowledge of results[9] is critical to learning. A study by Shohamy et al[18] indicated that PD patients might perform better when they learn information through observation rather than through verbal feedback. When we repeatedly provide the patient with knowledge of results, performance is enhanced but retention is impeded. Schmidt[13] suggested that, with normal subjects, one should initially give feedback frequently, but not on every trial, and to avoid going for long periods of time without providing any feedback at all. As skills develop, we reduce the frequency of feedback to allow for the transfer of motor skills to other activities. This transfer of learning allows the patient to draw on past experience such as tying shoes to perform a new task such as tying a scarf. However, in a recent study Guadagnoli and colleagues,[19] found that Parkinson's subjects depended on knowledge of results more than the control subjects, thus patients with PD may require feedback for a longer time period.

There is increasing evidence to suggest that patients with PD are capable of improving their performance on a task, but require more practice than normal subjects.[20-22] Nutt and colleagues[23] studied the effects of practice on tapping speed in normal and PD subjects and found that the PD patients benefited from short-term practice but did not improve with continued practice. Agostino et al[24] also found that PD patients did not benefit from prolonged practice and recommended that training time be spent by training more tasks for a shorter time rather that fewer tasks for a long time. Behman et al[22] suggested that practice of fast movements might increase performance speed and have long-lasting effects upon motor performance. While Soliveri et al[21] argued that PD patients have the ability to acquire new motor skills, the research is still limited as to if and to what extent new learning is possible[25] (Sidebar 9-1).

OCCUPATIONAL THERAPY ASSESSMENT

Identifying Deficits That Affect Occupational Performance

Patients with Parkinson's disease face numerous challenges and obstacles in their daily lives depending on the disease state and degree of impairment. Those in the early stage may experience difficulty with fine motor tasks such as fastening the top or cuff button on a shirt, and complain of writing changes and excessive fatigue. Although a resting tremor may be present, it subsides with action. It may, however, prove embarrassing for the patient, particularly in social situations. Patients may complain of mild gait or balance problems, slowness of movement (bradykinesia), and difficulty performing repetitive movements.[26] In the early stage, patients are still independent in their daily activities, although they may need more time to dress, bathe, and perform other ADL. They may find themselves spending less time playing golf and more time engaging in more pas-

---

Sidebar 9-1: Incorporating Learning Theory into Treatment

- Move from blocked practice to random practice
- Tell patients when they are successful with a task and when they are not (knowledge of results)
- Reflect the patient's actual performance when giving feedback (be truthful)
- Tell patients how to correct problems
- Tell patients how they can improve performance
- Move from giving the patient frequent feedback to delayed feedback
- Withdraw all feedback gradually as performance improves
- Attempt to simulate the real word in practice sessions
- Avoid use of drill or rote forms of practice

---

sive pursuits such as reading, watching sports, and attending films. Patients who are not retired by reason of age or choice are most often working.

In the middle stages patients may experience dyskinesias (a side-effect of levadopa therapy), which can interfere with function, and their ability to engage in normal activity can fluctuate, sometimes dramatically, due to the on/off effect of medication.[27] They tend to be less active. They experience loss of automatic movement (ie, facial expression, swallowing) increased episodes of freezing (especially in doorways and turning), and exhibit problems performing sequential and simultaneous movements and planning and executing movements.[28] Musculoskeletal changes occur that further contribute to reduced speed and increased stiffness, thereby increasing the patient's fall risk. Patients may exhibit problems with memory and executive functioning and complain of slowness of thought (bradyphrenia). Autonomic dysfunction may become more pronounced, resulting in excessive sweating, which can further interfere with hand function.[29] With the worsening of the disease comes increased difficulty performing ADL and IADL. As speech becomes more impaired, patients become more socially withdrawn. The patient, at this point, usually requires some assistance from others, especially for activities such as socializing with friends, gardening, grocery shopping, meal preparation, laundry and other household tasks, and leisure activities. Hand skills are increasingly impaired for hygiene, dressing, eating, and writing. Safety becomes an issue, and driving becomes more problematic. With progression of symptoms, patients are no long able to continue working outside the home.[30]

In the advanced stage of PD, patients are often wheelchair- or bed-bound and gradually require maximum to total assistance with all activity. Cognition, speech, and swallowing become more impaired. Forty to 75% of PD patients experience pain, frequently in the back and neck and sometimes in the legs.[31] Some patients may lose the ability to communicate verbally, and social isolation is common. The patient's quality of life issues now become paramount as does training the caregiver to most effectively perform his or her role, and treatment focuses on palliative care.[32]

Patients with PD find their symptoms fluctuating hourly and daily. Occupational performance depends on the medications on/off state as well as the patient's physical condition, a situation that often frustrates patients and families alike. A spouse will typically comment, "He was able to brush his teeth yesterday. I don't know why he can't today." Or, "She was walking fine this morning. Now she claims she can't move." Thus it is crucial for members of the health care team to educated patients, families, and caregivers about all aspects of the disease, including the effects of medication, and to provide the physician with feedback on the patient's functional performance.

It is important to keep in mind that all of the issues and challenges that affect an aging population, such as visual impairment, role changes, reduced strength and endurance, reduced activity, and changes at the cellular level are also applicable to the majority of PD patients.[33]

Assessment Tools

Before deciding on assessment tools, the occupational therapist should consider the patient's goals, treatment setting, stage of PD, the patient's age and environment, and how the information will be used. The spouse, companion, family member, or care partner should be included in the process. The occupational therapy assessment of any patient should always include the social context as well as the physical context of activity and skill.

In a medical climate of cost constraints and the limited time allocated for occupational therapy services, the practice setting requires the occupational therapist to move quickly from evaluation to treatment planning to intervention.[34] Strickland[34] points out that the evaluation process should be meaningful to the patient, the efforts relevant to treatment, and the intervention plan appropriate to the patient's occupation.

Trombly[6] suggested that one way to approach the evaluation is for the therapist to first determine the patient's roles and activities prior to the limitations imposed by the disease process and what those roles/activities will be in the future. The therapist must then determine the physical, cognitive, and social requirements needed to carry out these tasks and address those variables that have become problematic.

Knowledge about the patient's everyday activities can provide insight into his or her goals and motivations.[35] Much can be learn by simply asking the patient to describe his or her typical day or ask "How do you spend your day?" The interview and observation are essential to any occupational therapy assessment.

Four instruments frequently used to measure Parkinson's disease are useful tools for the occupational therapist and can be administered in most settings. The Unified Parkinson's Disease Rating Scale (UPDRS), was designed to follow the clinical course of PD over time.[36] It consists of subscales that include: 1) mentation, behavior, and mood; 2) activities of daily living; and 3) motor skills. Particularly applicable to occupational therapist are the ADL and motor sections of the instrument.

Another helpful measure is the Modified Hoehn and Yahr Staging,[37] which classifies PD into six stages with 0 being "no clinical signs evident" to 5 being "wheelchair bound or bedridden unless aided." The Schwab and England Activities of Daily Living Scale[38] is a disability scale that rates ADL ability from 100% (essentially normal) to 0% (vegetative). The Parkinson's Disease Questionaire-39 (PDQ-39)[39-41] measures eight quality of life dimensions specifically related to PD such as mobility, ADL, emotional well-being, and social support. (For more information-specific instruments for PD, see Chapter 3).

Another instrument that can be used to evaluate the PD patient is the Functional Neurological Screening for Basal Ganglia Disorders developed by Gutman and Schonfeld.[42] The Fatigue Severity Scale[43] and the Multidimensional Fatigue Inventory[44] are frequently used to measure fatigue in patients with PD.

Jette developed The Functional Status Index to screen ambulatory patients and established the reliability of its subcomponents.[45] It is useful as a brief self-report of physical, psychological, and social function.

The Kohlman Evaluation of Living Skills (KELS), although initially developed for psychiatric patients, is now widely used with other populations.[46] This interview and task performance test is a quick, effective tool to obtain information on a patient's ability to perform ADL/IADL. Seventeen living skills are tested under the areas of: 1) Self-Care, 2) Safety and Health, 3) Money Management, 4) Transportation and Telephone, and 5) Work and Leisure.

The Assessment of Motor and Process Skills (AMPS)[47] provides information by observing the person doing ADL and IADL and measures process skills (information on sequencing of actions, selection and appropriate use of tools and materials, and adaptation to problems) and motor skills (information on the actions done to move oneself or objects). It takes 30 to 60 minutes to administer and score.[48]

Based on client-centered practice, The Canadian Occupational Performance Measure (COPM)[49] administered as a semi-structured interview, measures occupational performance and satisfaction. Gaudet[50] reported that the COPM can be administered to PD patients in 30 to 40 minutes and recommends that the identification of issues be scored separately for both the on and off medication states.

Canadian occupational therapists also developed The Safety Assessment of Function and the Environment for Rehabilitation (SAFER), a functional and environmental assessment tool to be used with the over-65 age group in the home.[51,52] The SAFER addresses 14 areas of concern and is subdivided into 128 items or functions.

Three separate studies[53-55] validated the Berg Balance Scale[56] as an effective instrument to detect changes in balance in patients with PD.

For fine motor skills, the Pudue Pegboard[57] and the Nine-Hole Peg Test,[58] are effective tools for outcome measurement. The Mini Mental Status Exam[59] is a widely used global assessment to screen for orientation and cognitive deficits and was found by Stern to be a useful indicator of intellectual function in patients with PD.[60] (See Chapter 4 for more on cognitive and visual-perceptual motor assessments.)

Additional areas for evaluation include musculoskeletal, biomechanical, and behavioral factors,[8] passive and active range of motion, muscle tone and strength, transfers, sensation, and vision.

Another assessment method is the use of chronography (timing the activity using a stopwatch). Lyons and Tickle-Degnen recently measured expressive behavior of persons with PD using short segments of video-taped activity.[61] Likert-type scales can also be used (ie, on a scale of 0 to 10 with 0 being none and 10 quite severe, how you would rate your fatigue?).

Assessment and observation will coincide with treatment and is an ongoing process. Knowledge of the patient's medication regime is important and the patient's on or off status during the evaluation should be recorded.

OCCUPATIONAL PERFORMANCE ISSUES

Tremor

Tremor is an involuntary rhythmic oscillation observed in body segments and characterized by specific amplitudes and frequencies.[62] This type of activity has been recorded in the globus pallidus and the subthalamic nucleus of patients with PD who exhibit a

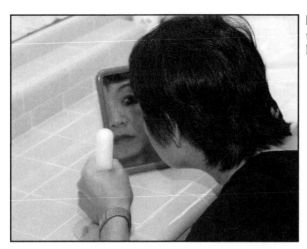

Figure 9-1. The handhold can be used to reduce tremor when performing a one-handed activity.

resting tremor.[63] Frequently disease onset begins with a resting tremor, one of the cardinal signs of the PD.[64,65] Tremors worsen with anxiety, stress, contralateral motor activity, and during ambulation. Because the resting tremor subsides during activity, it seldom interferes with voluntary movement or a patient's ability to perform ADL.[66] If it becomes problematic there are several strategies patients can use such as putting their hands in their pockets or grasping an object such as the "single handhold," (a plastic dowel with a suction cup that adheres to a hard surface) while performing a unilateral activity (Figure 9-1). The tremor responds to levodopa and surgical treatment[64] and is unlikely to lessen due to occupational therapy intervention techniques.[10]

The PD action tremor,[67,68] however, interferes with eating, dressing, grooming, and other tasks involving fine motor control.[69] It can be quite disabling and does not always respond to levadopa therapy.[70] Deuschl and Krack[62] defined the action tremor as "any tremor occurring during voluntary contraction of muscle." This can include the postural, isometric, and kinetic tremors. The postural tremor occurs when a person is voluntarily maintaining a position against gravity.

In a 2001 study of 197 PD patients, Louis and colleagues[71] found an action tremor present in 184 or 93.4%. Fossberg et al[72] suggested that the higher frequency action tremor impairs fine motor movements like buttoning. Other researchers[70] found that it affects dexterity when associated with severe akinesia although the exact relationship between tremor and bradykinesia is unknown. Another study[69] provided evidence that patients in the early stage of PD as well as those in the advanced stage have a voluntary tremor that can interfere with tasks such as using a spoon or drinking from a glass.

Raethjen and colleagues[70] also reported that the action tremor in PD can be quite disabling and found weights to be ineffective in reducing the tremor. In a 2002 study, Meshack and Norman[73] evaluated the effects of weights to reduce the postural tremor in 14 PD patients who were independent in daily activities and did not use assistive devices. For recording the tremor, three devices were used: a built-up spoon that weighed 108 g, a weighted spoon (248 g), and a weighted wrist-cuff (470 g), which was used with the built-up spoon. They found no support for the premise that weighted utensils or weight cuffs reduce the hand tremor in PD patients. (Note that people with PD do not exhibit the same type of postural tremor as found in cerebellar lesions such as multiple sclerosis.)

Figure 9-2. Supporting the arms on a countertop while seated facilitates grooming activities.

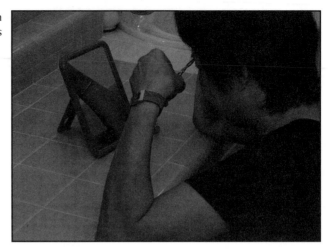

Opinions are mixed on the benefit of applying relaxation as a treatment modality for persons with PD. Although Schenkman and Butler recommend their use,[7] Carr and Shepherd[9] cite lack of evidence as to their effectiveness. In a 2004 study,[74] Ludervald and Poppen concluded that use of EMG biofeedback and relaxation training held promise for older adults with essential tremor (primarily postural and kinetic/action in nature) while performing ADL tasks. Progressive muscle relaxation techniques may also have some benefit for this group of patients, but the evidence is limited. Wood[75] looked at the effects of meditation/relaxation between meditators and nonmeditators on physiological responses during the performance of a fine motor and a gross motor task and found no significant difference.

The author has found that the most helpful intervention to reduce the effects of an action tremor with this patient population is to teach the patient compensatory hand/arm support techniques to eliminate the effects of gravity and to improve limb stability while decreasing the degrees of freedom (number of joints used) when performing ADL. Upper extremity function is usually enhanced with the person seated, especially when postural instability is present. A gross grasp or power grip can be substituted for a three-point grip. When possible, shoulders should be adducted and elbows flexed or the forearms supported on a table or other surface.[76] Both hands can be used to grasp tweezers or an electric shaver while propping the elbow on a sink or countertop (Figure 9-2). Commercial wrist supports, by stabilizing the wrist, sometimes facilitate activities such as applying make-up, brushing teeth, or peeling vegetables (Figure 9-3). When manipulating objects, the patient can maintain his or her hands in a position close to the body rather than handling them at a distance.[9] The occupational therapist can work with the patient to find body postures that limit involuntary movement and provide trunk support and proximal stability when performing ADL.[76]

Because stress is known to worsen tremors and neurological symptoms in general, the psychosocial aspects of the environment, especially for eating, should always be considered. Parkinson's disease can cause slowing of the gastrointestinal tract, resulting in severe constipation, affect swallowing, and lead to poor nutrition. The patient's lifestyle habits and preferences prior to the onset of PD should be considered when assessing the social environment most conducive to food intake. For some, mealtime is a pleasure, dining a leisure activity, whereas others could care less about what they eat. Options for meal-

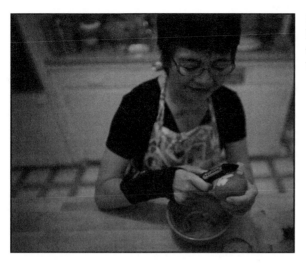

Figure 9-3. Patients with tremors or dyskinesias benefit from sitting with the arms supported to perform a task. A commercial wrist support is sometimes helpful.

time could include dining with family or friends, eating alone, or eating while watching a favorite television program or listening to music. Optimal seating and positioning and a pleasant, peaceful environment will further enhance the process and help make mealtime more enjoyable.[77] As with all activities, a person with PD should never be rushed, and all time constraints involving mealtime should be eliminated (see Sidebar 9-2).

SIDEBAR 9-2: TYPES OF TREMORS SEEN IN PD

- Resting tremor—The most common tremor seen in PD. It is most visible in the upper extremities and occurs when the body part is not voluntarily activated and is completely supported against gravity.

- Postural tremor—Occurs during a sustained muscle contraction and when the person voluntarily maintains a position against gravity.

- Kinetic tremor—Occurs during voluntary movement.

- Action tremor—An enhanced physiologic tremor; higher frequency than resting tremor, and postural and kinetic in nature. Can be very disabling. Occurs less frequently than resting tremor.

- Essential tremor—Dominantly inherited action tremor of the upper extremities that is predominantly postural. Absent at rest.

Dyskinesias

After 5 years of levadopa treatment, about 40% of PD patients will experience fluctuations (on/off effect) and dyskinesias,[78] although the dyskinesias can sometimes occur much earlier.[79] They often take the form of continuous single or mixed movements of chorea, ballism, dystonia, and myoclonus and can be stereotypic. These involuntary movements usually involve the head, trunk, limbs, and sometimes the respiratory muscles.[79] They typically occur when the patient is in the "on" state with levadopa treatment.

In a 1995 single case study, Chung and colleagues[80] found that a 63-year-old male with PD dyskinesias showed some improvement with ADL and reductions in tremor ratings after relaxation training. Shumway-Cook and Woollacott[12] recommended that patients be taught to perform functional movement with decreased effort, because increased effort tends to worsen the involuntary movement. The author has found that limiting the degrees of freedom and the effects of gravity and modifying the environment (ie, consider the type of cup, position of the cup, position of the arm, table height, seat height) are the most useful techniques to overcome the effects of involuntary movement upon ADL.

CASE STUDY 1: MR. SMITH

Mr. Smith was a 60-year-old man with a 12-year history of Parkinson's disease (PD). His neurologist referred him to occupational therapy for consultation, and the sessions occurred in the patient's home. Although Mr. Smith was independent in ADL and IADL, he had developed severe dyskinesias due to levodopa therapy, and he frequently dropped objects. Mr. Smith, who held a doctorate in economics, had adopted a cognitive approach to cope with the problems resulting from PD.

Mr. Smith led an active lifestyle—he operated his own business and enjoyed reading and gardening, and until his Parkinson's symptoms worsened, he had played racquetball and tennis. The nature of his work required him to conduct frequent business meetings with clients and attend formal social functions. He felt that his involuntary movements disconcerted other people and hindered his social life. In social situations people sometimes asked why he was nervous, asked him to be still, and made other comments about his dyskinesias. He was quite adamant that he did not want anyone outside his immediate family to know his diagnosis or even that he had a neurological condition.

Mr. Smith's goals for occupational therapy were twofold: to learn how to decrease spills in the kitchen and to develop a strategy to deal with his disability in social and business situations. When transporting a one-quart carton of milk from the refrigerator to the counter, Mr. Smith frequently dropped the carton due to involuntary twisting and jerking movements. Then, as he poured milk from the carton into a glass, his involuntary movements caused him to spill the liquid onto the floor or countertop. Solutions and strategies were as follows:

The occupational therapist explained the principles of task analysis and discussed how the concept could be use to analyze the problems Mr. Smith encountered in the kitchen and in other ADL/IADL situations.

As Mr. Smith performed these kitchen activities, both he and the occupational therapist analyzed the motions and steps involved in each task, and discussed how he might simplify the movements and position his arms to avoid dropping and spilling. For instance, they both observed that he held the milk carton with one hand at a distance from his body. When he used both hands to grasp the carton, adducted his shoulders, and maintained both arms close to his trunk, he lessened the likelihood of dropping the milk. They also observed that when he poured the milk, he again used his right hand to grasp the carton, extended his arm, and held the glass aloft with his left hand (Figure 9-4). To accomplish the task with greater ease, he set the glass in the sink (to avoid clean-up in case of a spill), adducted his shoulders, and used both hands to pour (Figure 9-5).

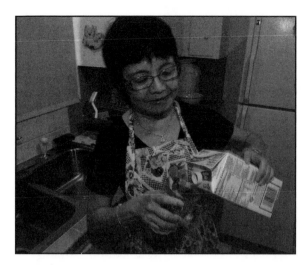

Figure 9-4. Pouring milk using one hand and with the arms extended increases the difficulty of the task.

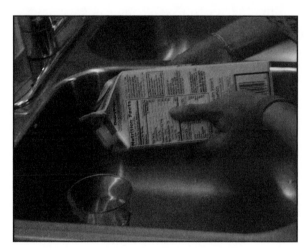

Figure 9-5. The patient sets the glass in the sink to avoid spills, and wears an apron with pockets to carry objects. She uses both hands to pour and supports her arms to reduce involuntary movements.

The occupational therapist asked Mr. Smith to perform the aforementioned tasks using mental rehearsal (he had used the technique in the past for racquetball). She suggested that he use this method daily before attempting kitchen work until mindful movements became routine.

The occupational therapist suggested that Mr. Smith develop stock phrases he could use in response to questions and comments about his involuntary movements. For instance, in response to "Why don't you relax," he might say, "It's out of my control," or "I try not to focus on it" or "I am relaxed." She suggested he use imagery to imagine himself in a social situation, relaxed, and without exhibiting the involuntary movements. He could also visualize himself at a party and responding to an inappropriate comment about his disability using a stock phrase with which he felt comfortable.

They discussed how he could apply task analysis, mental rehearsal, and imagery to his gardening activities.

The occupational therapist encouraged Mr. Smith to attempt more mindful deliberate actions and reduce automatic actions.

The essentials of Mr. Smith's occupational therapy treatment plan included: 1) task analysis, 2) simplification of movements and compensatory body techniques, and 3) use of mental rehearsal/imagery techniques. Upon discharge, it was agreed that Mr. Smith would contact the occupational therapist for follow-up as new/additional challenges occurred.

Dystonia

Dystonia is a "sustained muscle contraction associated with twisting, repetitive, and patterned movements, abnormal postures, or both"[61] and can interfere with all functional activity. Researchers estimate that it occurs in up to 30% of PD patients and is even more frequent in women and in those with young-onset disease. It is more common in the foot (with equinovarus posture and extension of the big toe) but can be seen in the limbs, eyes (blepharospasm), appear as writer's cramp, bent spine (camptocormia), and axial dystonia (scoliosis).[81] It may appear during the "on" or "off" state and can vary among individuals as to location and severity.

Zeuner and colleagues[82] developed a motor training program for treatment of hand dystonia or "writers' cramp." Depending on the pattern of dystonia, patients received flexor finger splints or extensor finger splints on all four digits, excluding the writing finger, to avoid co-contraction. They used a plastic splint with a pen attached for the training finger. In addition, they wore a wrist support and rested the elbow and forearm on a book or cushion. Each finger was training individually by making circles and letters. When patients experienced dystonic posturing, they changed positions or stopped writing. The training resulted in mild objective improvement of handwriting skills.

Handwriting

Patients with PD have difficulty performing well-learned motor tasks, particularly handwriting. Problems include lack of control, abrupt changes of direction, tremor, slowness, hesitation, variability of baseline, and micrographia.[83] Micrographia is a phenomenon whereby as the patient continues to write, the letters grow smaller, that is, stroke size is reduced, but the morphology and style remain intact. In some patients levodopa improves micrographia whereas anxiety and stress worsen the condition.[84,85] Longstaff et al[86,87] suggested the phenomenon is in part an adaptive strategy used to reduce movement variability.

Among the 800 PD patients in the DATATOP cohort, 90 patients reported problems with handwriting and listed handwriting as their most troubling PD symptom.[87] In a study of 27 PD patients and 12 elderly controls, Teulings and colleagues[83] detected incoordination in PD patients involving the finger and wrist, which they concluded might contribute to the handwriting difficulties these patients experience.

Arend et al[85] found that PD patients reduced the stroke size when processing demands (the number of words written) increased. From another study[88] they concluded that PD patients' handwriting performance deteriorated with increased motor load (writing while speaking and performing a subtraction task), and a third study[86] supported their premise that PD patients are unable to modulate force to meet size demands when writing or performing other graphic tasks such as drawing.

Oliveira and colleagues[89] compared 11 PD patients with 14 controls under three conditions: free writing, writing with dots to indicate the required size (visual cues), and writing with verbal reminders ("big"). The PD group increased their letter size significantly with visual cues and auditory reminders.

Teulings and Stelmach[90] found that PD patients without micrographria changed letter size and movement velocity when encouraged to write faster or bigger. In another trial, PD patients increased letter size when writing between parallel lines.[84]

Recently, researchers have applied The Lee Silverman Voice Treatment Technique (LSVT)—which focuses on vocal loudness as a therapeutic intervention for PD patients with dysarthria[91]—to limb movement.[92] This approach, Think Big, teaches patients to perform large amplitude limb movements while focusing on the largeness of the movement.

Preminger et al[93] examined the relationship between keyboarding ability and handwriting proficiency among 63 fifth grade students and found that keyboarding and handwriting might entail different skills. They proposed that using a computer might be a viable alternative for individuals who have difficulty writing.

To determine the proportion of patients who are able to perform basic computer skills and to measure the accuracy of those skills (mouse and keyboard use), Beck et al[94] studied 104 patients diagnosed with PD and other movement disorders. Ninety-six subjects successfully completed data entry tasks and over 70% displayed basic e-mail and Internet skills. Computer data entry was more accurate than handwritten entry. Patients with poorer computer skills were older, less educated, and exhibited more cognitive impairment whereas patients diagnosed with PD did not do as well as those with other movement disorders. However, the results suggested that computer use might be an alternative to handwriting (Sidebar 9-3).

Bradykinesia (Hypokinesia), Akinesia, and Freezing

Bradykinesia/hypokinesia, another cardinal sign of PD and the most disabling symptom in the early stages[64,95] refers to slowness or poverty of movement whereas akinesia is the absence of movement. It represents the loss of automatic movements.[96] Berardelli et al[97] hypothesized that bradykinesia results from a failure of the basal ganglia output to reinforce the cortical mechanisms that prepare and execute the commands to move. Repetitive movements such as brushing teeth, combing hair, and washing the hands tend to slow in amplitude and eventually fade out.[26,98]

Fine motor movements such as buttoning or manipulating small objects are more affected than gross motor movement. Other manifestations occur when the patient is rising from a chair, turning in bed, and transitioning from supine to sit. The classic shuffling gait, reduced arm swing, micrographia, hypophonia, decreased blink, and masked facies are other expressions of bradykinesia.[99,100] Generally, the execution of movement is more impaired than initiation, and problems with initiation are greater when the patient has to self-initiate the movement rather than respond to external stimuli.[101]

Stanley et al[15] suggested a quick method to assess bradykinesia by having the patient sit with both hands resting in his or her lap. Ask him or her to supinate/pronate the forearm as rapidly as possible for about 30 seconds. When bradykinesia is present the movement will slow and break down after a few seconds.

Freezing (motor blocks) refers to the sudden suspension of movement that usually involves gait. It is unknown if this phenomenon represents a severe form of akinesia or is physiologically separate.[95] Patients complain that their feet feel "stuck to the floor," and they experience problems such as walking in crowds, passing through doorways, entering elevators, turning, and walking down narrow isles, such as in a theater or church. Commonly used external cues to overcome freezing include: 1) have the patient visualize a line, a log, or a common object and try to step over it; 2) count aloud and try to move or say "go" before initiating movement; 3) shine a pen light on the floor and try to step over the beam of light; 4) rock back and forth before attempting to move, such as before

SIDEBAR 9-3: TIPS FOR HANDWRITING

- Assume a comfortable writing position and allow plenty of time.
- Eliminate distractions, and avoid talking or engaging in a secondary activity.
- Think "big strokes" when writing.
- Use lined paper.
- Vary the size, shape, and weight of the pen. Try pens with fat grip surfaces and thin grip surfaces. Change pens when your hand tires or your writing becomes increasing illegible. (It's like changing shoes when your feet hurt or tire.)
- Try pens with different types of textured grip surfaces and those with a slick surface. Which ones feel most comfortable between your fingers?
- Change your grip on the pen. Place the pen between your index and middle finger and wrap your thumb around the bottom of the pen for better stabilization and support.
- Is it easier to write with a fine point? A medium point? Practice with a roller pen, ball point pen and felt tip pen. Decide which one works the best.
- Support the elbow. Try supporting the wrist with a commercial support. Remove the metal insert for more flexibility.
- Practice forming big letters prior to writing using mental rehearsal for two or three minutes.
- Try writing between vertical lines or dots drawn on paper.
- Try writing to music. Try both waltz and march tunes and see which works best.
- Try keyboarding or typing instead of writing.

rising from a chair; 5) take a step backward or change directions; 6) Hum a march tune and move to the beat or wear a CD Walkman or MP3 player and activate the music when situations that cause freezing arise; and 7) use a mirror.[7,9,10] Patients with PD frequently report that they find it easier to go up or down stairs rather than walk across a flat surface due to the visual input provided by the stairs.

A study by Bernatzsky and colleagues[102] gave evidence that receptive listening to specific music (drumming) improved the precision of arm and finger movements in patients with PD. In another study,[103] PD subjects who underwent weekly sessions of music therapy for three months showed significant improvement in hypokinesia and significant trends for cutting food, dressing, falling, and freezing at the end of each session.

In a recent study, Hi et al[104] tested 16 PD patients and 16 age-matched controls initiating a task (reaching for a pen and bringing pen to paper) with an auditory cue (bell ring) and without. The cue affected movement kinematics of the PD patients but not the controls. Although their movements were not as smooth, the patients with PD elicited faster, more forceful and more efficient movement with the auditory cue.

In a study of hand preshaping while grasping objects of different shapes of 10 PD patients and 8 age-matched controls,[105] the PD patients delayed grasping the objects until they could actually see their hands.

Most of the studies involving external cuing have been done on gait, but the same techniques can be applied to upper extremity tasks as well. In a 2005 systematic review, Lim and colleagues[106] found only 2 of 24 studies to be randomized controlled trials. They reported that only one "high-quality" study, which focused on auditory rhythmical cueing, indicated that walking speed can be positively influenced. It is also unclear if techniques performed in the clinic transfer to the home and community. In the studies they examined, types of cues used included floor markers (lines, stripes), verbal cues/ instructions, auditory rhythms, metronomes, march music, strobe lights, and a laser beam stick.

Recently, Suteerawattananon et al,[107] in a study of 24 PD patients, found that auditory cues (a metronome beat) improved cadence, but visual cues (brightly colored parallel lines on the floor) improved stride length. Combined auditory and visual cues showed no improvement over using each cue alone. Morris et al[108] found that PD patients demonstrated the ability to maintain a normal gait with both visual and attentional strategies.

To be of benefit, external cues and attentional strategies should carry over outside the clinic and into everyday life. Melnick[109] reported that one of her patients tossed pennies on the ground in front of him and stepped over them as he walked. Another observed the movement of a person walking beside him as a cue to move his feet.

Turnbull[110] related how the comedian Terry Thomas hid chocolate around his house, so that when he froze at a doorway he would think about the candy on the other side of the door, "unsticking" himself so he could pass through. Turnbull described other patients who carried objects such as rocks or crushed paper they could toss on the ground to step over should the need arise.

The major drawback with all of these techniques is that the benefits cannot be sustained unless the patient integrates them into his or her movement patterns and thus into daily activities. Turnbull[110] pointed out that because more permanent gains occur when the techniques are "learned," as ADL skills deteriorate, components of the activity (ie, tying shoes, buttoning, dressing, standing, rolling) can be practiced and relearned in accordance with Schmidt's learning theory.[13] This involves the cognitive phase (the therapist explains the skill such as rising from a chair) and the practice phase (repetition of the movement) whereby the therapist provides feedback so that motor learning can occur. Only movement components the patient performs incorrectly need be practiced and then reintegrated into the overall movement. Turnbull[110] emphasized that the patient must be convinced the new skills are worth acquiring and be involved in the decision making and goal setting aspects of the treatment program.

Carr and Shepherd[9] recommended that PD patients practice difficult tasks by cognitively "getting the idea of the movement" so they can develop strategies to overcome the problem.

Occupational therapists can play a major role in adapting the home and work environment to facilitate normal movement and promote safety. Beyond recommending durable medical equipment such as tub transfer benches and raised toilet seats and freeing the space of environment hazards such as throw rugs and other obstacles, patients and their families can be taught to use floor tiles for stepping, place lines on the floors to provide visual cues and post signs near doorways to provide attentional reminders or cues (such as visualize stepping over a log) to facilitate functional movement in the home. Risers under chairs and beds, lift chairs and lift cushions, and armchairs (Figure 9-6) can ease the transition from sit to stand. Patients frequently report that satin sheets and/or pajamas make it easier for them to move in bed (Sidebar 9-4).

Figure 9-6. A high chair with arms eases sit to stand.

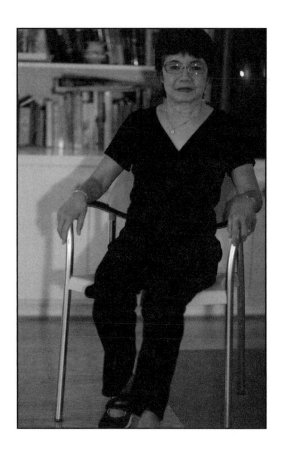

Dual Task Performance

People with PD typically have difficulty performing two tasks at the same time such as walking and carrying on a conversation, ironing and watching television, walking and removing a wallet from a purse or pocket, styling the hair with a brush while using a hair dryer, and flexing the elbow and squeezing the thumb and index finger at the same time.[7,9,111-113] This deficit causes frustration and stress for patients, and increases the length of time necessary to perform combined activities such as eating, dressing, bathing, and toileting. Bond and Morris[112] found that PD patients with moderate disability experienced difficulty and showed deterioration in gait speed when they were required to walk and attend to a complex visual motor task involving the upper extremities (carrying a tray with four plastic glasses). The beneficial effects of visual and attentional cueing disappeared with the performance of added tasks and patients required constant oversight to sustain the effect.

Rochester and colleagues[114] indicated that other factors compound the problems with dual and multiple task performance such as impaired executive function, depression, anxiety, and fatigue. Maintaining balance and coping with environmental distractions (furniture, floor coverings, obstacles, people, etc) place increased demands upon attentional resources. In their study of 20 PD patients and 10 controls, the PD subjects demonstrated significantly slower gait speed and reduced step length when performing concurrent cognitive and multiple tasks in a home environment that increased their fall risk. In a follow-up study,[115] PD subjects benefited from external auditory cues (a device worn on a belt delivering an auditory tone via an earphone) while performing more complex functional activities. Arend and colleagues[88] found that PD patients were more affected by the motor component of a dual task than by the mental component.

SIDEBAR 9-4: HOME SAFETY TIPS

- Install illuminated light switches. Light floors or stairways and use nightlights. Arrange furniture so that lamp switches/light switches are within easy reach.

- Decrease the temperature setting on hot water heaters to 120 degrees or lower or install temperature-limiting mixer valves on tubs and showers. Check water temperature by hand before entering the bath or shower.

- Install touchless faucets with preset temperatures.

- Keep a fire extinguisher in the kitchen, and learn how and when to use it. Install smoke detectors.

- Avoid wearing loose clothing when cooking. Long sleeves are more likely to catch on pot handles and are more like to catch fire than short sleeves.

- Arrange for good lighting over stove, sink, and kitchen work areas, especially where food is cut or sliced.

- Post emergency numbers in visible areas and near the telephone.

- Make sure you have access to a telephone if you fall. If possible, carry a cell phone in your pocket. Arrange furniture so you can reach the telephone without getting out of bed.

- For those who live alone, an emergency response service provides a safety net.

- Keep a flashlight handy.

- Place switches and thermostats no higher than 48" from the floor, electrical outlets no lower than 27".

- Install grab bars in bathrooms and hand rails along hallways and on both sides of stairways.

- Lower or remove thresholds.

- Arrange furniture to avoid the use of extension cords. Arrange cords against walls where people can't trip over them.

- Remove throw rugs and/or use only those with slip-resistant backing.

Wu and Hallett[116] presented PD patients with a dual task involving letter counting and found that after training, most of them could perform at the level of normal subjects. They concluded that the ability to perform the dual task is not totally lost and, with proper training patients can execute some simultaneous movements correctly.

O'Shea et al[111] suggested teaching PD patients to avoid performing dual tasks involving gait and to teach them about the safety risks involved in performing a complex activity while walking. Some actions are obviously hazardous—such as walking across a street and searching for one's car keys in a purse or pocket—and should be avoided. When objects must be carried, patients can be taught to adapt compensatory methods such as placing items in a back pack, waist pack, or pocket. Therapists can teach their patients attentional strategies—focusing on taking big steps, focusing attention on the task, not letting the mind wander, and avoid talking while performing a dual task. Simultaneous tasks involving the upper extremities (shaving, styling hair, grooming) can be performed more effectively and safely in a seated position.

Therapists can help patients and their families analyze dual and multiple tasks that are essential to daily living and determine the most efficient and safest techniques to aid performance. When appropriate, treatment can focus on having the patient practice performing activities while using compensatory strategies, although to date no research has been conducted to determine if this method is effective. At the very least, PD patients and their families can profit from being made aware of the difficulties and potential hazards posed by executing simultaneous tasks.

Sequential Movements

Motor sequencing, "a complex action involving the execution of different movements in a prescribed temporal sequence,"[117] is also impaired in patients with PD. Patients have difficulty executing sequential actions such as moving from sit to stand, rolling in bed, dressing, and making a salad.[8,60,118-120] When a person with PD performs a sequential movement, the interval between movements takes longer and sometimes he or she is unable to perform the shift from one movement to the next.[118]

There is evidence to suggest[60] that the sequencing problems might be an intellectual impairment associated with higher-order motor control of sequential and predictive voluntary movement and not just related to the motor symptoms of PD. Furthermore, the basal ganglia might aid in the monitoring of ongoing movement and may inform the patient when to move from one portion of the motor plan to the next. However, Benecke et al[118] suggested that the difficulty experienced by PD patients when trying to perform two rapid sequential movements is a deficit in the capacity to switch from one motor program to another within an overall motor plan. Work by Samuel and colleagues[121] hypothesized that PD patients can switch to circuits involved in facilitating cued movement to overcome difficulties in generating volitional movements.

Cahn et al[122] found in a study of 39 PD patients that executive functioning, in particular sequencing, was an independent predictor of their ability to perform IADL. In a study looking at the practice effects of a three-dimensional sequential task, Smiley-Oyen et al[123] found that PD patients improved their performance both in planning and executing the movements, and movement time for the overall sequence improved, although not as much as in the control group. Wu and Hallett[116] also found that PD patients could improve their ability on a sequencing task after training.

Curtis et al[124] looked at the effects of an exercise training program on the performance of a functional task that involved sequential and simultaneous movement components. The program consisted of exercises that challenged postural control and coordination of multiple movement components. Some of the exercises combined movement of multiple body parts such as arm elevation and neck/trunk extension, others involved transitional movements, and others emphasized balance, coordination, strength, and endurance. Performance improvements in the patients (particularly those with bradykinesia) appeared to indicate "enhanced postural control or coordination of sequential and simultaneous movement components."

Yekutiel[125] pointed out that PD patients have difficulty with whole body movement. In a non-randomized clinical control trial, she had patients practice whole body movement while throwing and catching, sitting, kneeling, and half-kneeling and had them develop and practice strategies for difficult activities such as getting up in the night. She also taught biomechanical explanations for normal movement and instructed patients in new movement strategies such as visualizing the corner of a bed as a continuous curve instead of two paths at right angles. Results of the program indicated improvement in speed on mobility tasks such as sit to stand. Elements of this program can be incorporated into a therapy plan for patients exhibiting the above type of deficits.

Agostino and colleagues[126] found that PD patients were slower in execution of movements and had problems transitioning from one movement to the next. The PD patients also had more difficulty with individual finger movement than with gross hand grasp movement. These findings indicate that occupational therapists can train patients who demonstrate problems with finger tapping to use a gross grasp or power grip instead of a three-point grip involving only the first three digits. In the home, lever handles can be placed on faucets and doors, and other adaptations can be made as needed. An adapted key hold or pliers might aid in key turning and a button hook can hasten dressing.

Georgiou et al[127] reported that patients with PD were best able to shift between subcomponents of a movement sequence when auditory cues (use of a metronome) were given late in the movement cycle. Other researchers[128] suggested that the best methods to facilitate sequencing are modeling and verbal and mental rehearsal.

Schenkman[129] recommended teaching a single strategy, break the task into manageable parts, provide simple verbal cues, and use frequent repetitions without attempts to generalize the learning to another activity. Instructions for rolling in bed might include, "Bend your hips and knees, drop your knees to the side, reach across your body with your arm, and roll on to your side."

Swinnen et al[20] in a study where PD subjects performed a bilateral triangle drawing task involving the sequential performance of subcomponents, found that patients made substantial improvements in movement as a result of practice. Researchers in the Netherlands[130] developed a protocol to teach PD patients alternative strategies to rise from a chair, turn while walking, turn in bed, and getting in and out of bed. They broke complex movement patterns into separate, simple sequential movements and taught the patients to consciously execute the movements without time constraints. During training, the researchers required the patients to memorize the separate steps in detail and to verbalize the strategies without performing them. The patients used mental practice before physically practicing the task. Verbalizing each step prior to execution required them to perform the movements more consciously, and when they made errors, they analyzed their actions. Results proved the training successful, but the positive effects were activity specific and did not transfer to other activities of daily living. The researchers concluded that functional gains can be accomplished when training is task specific (Sidebar 9-5).

Rigidity

Rigidity, one of the cardinal features of PD, is the increased resistance of a joint to passive movement. Although patients complain of stiffness and an inability to relax their muscles, rigidity does not appear to play a large role in the disability experienced by persons with PD,[101] although it may increase energy expenditure and be involved in feelings of fatigue.[43]

Henneberg[131] evaluated the effects of low-frequency muscle stimulation (15 minutes of treatment 2 times a day for 4 weeks) on 180 PD patients who experienced pain and tension due to rigidity in the neck muscles. Improvement occurred in 82% of the cohort, indicating this might be a viable treatment intervention.

Although treatment methods such as PNF patterns,[132] Bobath therapy,[133] relaxation, rhythmatic and auditory cues have been used to treat rigidity, there is no evidence for their effectiveness beyond an immediate one, and there is no evidence of carry-over into functional performance.[9,134] Morris[10] pointed out that the neural component of rigidity does not appear to compromise voluntary movement and suggested that therapists should not spend treatment time directed at attempting to reduce it—as was done in the 1950s and 1960s. The extent to which it contributes to overall movement dysfunction is

SIDEBAR 9-5: TIPS FOR TRAINING PD PATIENTS IN ADL STRATEGIES

- Reorganize the movement into steps that require simple single movements or combinations of simple movements.
- Demonstrate the correct movements and actions for the patient.
- Ask the patient to verbalize each step as he/she observes the therapist perform the action.
- Have the patient mentally rehearse the task prior to attempting it physically. This will also aid in cognitive execution of the activity.
- Discuss difficulties the patient experiences when attempting the task. Have the patient analyze mistakes before attempting the movement a second time.
- Allow adequate time for performance of the activity. PD patients should not be made to feel hurried or rushed.
- For maximum learning to occur, alternate practice of one task, such as donning a shirt, with another, such as donning shoes.
- Work with patient and family to plan ADL's during medication "on" time.

undetermined.[8] Fortunately, levodopa is an effective treatment.[135] Instructing the patient and family in an exercise program emphasizing flexibility and encouraging other types of exercise such as swimming, Tai Chi, and yoga are perhaps the most effective nonpharmachological interventions.

Hand Skills

In addition to exhibiting reduced wrist and finger coordination,[83] studies have shown that PD patients have abnormally high grip forces (holding a cup) and require more time than normal subjects to lift an object (bringing the cup to the mouth), particularly lighter loads.[136] Bradykinesia affects hand function, and the PD patient's difficulty performing sequential movements impedes many daily activities noted previously. Treatment strategies can include having the patient mentally rehearse the action, verbalizing the steps involved in the action, performing parts of the action before moving to whole performance, and providing visual input. Practice to improve hand skills should involve the ADL task itself (ie, fastening buttons, zipping zippers, tying shoes, writing practice) as there is no evidence in the literature that skills gained from performing tabletop activities and pegboard tasks transfer to the real world.

Striatal Hand

In the hand, dystonia can result in the striatal hand deformity,[137] a deformity involving the wrist and fingers. This condition is very disabling and is sometimes mistaken for rheumatoid arthritis (RA), however, unlike RA, there is no swelling, stiffness, or inflammation.[138,139] Typically, the fingers ulnarly deviate, flex at the metacarpophalengal joints,

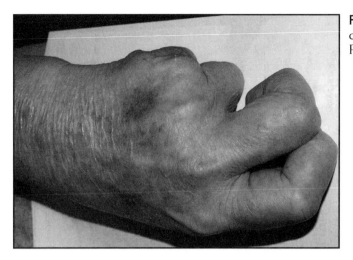

Figure 9-7. "Striatal hand" is a common deformity associated with Parkinson's disease.

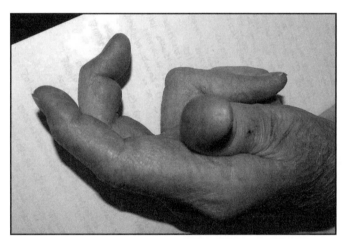

Figure 9-8. "Striatal hand" is often mistaken for arthritic joint deformities.

and hyperextend at the proximal interphalangeal joints, limiting normal function. Fixed, painful contractures frequently develop, most often in the advanced stages of PD, but they can occur relatively early. Despite the distorted posture, the joints themselves remain unaffected. Clawlike hand deformities and boutonniere deformities have been described. The malformations have also been linked to spasm and rigidity, but the exact mechanism remains unclear[137] (see Figures 9-7 through 9-9).

Prevention of hand deformity involves training the patient and family in stretching methods for the wrist and hand. Aggressive intervention should occur as soon as the distorted posture first manifests itself. When the therapist explains the phenomenon, its consequences, and the rationale for treatment to the patient and family, there is greater potential for compliance. The patient should be fit with a functional position splint and

Figure 9-9. "Striatal hand" is a common deformity associated with Parkinson's disease.

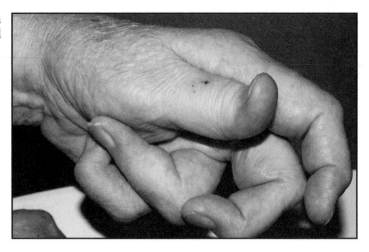

provided with a wearing schedule that is compatible with his or her lifestyle and environment. The patient and family should continue with active and passive range of motion for the wrist and hand and perform other stretching exercises as instructed (see the next section on Musculoskeletal Limitations).

If the patient resides in a nursing facility, the application of a splint is more problematic. Unless the staff is trained in the proper application and can be counted on to apply the splint properly and observe skin precautions, another positioning device such as a hand cone and an intension range of motion program (with family involvement) might be an (albeit lesser) option. It goes without saying that the patient should always be encouraged to actively use the affected hand as much as possible, and the occupational therapist can suggest functional activities to facilitate wrist and finger extension.

Musculoskeletal Limitations

The effects of normal aging include loss of both the number and size of muscle fibers and an increase in connective tissue and fat within the muscles resulting in reduced strength, flexibility, and reaction time. The forward head posture and rounded shoulders typically seen in PD patients are also common age-related changes that occur in the axial skeleton.[140] Typically, as PD patients experience disease progression, there is loss of range of motion (ROM) of the extremities and mobility of the truck.[141] In a survey of 150 patients with PD and 60 matched controls,[142] 43% of the PD patients reported a history of shoulder disturbance. Frozen shoulder occurred in 12.7% of the study patients, and in 8% of the patients frozen shoulder was a presenting feature of PD which the researchers postulated was secondary to akinesia. Patients with bradykinesia and tremor were more likely to have limitations in both upper and lower extremity range of motion, and these limitations were correlated with difficulty performing ADL.

The typical stooped posture assumed by PD patients and their increasingly sedentary lifestyle contribute to postures of flexion, which in turn lead to muscle length changes and loss of musculoskeletal flexibility.[7] These impairments affect the patient's mobility, balance, respiration, swallowing, cardiovascular output, ability to perform ADL/IADL, and contribute to their total physical disability.[143]

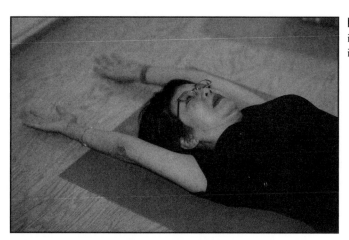

Figure 9-10. Therapists should instruct patients with "striatal hand" in range of motion techniques.

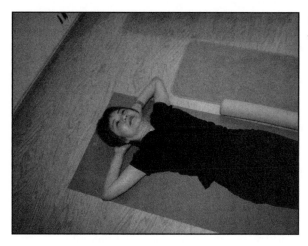

Figure 9-11. Mrs. W. performs shoulder stretches as part of her daily routine.

The occupational therapy treatment plan should include patient/family education about the consequences of reduced flexibility and a preventive exercise program designed to enhance flexibility and incorporate postures that promote extension, thoracic expansion, and deep breathing. To counter the overall flexed posture, Carr and Shepherd[9] recommended having the patient lie in supine on a firm surface and stretch the upper extremities and trunk flexors by actively raising and lowering the arms, using a roll along the spine to encourage extension. The author has successfully used this technique with motor neuron disease patients by additionally having the patient hold his or her arms fully extended for thirty seconds (Figure 9-10). Another useful stretch is to have the patient lie in supine and clasp the hands, extend the arms, and abduct the shoulders (Figure 9-11). A vertical roll placed under the cervical and thoracic spine while the patient is resting provides passive scapular abduction.[144,145] A home program should include instructing the family in upper quadrant stretches. (For more information, see Chapter 6.)

Driving

A number of studies have looked at the driving ability of persons with PD. Zesiewicz et al[146] tested 39 PD patients and 25 controls on a driving simulator. Findings showed that the PD patients had significantly more driving simulator collisions than age-matched controls. Patients with more severe disease were more likely to have accidents. The researchers postulated that cognitive as well as motor decline may have contributed to driving difficulties.

Grace and colleagues[147] found that drivers with PD "distinguished themselves from other drivers by a head turning deficiency," and that driving performance in the PD patients was related to disease severity, neuropsychological measures, and specific motor symptoms—axial rigidity and postural instability.

In another study to determine how PD affects driving performance, Wood and colleagues[148] assessed 25 PD patients and 21 age-matched controls in an automatic dual brake vehicle on the open road in traffic conditions with a driving instructor and an occupational therapist. The PD subjects were less safe than the controls and made significantly more errors in lane keeping and lane changing, reversing, parking, monitoring of their blind spot, and negotiating traffic light–controlled intersections. They exhibited more problems with steering and moving their feet between pedals and demonstrated poor attention at traffic junctions, poor road positioning, and poor negotiation of roundabouts. The authors concluded that currently used clinical disease markers do not adequately reflect features of PD that are associated with unsafe driving.

The authors made several recommendations applicable to occupational therapy intervention. The therapist can: 1) Advise the patient and family about the potential impact of PD on driving performance, 2) Monitor patients regularly and teach compensatory strategies, 3) Perform driving assessments to determine fitness for driving and/or the need for driving rehabilitation, and 4) Use targeted interventions that address specific areas of difficulty known to be associated with PD.

Stolwyk et al[149] and colleagues tested 18 patients in the mild to moderate states of PD and 18 controls in a driving simulator under 4 experimental conditions. Patients with PD demonstrated problems with using advanced information to internally adjust their driving performance and relied on external cues. They also had more difficulty adapting their driving behavior to changing road and traffic conditions. The PD patients, as compared to the controls, approached traffic signals at lower speeds, decelerated later, and had more difficulty stopping in time. They drove around curves at a slower speed, had difficulty maintaining a constant lateral position, and were more likely to run through traffic signals.

In a 2003 paper, Homann et al[150] reviewed the literature on driving and PD and found that patients' most commonly perceived problems while driving included motor fluctuations, dyskinesias, difficulties with managing pedals, and difficulties assessing distance proportions. But patients often claimed that tremor and dyskinesias lessened when they focused their attention on driving, thus (they felt) made driving safer and easier.

Homann's review[150] revealed that driving is a complex activity performed in an ever changing environment and requires cognitive and psychomotor functions affected by PD including perception, information processing, decision making, and maintaining attention. Driving is particularly problematic for PD patients who have difficulty with dual task performance, which taxes short term and non-verbal memory, vision, and visual-spatial-perceptual functions.

Parkinson's disease also causes visual dysfunction, which is likely to further compromise a patient's ability to drive safely.[151] Problems include specifically reduced spatial contrast sensitivity as well as impairment of the central visual system, and this dysfunction may worsen performance on cognitive tasks. Uc and colleagues[151] found that PD patients scored significantly worse on visual and cognitive tests as compared with an elderly control group. Furthermore, reduced contrast sensitivity contributed to deficits in perceptual motor skills and attention. These results suggest that a visual screening should be included in an initial occupational therapy assessment. Depth perception, which is critical for driving, can be screened by holding two identical objects at eye level and moving one in relation to the other. Ask the patient to designate which one appears closer.[12] Patients who require comprehensive visual testing should be referred to their neurologist or ophthalmologist.

When concerns about safe driving arise, the patient can be referred to an occupational therapist trained in driver rehabilitation. In addition, the American Association of Retired Persons (AARP) conducts driver safety programs in most cities and the state Department of Motor Vehicles may have a drivers' evaluation program or offer special licensing alternatives. The American Automobile Association (AAA) offers senior drivers a computer program called Roadwise Review: A Tool to Help Seniors Drive Safely Longer. It allows older drivers to test mental and physical abilities required for safe driving and helps them determine changes they might make in their driving. It also offers tips for improving skills needed to operate a vehicle and provides suggestions to address more serious issues. In addition, the program suggests ways to compensate for declining functional abilities.

The occupational therapist can initiate discussions with the patient and family about alternative methods of transportation and provide them with a list of community resources such as services for senior citizens, public transportation—including those services for the disabled—and taxi services, and organizations that provide volunteer drivers for grocery shopping, medical appointments, and other necessities. For many, driving symbolizes independence, and most US residents rely on the automobile to engage in the life of the community and carry out their instrumental activities of daily living. A study by Elliott and Velde[152] revealed that driving was one of the significant occupational losses reported by PD patients. Before recommending driving cessation, every effort should be made to help patients compensate for the limitations imposed by Parkinson's disease. (For more information, see Chapters 5 and 14.)

SELECTED TREATMENT INTERVENTIONS

Mental Imagery

Mental imagery, also referred to as mental rehearsal, mental practice, and creative visualization, is the act of cognitively reproducing or visualizing a physical activity or scene without any corresponding motor output.[153] Findings by Jackson and colleagues using positron emission tomography demonstrated that learning a sequential motor task through motor imagery practice produces cerebral functional changes similar to those observed after physical practice of the same task.[153] That is, cortical areas activated during the imagination of a movement are similar to those activated during its actual performance.[154]

Mental practice, whereby the internal reproduction of a motor act is repeated over time with the intent of improving performance, has long been used by athletes, pianists, and even surgeons. Health care practitioners have used the techniques with cancer patients, and it is frequently a component of alternative and complementary medicine. Few attempts have been made to apply the technique to rehabilitation.[155] Results of a 1985 study by Fansler et al[156] of community elderly women found that mental practice combined with physical practice significantly improved their balance time. Yue and Cole[157] reported improved isometric muscle strength in healthy individuals after mental practice. Although studies show that physical practice is superior to mental practice, there is evidence that mental practice is superior to no practice at all and that physical and mental practice combined can yield the best results.[155]

Mental imagery techniques can be practiced externally, from a third person viewpoint (like watching home movies), or internally (from a first person viewpoint), which promote kinesthetic feelings of movement.[158] Jackson et al[155] and others[159] suggested that internally driven images may be more effective and yield better results.

Morris,[10] Turnbull,[110] and Carr/Shepherd[9] all recommended mental rehearsal as a therapeutic intervention for patients with PD. Patients need to be cognitively intact with adequate abstraction and visual spatial function. To date, few studies have been conducted using mental practice techniques with PD patients,[160,161] and both indicated that although PD patients can generate conscious motor representations, they might have difficulty maintaining the mental images and translating them into motor actions. However, Yaguez and colleagues presented their subjects with a new rather than a familiar task and provided only ten minutes of training rather than training and repetitive practice over time.[161] In another study of 23 PD patients, Tamir et al[162] compared the results of physical therapy only with a combination of physical therapy and mental practice. The combined treatment group made more gains, especially in the reduction of bradykinesia.

Interestingly, in a study of hemi-Parkinson's patients, Dominey and colleagues found that patients exhibited both motor imagery asymmetry and motor asymmetry, that is their imagined movement was slowed as well as the executed movement.[160] In another study of stroke patients, both executed and imagined movements took longer with the affected limbs than with the unaffected limbs.[163] Both studies reinforce the belief that motor execution and motor imagery share common motor circuits.[155]

Suinn[164] raised the question as to whether mental practice extends physical practice by involving the right hemisphere in acquisition-storage that might lead to automatic performance. If this is the case, mental practice would have increased significance for PD patients because they have particular difficulty with automatic movements.

There are multiple benefits to using mental imagery as a therapeutic strategy. Mental imagery is a cost effective intervention that allows patients to practice exercises and activities at home and between therapy visits without the need for specialized equipment.[155] The technique allows the patient to rehearse a task without the threat of incurring fatigue or risking a fall. For immobile patients, it is a means of exercise/activity that increases the possibility of keeping the neuroanatomical circuits functional. It is an effective means of practice when a therapist, a family member, or a caregiver is unavailable to assist or supervise the patient.[165] Mental imagery provides a holistic approach to treatment, a method occupational therapists have long championed, recognizing that the mind can not be separated from the body. There is evidence that humans thought in images long before the development of language.[166]

The Movement Imagery Questionnaire—Revised[167] is an effective instrument therapists can use to test a patient's ability to visualize. Additionally, Jackson et al[155] suggested two techniques clinicians can use to assess a patient's ability to perform mental rehearsal. The time it takes for the patient to perform the imagined task should reflect his or her motor deficit, and the time it takes for the patient to perform the imagined task or movement should be the same from one trial to the next. He proposed that mental practice might enhance long-term retention of a skill.[168]

Imagery techniques can be applied and if necessary, modified, for patients with Parkinson's disease. In most studies, the participants practiced mental imagery only on one occasion and for a brief period of time. Many of the studies have focused on physical exercise or graphic activities such as drawing, but the techniques can be applied to a medley of tasks and situations such as ADL/IADL, social interactions, relaxation, pain control, memory enhancement, and freezing episodes. The author has successfully used imagery to facilitate tasks such as bathing, hygiene, and meal preparation, to address fatigue issues, and to help patients deal with situations involving social embarrassment. Mental imagery can be a particularly potent tool when combined with task analysis.

To date, there are no studies that support the optimal length of time for practice or a specific protocol to facilitate performance, but there are suggestions from the literature to apply when using mental imagery. Warner and McNeill[169] pointed out the need, frequently cited,[13,159] for vivid color images, visualizing a positive outcome, an active rather than passive mental process, and imagining the movement/task properly. Schmidt recommended having the learner imagine several different tasks in the same session and to use random imagery for optimal learning. The movement should always unfold in real time.[13] Jackson et al[168] suggested that, for people with motor deficits, a simple task is easier to learn than a complex one, and that patients should first practice the task correctly so they can develop a good motor representation of the skill.

Murray[170] offers specific mental imagery for tennis players that can be adapted by occupational therapists teaching patients a skill such as walking from the refrigerator to the kitchen counter while carrying a carton of milk. He recommends lying in a quiet room and looking at pictures or videos of the movement(s) prior to using imagery. Other suggestions include: 1) Make the images as realistic as possible and include all of the senses and the emotional context, 2) Practice regularly and maintain a positive attitude that imagery works, 3) Stay focused and picture yourself accomplishing the feat from the mind's eye, and 4) Imagine perfection.

When learning a new skill the patient can, if necessary, break the task into key parts, pay special attention to those that pose more difficulty, and attend to transitions before moving as soon as possible to whole task performance. The goal is to reach the point where the patient is kinesthetically rehearsing the entire performance sequence in real time from inside his or her own body.

The author recommends that the initial session be no longer than 2 or 3 minutes. Depending on the patient's endurance, ability to attend, and his or her motivation, the practice time can be increased to ten minutes. Korn[166] advises using all five senses rather than visualization alone to create the image and recommends daily practice. The image should be dynamic (moving) rather than static (still).

Adaptive Strategies

Adaptive strategies are a means to help patients deal with the physical, cognitive, and psychosocial limitations imposed by PD. Poole[171] categorized adaptive strategies as techniques and equipment and routines and social supports. Kielhofner,[172] in his *Model of Human Occupation*, pointed out that environmental factors are critical to whether and how impairments affect performance. The physical environment can be adapted to facilitate patients' independence in ADL and IADL and allow them to participate in the life of the community. Environmental modifications can be simple (moving a piece of furniture) or more complex (widening a doorway). Poole[171] pointed out that the environment can support or hinder a patient's ability to engage in daily occupations, and that there are multiple factors—from social supports to environmental designs—involved in determining the patient's level of engagement in everyday occupations. Christiansen[173] emphasized that the rehabilitation team and the person receiving the care must decide which approaches to employ based on the patient's abilities, values, and personal and social circumstances.

A study by Cumming et al[174] found that visits by occupational therapists to the home to assess for environmental hazards and recommend home modifications can help prevent falls among older persons. Two prospective studies of falls in PD patients found the fall rate to be 68% and 51%, respectively.[175,176] Patients with PD had a nine-fold increased fall risk over healthy controls,[176] and usually fell indoors. Grimbergen et al[177] found that PD patients often fall during transfers and while performing simultaneous tasks. Yekutiel[125] had patients record the time and location of falls on maps of their apartments and consequently directed therapy toward the circumstances and locations of the falls and helped patients develop visual strategies to negotiate furniture. (For more information on falls, see Chapter 8).

Equipment for safety and mobility can reduce falls and minimize the patient's reliance on a caregiver or significant other. Doorways can be widened to accommodate walkers and wheelchairs. Substituting a pocket door for a swing door can increase the maneuvering space in the bathroom. A swing away door hinge increases the door width by about 2", or an additional 1" clearance can be achieved by removing the lower portion of the door stops from the jam.[178] Prefabricated ramps are available through some companies, or ramps can be constructed.

Many institutions and even communities are implementing universal design. The Rehabilitation Engineering and Research Center on Universal Design at the University at Buffalo, SUNY, has a comprehensive exhibit, including designs for the home and community and adaptive aids that can be viewed at www.ap.buffalo.edu/idea/ubweb/page1.htm.

Several studies have been done to determine PD patients' use of adaptive equipment. In a study following up on 62 patients with PD 10 months after they had received adaptive devices, Beattie and Caird[179] found that most patients thought them helpful. Aids for bathing (rails, mats, bathboards, bathseats) were reported as being most necessary. Few patients used aids for feeding (plates, cups, utensils, Dycem), but the majority who did found them useful. Clarke and colleagues[180] surveyed 72 PD patients and found that 64% used some type of assistive device, the most common being mobility and bathing aids. Clausen[181] surveyed 30 PD patients on the use of adaptive devices and found an 86% usage rate. Patients were more likely to use bathing equipment (25 of 30 patients) and ambulation devices (13 of 30 patients) and less like to use aids for toileting, eating, and dressing.

Patients are more likely to use a piece of equipment if they perceive both a need and a benefit and if they have been properly trained in its use. Assistive devices such as button hooks and reachers can be advantageous for some PD patients. Other items such as plate guards, curved utensils, scoop plates, and pizza cutters are sometimes helpful (Figure 9-12).

Because fatigue occurs in 40 to 56% of PD patients,[182] motion economy and energy conservation training are integral to the treatment plan. Patients and their families can be taught motion analysis to reduce the number of movements necessary to perform a task. Poole[171] recommended that patients with movement disorders who fatigue easily may need to plan three different strategies for toileting. For example, one for getting on the toilet using grab bars, another using a sliding board transfer, and another using a spouse or caregiver for physical support.

Because patients with PD tend to move slowly and need longer periods of time to carry out their daily activities, they can also benefit from time management concepts and suggestions on how to organize their space for maximum efficiency. This should include finding a table or counter that will allow them to rest their forearms and/or prop their elbows to perform upper extremity activities at an optimum work height. The occupa-

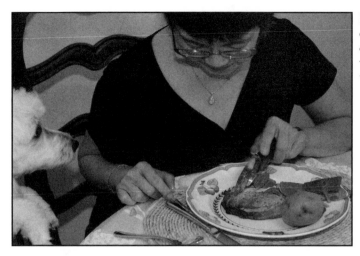

Figure 9-12. Although a pizza cutter can sometimes help with cutting meat, asking the person with PD to hurry can make the task more difficult to perform.

tional therapist can work with patients and their families to help them plan their basic ADL during their "on" medication times.

For patients with visual deficits, adaptations can be made in accordance with low vision protocols such as appropriate lighting, color contrasts, clocks with large dials, large print telephones, and so on.

The National Parkinson Foundation offers a myriad of patient publications, including booklets on activities of daily living,[183] medications, speech, and psychosocial issues that can be ordered from their Web site at www.parkinson.org.

Gardening

Gardening offers opportunities for patients with PD to remain active, increase flexibility, and improve strength, coordination, and balance. Gardening also provides an outlet for creativity, stress relief, and offers other untold benefits. Relf[184] points out that Benjamin Rush advocated digging in the soil in the 18th century, and horticulture therapy was first widely used as a treatment for emotional disorders in the United States and Europe.

VandenDolder and colleagues[185] reported on a horticulture therapy program created for patients with PD in an outpatient day center. Raised flower beds and adapted garden tools helped patients with limited mobility compensate for lack of reach, and graded activities with sensory and tactile cueing assisted cognitively impaired clients. Indoor activities included cooking produce, flower arrangements, and fabricating garden decorations. Other program components consisted of educational lectures and field trips.

A gardening program can be created in a limited environment. In lieu of a sunny window, special lights can be installed for growing plants, and in lieu of a garden, potted plants, dish gardens, and terrariums can be used.[186] Raised beds or containers are ideal for those with limited mobility. They can be adapted to an outdoor garden, a balcony, an indoor room, or the corner of an occupational therapy clinic. One innovative occupational therapist takes her patients to the hospital lawn to dig in the soil and plant flowers. There are a variety of commercially available garden tools for persons with limited reach and grip in addition to numerous Web sites that provide detailed information on gardening techniques, adaptations, and tools for the elderly and people with special needs.[186-191]

Kitchen Work

For those patients for whom meal preparation is a necessity or for those who enjoy the culinary arts, kitchen work and training as a therapeutic intervention provide opportunities to activate normal movement patterns, exercise visual perceptual skills, improve strength and endurance, maintain or improve mobility, maintain or improve coordination and balance, and stimulate cognition. Kitchen work is task-specific, functional, and goal oriented, and tasks can be graded in all of the aforementioned categories.[192]

Kitchen work as a therapeutic activity also offers multiple opportunities both for retraining and teaching compensatory strategies for PD patients who demonstrate problems with dual tasks and sequential movements. Observing the patient performing cooking related activities provides the therapist with an excellent venue to assess for and train in safety-related issues.

Meal preparation, while a necessity for most and a chore for others, can also serve as a source of creative endeavor, leisure, and recreation. It is a therapeutic intervention that can be used in the clinic, home, or institutional setting. It can take place during an individual treatment session or as a group activity. It can stimulate memories of the past and conversations about the present. For many, the kitchen is the heart of the home, and for some patients (though not all), engaging in kitchen work can be a life affirming activity.

For patients with reduced grasp, reach, strength, and endurance, utensils, wares, and appliances can be found in grocery, discount, and department stores as well as specialty shops and catalogues. Often, simple environmental modifications can allow patients with PD to maintain their independence in the kitchen.[193]

Tai Chi and Yoga

Tai Chi Chuan is an ancient martial art practiced for centuries in China for flexibility, strength, balance, posture control, relaxed breathing, and mind–body interaction. It can be performed alone or in a group, relies on internal rather than external feedback, and requires no equipment.[194] Wolf and colleagues have reduced the 108 forms of Tai Chi to 10 composite forms for use by older individuals.[195-197]

In a 2002 study by Marjama-Lyons et al,[198] PD patients who participated in weekly Tai Chi classes demonstrated improved motor function and reduced falls and in a recent case study,[199] two PD patients showed improved balance skills following an 8-week Tai Chi class.

Although to date there are no studies on the benefits of yoga for PD patients, the emphasis on flexibility and deep breathing seems tailored for this population, although patients should avoid inverted positions and be cautious with postures involving extreme hyperextension.

Patients with PD should engage in these alternative forms of exercise under the supervision of a qualified Tai Chi or yoga instructor familiar with the special needs of this population. Local Parkinson's organizations, senior citizen centers, and other community organizations frequently offer Tai Chi and yoga classes. For patients with PD, exercise needs to be a regularly scheduled activity, incorporated into daily life, and continued over a lifetime.

ACTIVITY AND OCCUPATION

A recent study suggests that higher levels of physical activity may lower the risk of PD in men and found that men with PD were less physically active up to 12 years prior to their diagnosis.[200] Other studies have indicated that regular exercise is associated with a delay in the onset of dementia and Alzheimer's disease,[201] and that older women with higher levels of physical activity are less likely to develop cognitive decline.[202] Leisure activities, particularly those that involve cognitive skills such as crossword puzzles, reading, board games, and playing musical instruments, have also been associated with maintenance of cognitive function,[203-205] whereas television viewing has been associated with an increased likelihood of dementia.[206,207]

The definition of exercise has broadened to encompass activities, occupations, and leisure pursuits. The World Health Organization defines exercise as "all movements in everyday life, including work, activities of daily living, recreation, exercise, and sporting activities," and recommends that every adult accumulate 30 minutes of moderate-intensity physical activity daily, regardless of health status or disease state.[208] The American Heart Association's[209] includes gardening, yard work, dancing, mowing, pruning, digging, raking leaves, walking the dog, and housework as physical activities that promote a healthy lifestyle.

In 1991, nearly 60% of adults in the United States reported little or no leisure-time physical activity.[210] Two separate studies looking at the daily life of the elderly found that television viewing occupied most of the participants' free time.[35,211]

Given that approximately 40% of patients with PD suffer from depression,[212] and that in general, active people have greater life satisfaction and less depression than those who are inactive and isolated,[213] helping patients explore ways to move from sedentary to more active lifestyles and to establish meaningful patterns of activity and occupational engagement is a challenge for the occupational therapist. The evidence is building and clearly indicates that sedentary behavior is a major risk factor for chronic disease morbidity and mortality[210] and that regular engagement in a variety of activities and roles has a positive influence on well-being. Those occupations that involve socializing, work, and leisure appear to be particularly important.[214]

The presence or absence of activity in our lives influences not just the physical domain, but the emotional and social as well, and serves as a link to our identity. A prospective longitudinal study of quality of life in 111 PD patients over a 4-year period found a significant decrease in health-related quality of life not only in physical mobility but in emotional reactions, pain, and social isolation.[215]

When planning activity, the therapist must take into account the patient's interests, roles, expectations, occupational history, environment, social supports, cognitive status, community participation, and medication cycles. Time and the environment exert the most influence on a patient's participation in activities, and socioeconomic and marital status, gender, and age can help or hinder the process.[35]

In a 2006 prospective study of 437 community-residing older adults, Varghese et al, found that high levels of participation in cognitive leisure activities is associated with reduced risk of mild cognitive impairment.[216] There are a number of leisure activity checklists, such as the Leisure Satisfaction Scale,[217] the Meaningfulness of ActivityScale,[218] and the Minnesota Leisure Time Physical Activities Questionnaire[219] that can be used to facilitate ideas about use of free time. Bundy[220] recommends asking the patient about activities he or she has done in the past and found totally absorbing rather than asking, "What do you do in your leisure time?"

Decker[221] viewed leisure as an opportunity to "rejuvenate spirits, enjoy interests, build relationships, make memories, and make life's difficult moments more bearable for everyone involved." She categorized leisure into five domains of activity: physical, intellectual, emotional/expressive, social, and spiritual. To gather information and facilitate discussion on leisure activities and interests, Decker developed the Checklist of Leisure Favorites, which is a useful tool for patients with PD.

There are surveys validated with adult population for measuring participation in activities and occupations such as and the National Institutes of Health Activity Record (ACTRE), which can be used to document daily activities and quantify the amount of time spent between rest and physical activity and the intensity of pain and fatigue associated with activities.[222] The Occupational Questionnaire, a shortened version of the ACTRE, is another self-report form.[223]

Using the Yesterday Interview with patients diagnosed with neurodegenerative disease, including PD, and controls, Lomax and colleagues[214] found that the patient group spent more time in bed, in self care, and in passive activities. Almost one-third of the patients stayed indoors the entire 24-hour period and overall, patients spent much more time in the home per day as compared to the controls. The Yesterday Interview[224] is a semi-structured interview used to reconstruct the preceding 24 hours of a person's life and provides information on the frequency and duration of activities, the richness of activities, and the breadth of the activity contexts in terms of the physical and social environments,[35] and can be useful tool for the occupational therapist to engage the patient in discussion about the presence of activity in his or her life.

Occupation is a synthesis of doing, being, and becoming.[225] Engaging in occupation allows patients to explore new possibilities for activity within the constraints of their illness. Involvement in meaningful tasks can help patients transcend difficult circumstances and find new avenues for life satisfaction. By helping our patients explore new ways to engage in valued activities we can also help them develop the potential to transform their lives.

CONCLUSIONS

Patients with PD contend with an array of deficits that affect their ability to engage in daily activities and life enhancing occupations and participate in the life of the community. Because patients' impairments are typically individualized, therapy needs to be customized to each person's specific problems and needs. This chapter described the nature of the deficits and presents strategies and suggestions for interventions that occupational therapists can use when working with these individuals. Presently, there are few studies to document the efficacy of occupational therapy as an effective supplement to the pharmacological treatment of patients with PD. We need to promote and engage in research in the form of randomized controlled trials to build the evidence base for effective interventions for patients living with this disabling and progressive disease.

CASE STUDY 2—MRS. JONES

Mrs. Jones is a 58-year-old widow and retired teacher diagnosed with Parkinson's disease for about 5 years. Her neurologist referred her for one occupational therapy session for education and home program instruction with a 1-month follow-up visit. Mrs. Jones described herself as independent, fairly active, and involved in her book and gardening clubs. She presented with a resting hand tremor, problems with writing, and episodic freezing, especially upon entering elevators and walking through doorways. She admitted to mild fatigue and sometimes felt "unsteady" but denied falls. She disclosed that during her medication's (levodopa) "off periods" she felt as if she were in "slow motion," and it took her longer to accomplish tasks such as showering and meal preparation. She complained of mild forgetfulness and distractibility. She exhibited the beginning of a forward head, flexed posture. She voiced her goal of remaining in her home for as long as possible.

The occupational therapist instructed Mrs. Jones in mental imagery techniques and task and activity analysis to ease performance while engaging in valued occupations. Task analysis consisted of analyzing each phase of the task or movement by breaking it into sequences and examining the biomechanics of the movements involved. For instance, Mrs. Jones liked to shower and wash her hair daily, but she dreaded doing so because it took 2 hours from her day and resulted in significant fatigue.

The occupational therapist suggested that Mrs. Jones prepare a list of all the steps involved in showering and washing her hair: removing her nightgown, washing, rinsing, drying, combing, and dressing. Next, Mrs. Jones broke each step into its component parts and listed the movements involved (eg, doffing her nightgown required flexing her shoulders and elbows and extending her arms to pull it over her head). As she analyzed the steps and movements with the aid of the occupational therapist, Mrs. Jones discovered that she could eliminate some unnecessary motions and sit to do some tasks, thus reducing fatigue and fall risk. The occupational therapist suggested that she purchase a shower seat and install grab bars.

Mrs. Jones practiced grooming, showering, and washing her hair through mental rehearsal so that she was able to complete the task in 45 minutes. During practice, Mrs. Jones incorporated all five senses into the visualized activities. She imagined the sound of the running water, the smells of the toothpaste and soap, the taste of the mouthwash and toothpaste, the sensations of the toothbrush bristles on her teeth and the water hitting her skin, the texture of the soap, and the feel of the lather. She conjured vivid color images of each action.

A month later she reported having reduced the time by laying out her clothes and other necessary items the night before and by further economizing on her motions. She said she felt "as efficient as an assembly line worker." She had begun to intentionally use cognitive strategies to elicit more effective motor patterns.

To prod her memory, Mrs. Jones wore a watch with an alarm as a medication reminder. She also kept an appointment calendar handy and carried it in her pocket so she could refer to it throughout the day, and she habitually made "to-do" lists on a kitchen blackboard.

Mrs. Jones practiced using visual (tape placed on the floor at step length) and auditory (counting) cues to facilitate movement during freezing episodes. The occupational therapist instructed her in motion economy and energy conservation techniques and recommended that she schedule her activities during the "on" phase of her medication. She referred her to the community Parkinson's disease Tai Chi exercise class and support group. In addition, she instructed Mrs. Jones in stretching to the shoulder complex and anterior chest musculature, chin tucks and scapular retractions and depressions, and passive positional stretching with a towel roll to the cervical and thoracic spine. She also recommended a lumbar support for Mrs. Jones' favorite chair.

Mrs. Jones was advised that when dual tasks such as walking and carrying objects at the same time presented a problem, she should attend to the object cognitively and think "big steps" while walking and avoid talking and other distractions. She also could use compensatory measures such as placing the objects in a backpack or fanny pack, leaving her hands free.

Visual imagery techniques which included imagining large movements, use of lined paper, and writing to music improved Mrs. Jones micrographic handwriting.

ACKNOWLEDGMENTS

The author thanks friends Jim Babcock, MD, for his photographic expertise, Betty Baer, OTR and Helen Cohen, EdD, OTR, FAOTA, for their professional insights, and Dorothy Wong, PhD, for sharing her thoughts about living with Parkinson's disease. She is an inspiration to us all.

REFERENCES

1. Physical and occupational therapy in Parkinson's disease. *Mov Disord.* 2002; 17(4):5156-5159.
2. Deane KHO, Ellis-Hill C, Playford ED, Ben-Shllomo Y, Clarke CE. Occupational therapy for Parkinson's disease. *Cochrane Database Syst Rev.* Vol 3CD.002813. 2005; 3.
3. Murphy S, Tickle-Degnen L. The effectiveness of occupational therapy-related treatments for persons with Parkinson's disease: a meta-analytic review. *Am J Occup Ther.* 2001;55(4):385-392.
4. Deane KHO, Ellis-Hill C, Dekker K, Davies P, Clarke CE. A Delphi survey of best practice occupational therapy for Parkinson's disease in the United Kingdom. *British Journal of Occupational Therapy.* 2003;66(5):193-200.
5. Tse DW, Spaulding SJ. Review of motor learning: implications for occupational therapy for individuals with Parkinson's disease. *Phys Occup Ther Geriatr.* 1998;15(3):19-38.
6. Trombly CA. Theoretical foundations for practice. In: Trombly CA, ed. *Occupational Therapy for Physical Dysfunction.* Baltimore, MD: Williams & Wilkins;1995:15-37.
7. Schenkman M, Butler RB. A model for multisystem evaluation and treatment of individuals with Parkinson's disease. *Phys Ther.* 1989;69(11):932-943.
8. Rogers MW. Motor control problems in Parkinson's disease. From: Contemporary Management of Motor Control Problems: Proceedings of the II Step Conference. Foundations for Physical Therapy, Alexandria, VA:1991.
9. Carr J, Shepherd R. Parkinson's disease. In: Carr J, Shepherd R, eds. *Neurological Rehabilitation: Optimizing Motor Performance.* Oxford: Butterworth Heineman; 1998:305-331.
10. Morris ME. Movement disorders in people with Parkinson disease: a model for physical therapy. *Phys Ther.* 2000;80(6):578-597.
11. Mathiowetz V, Haugen JB. Motor behavior research: implications for therapeutic approaches to central nervous system dysfunction. *Am J Occup Ther.* 1994; 48(8):733-745.
12. Shumway-Cook A, Woollacott MH. *Motor Control.* 2nd ed. Philadelphia: Lippincott Williams & Wilkins, 2001.
13. Schmidt RA. *Motor Learning and Performance: From Principles to Practice.* Champaign, IL: Human Kinetics Books, 1991.
14. Poole JL. Application of motor learning principles in occupational therapy. *Am J Occup Ther.* 1991;45(6):531-537.
15. Stanley RK, Protas EJ, Jankovic J. Parkinson's disease. In: Myers JN, Herbert JG, Humphrey R, eds. *ACSM's Resource for Clinical Exercise Physiology.* Philadelphia: Lippincott Williams & Wilkins; 2002:38-47.
16. Schmidt RA. *Motor Control and Learning: A Behavioral Emphasis.* 2nd ed. Champaign, IL: Human Kinetics, 1988.
17. Ma HI, Trombly CA. The comparison of motor performance between part and whole tasks in elderly persons. *Am J Occup Ther.* 2001;55(1):62-67.
18. Shohamy D, Myers CE, Grossman S, Sage J, Gluck MA, Poldrack RA. Cortico-striatal contributions to feedback-based learning: converging data from neuroimaging and neuropsychology. *Brain.* 2004;127(Pt 4):851-859.
19. Guadagnoli MA, Leis B, Van Gemmert AW, Stelmach GE. The relationship between knowledge of results and motor learning in Parkinsonian patients. *Parkinsonism Relat Disord.* 2002;9(2):89-95.
20. Swinnen SP, Steyvers M, Van Den BL, Stelmach GE. Motor learning and Parkinson's disease: refinement of within-limb and between-limb coordination as a result of practice. *Behav Brain Res.* 2000;111(1-2):45-59.
21. Soliveri P, Brown RG, Jahanshahi M, Marsden CD. Effect of practice on performance of a skilled motor task in patients with Parkinson's disease. *J Neurol Neurosurg Psychiatry.* 1992;55(6):454-460.
22. Behrman AL, Cauraugh JH, Light KE. Practice as an intervention to improve speeded motor performance and motor learning in Parkinson's disease. *J Neurol Sci.* 2000;174(2):127-136.
23. Nutt JG, Lea ES, Van Houten L, Schuff RA, Sexton GJ. Determinants of tapping speed in normal control subjects and subjects with Parkinson's disease: differing effects of brief and continued practice. *Mov Disord.* 2000;15(5):843-849.

24. Agostino R, Curra A, Soldati G, Dinapoli L, Chiacchiari L, Modugno N et al. Prolonged practice is of scarce benefit in improving motor performance in Parkinson's disease. *Mov Disord.* 2004;19(11):1285-1293.
25. Morris ME, Collier JM, Matyas TA, Summers JJ, Iansek R. Evidence for motor skill learning in Parkinson's disease. In: Piek JP, ed. *Motor Behavior and Human Skill: A Multidisciplinary Approach.* Champaign, IL: Human Kinetics Books, 1998: 312-329.
26. Nutt JG, Wooten GF. Clinical practice. Diagnosis and initial management of Parkinson's disease. *N Engl J Med.* 2005;353(10):1021-1027.
27. Fahn S. Description of Parkinson's disease as a clinical syndrome. *Ann N Y Acad Sci.* 2003;991:1-14.
28. Poewe WH, Wenning GK. The natural history of Parkinson's disease. *Ann Neurol.* 1998;44(3 Suppl 1):S1-S9.
29. Adler CH. Nonmotor complications in Parkinson's disease. *Mov Disord.* 2005;20 Suppl 11:S23-S29.
30. Playford D. *Neurological Rehabilitation of Parkinson's Disease.* London: Taylor and Francis, 2003.
31. Djaldetti R, Shifrin A, Rogowski Z, Sprecher E, Melamed E, Yarnitsky D. Quantitative measurement of pain sensation in patients with Parkinson disease. *Neurology.* 2004;62(12):2171-2175.
32. Bozi M, Bhatia K. The pharmacological management of Parkinson's disease. In: Playford D, ed. *Neurological Rehabilitation of Parkinson's Disease.* London: Taylor and Francis; 2003:1-24.
33. Chodzko-Zajko WJ. Biological theories of aging: implications for functional performance. In: Bonder BR, Wagner MB, eds. *Functional Performance in Older Adults.* Philadelphia: F.A. Davis Company; 2001:28-41.
34. Strickland LS. Evaluation issues in today's practice. In: Hinojosa J, Kramer P, Crist P, eds. *Evaluation: Obtaining and Interpreting Data.* Bethesda, MD: AOTA Press; 2005:51-59.
35. Horgas AL, Wilms HU, Baltes MM. Daily life in very old age: everyday activities as expression of successful living. *Gerontologist.* 1998;38(5):556-568.
36. UPDRS Development Committee. Unified Parkinson's Disease Rating Scale. In: Fahn S, Elton RL, eds. *Recent Developments in Parkinson's Disease*, Vol 2. Florham Park, NJ: MacMillan Healthcare Information; 1987:153-163.
37. Hoehn MM, Yahr MD. Parkinsonism: onset, progression, and mortality. *Neurology.* 2001;57(10 Suppl 3):S11-S26.
38. Schwab R, England A. Projection technique for evaluating surgery in Parkinson's disease. In: Gillingham FJ, Donald IML, eds. *Third Symposium on Parkinson's Disease.* Edinburgh: Liningstone, 1969.
39. Jenkinson C, Fitzpatrick R, Peto V, Greenhall R, Hyman N. The Parkinson's Disease Questionnaire (PDQ-39): development and validation of a Parkinson's disease summary index score. *Age Ageing.* 1997;26(5):353-357.
40. Peto V, Jenkinson C, Fitzpatrick R. PDQ-39: a review of the development, validation and application of a Parkinson's disease quality of life questionnaire and its associated measures. *J Neurol.* 1998;245 Suppl 1:S10-S14.
41. Ramaker C, Marinus J, Stiggelbout AM, Van Hilten BJ. Systematic evaluation of rating scales for impairment and disability in Parkinson's disease. *Mov Disord.* 2002;17(5):867-876.
42. Gutman SA, Schonfeld AB. *Screening Adult Neurologic Populations: A Step-By-Step Instruction Manual.* Baltimore, MD: American Occupational Therapy Association, 2003.
43. Friedman J, Friedman H. Fatigue in Parkinson's disease. *Neurology.* 1993; 43(10):2016-2018.
44. Smets EM, Garssen B, Bonke B, De Haes JC. The Multidimensional Fatigue Inventory (MFI) psychometric qualities of an instrument to assess fatigue. *J Psychosom Res.* 1995;39(3):315-325.
45. Jette AM. Functional Status Index: reliability of a chronic disease evaluation instrument. *Arch Phys Med Rehabil.* 1980;61(9):395-401.
46. Zimnavoda T, Weinblatt N, Katz N. Validity of the Kohlman Evaluation of Living Skills (KELS) with Israeli elderly individuals living in the community. *Occup Ther Int.* 2002;9(4):312-325.
47. Fisher AG. *Assessment of Motor and Process Skills.* Ft. Collins, CO: Three Star Press, 1999.
48. Kielhofner G, Forsyth K, de las Heras CG, Hayashi MJ, Raymond L. Observational assessments. In: Kielhofner G, ed. *Model of Human Occupation.* Baltimore, MD: Lippincott Williams & Wilkins; 2002:191-212.
49. Law MC, Baptiste S, Carswell A, McColl MA, Polatajko H, Pollock N. *The Canadian Occupational Performance Measure.* 3rd ed. Toronto, Ontario: Canadian Association of Occupational Therapy, 1998.
50. Gaudet P. Measuring the impact of Parkinson's disease: an occupational therapy perspective. *Can J Occup Ther.* 2002;69(2):104-113.
51. Oliver R, Blathwayt J, Brackley C, Tamaki T. Development of the Safety Assessment of Function and the Environment for Rehabilitation (SAFER) tool. *Can J Occup Ther.* 1993;60(2):78-82.
52. Oliver R, Balthway J, Brackley C, Tamaki T. *Functional Assessment and Safety Tool User's Manual.* 1994. McMaster University/Hamilton Civic Hospitals, Hamilton.
53. Nova IC, Perracini MR, Ferraz HB. Levodopa effect upon functional balance of Parkinson's disease patients. *Parkinsonism Relat Disord.* 2004;10(7):411-415.
54. Qutubuddin AA, Pegg PO, Cifu DX, Brown R, McNamee S, Carne W. Validating the Berg Balance Scale for patients with Parkinson's disease: a key to rehabilitation evaluation. *Arch Phys Med Rehabil.* 2005;86(4):789-792.

55. Brusse KJ, Zimdars S, Zalewski KR, Steffen TM. Testing functional performance in people with Parkinson disease. *Phys Ther.* 2005;85(2):134-141.

56. Berg KO, Wood-Dauphinee SL, Williams JI, Maki B. Measuring balance in the elderly: validation of an instrument. *Can J Public Health.* 1992;83 Suppl 2:S7-11.

57. Buddenberg LA, Davis C. Test-retest reliability of the Purdue Pegboard Test. *Am J Occup Ther.* 2000; 54(5):555-558.

58. Mathiowetz V, Weber K, Kashman N, Volland G. Adult norms for the Nine Hole Peg Test of Finger Dexterity. *Occup Ther Journal of Res.* 1985;5:24-38.

59. Folstein MF, Folstein SE, McHugh PR. "Mini-mental state". A practical method for grading the cognitive state of patients for the clinician. *J Psychiatr Res.* 1975; 12(3):189-198.

60. Stern Y, Mayeux R, Rosen J, Ilson J. Perceptual motor dysfunction in Parkinson's disease: a deficit in sequential and predictive voluntary movement. *J Neurol Neurosurg Psychiatry.* 1983;46(2):145-151.

61. Lyons KD, Tickle-Degnen L. Reliability and validity of a videotape method to describe expressive behavior in persons with Parkinson's disease. *Am J Occup Ther.* 2005;59(1):41-49.

62. Deuschl G, Krack P. Tremors: Differential diagnosis, neurophysiology, and pharmacology. In: Jankovic J, Tolosa E, eds. *Parkinson's Disease and Movement Disorders.* Philadelphia: Lippincott Williams & Wilkins; 1998:419-452.

63. Beuter A, Barbo E, Rigal R, Blanchet PJ. Characterization of subclinical tremor in Parkinson's disease. *Mov Disord.* 2005;20(8):945-950.

64. Samil A, Nutt JG, Ransom BR. Parkinson's disease. *Lancet.* 2004; 363(9423):1783-1793.

65. Stern MB, Koller WC. Parkinson's disease. In: Stern MB, Koller WC, eds. *Parkinsonian Syndromes.* New York: Marcel Dekker, Inc.; 1993:3-29.

66. Gauthier L, Gauthier S. Functional rehabilitation of patients with Parkinson's disease. *Physiotherapy Canada.* 1983;35:220-222.

67. Lance JW, Schwab RS, Peterson EA. Action tremor and the cogwheel phenomenon in Parkinson's disease. *Brain.* 1963;86:95-110.

68. Findley LJ, Gresty MA, Halmagyi GM. Tremor, the cogwheel phenomenon and clonus in Parkinson's disease. *J Neurol Neurosurg Psychiatry.* 1981;44(6):534-546.

69. Duval C, Sadikot AF, Panisset M. The detection of tremor during slow alternating movements performed by patients with early Parkinson's disease. *Exp Brain Res.* 2004;154(3):395-398.

70. Raethjen J, Pohle S, Govindan RB, Morsnowski A, Wenzelburger R, Deuschl G. Parkinsonian action tremor: interference with object manipulation and lacking levodopa response. *Exp Neurol.* 2005;194(1):151-160.

71. Louis ED, Levy G, Cote LJ, Mejia H, Fahn S, Marder K. Clinical correlates of action tremor in Parkinson disease. *Arch Neurol.* 2001;58(10):1630-1634.

72. Forssberg H, Ingvarsson PE, Iwasaki N, Johansson RS, Gordon AM. Action tremor during object manipulation in Parkinson's disease. *Mov Disord.* 2000; 15(2):244-254.

73. Meshack RP, Norman KE. A randomized controlled trial of the effects of weights on amplitude and frequency of postural hand tremor in people with Parkinson's disease. *Clin Rehabil.* 2002;16(5):481-492.

74. Lundervold DA, Poppen R. Biobehavioral intervention for older adults coping with essential tremor. *Appl Psychophysiol Biofeedback.* 2004;29(1):63-73.

75. Wood CJ. Evaluation of meditation and relaxation on physiological response during the performance of fine motor and gross motor tasks. *Percept Mot Skills.* 1986;62(1):91-98.

76. Gillen G. Improving activities of daily living performance in an adult with ataxia. *Am J Occup Ther.* 2000;54(1):89-96.

77. Trail M. Activity affects quaility of life. 2002. Vicki Appel Patient/Family Conference, Baylor College of Medicine, Houston, TX.

78. Ahlskog JE, Muenter MD. Frequency of levodopa-related dyskinesias and motor fluctuations as estimated from the cumulative literature. *Mov Disord.* 2001; 16(3):448-458.

79. Jankovic J. Motor fluctuations and dyskinesias in Parkinson's disease: clinical manifestations. *Mov Disord.* 2005;20 Suppl 11:S11-S16.

80. Chung W, Poppen R, Lundervold DA. Behavioral relaxation training for tremor disorders in older adults. *Biofeedback Self Regul.* 1995;20(2):123-135.

81. Jankovic J, Tintner R. Dystonia and parkinsonism. *Parkinsonism Relat Disord.* 2001;8(2):109-121.

82. Zeuner KE, Shill HA, Sohn YH, Molloy FM, Thornton BC, Dambrosia JM et al. Motor training as treatment in focal hand dystonia. *Mov Disord.* 2005;20(3):335-341.

83. Teulings HL, Contreras-Vidal JL, Stelmach GE, Adler CH. Parkinsonism reduces coordination of fingers, wrist, and arm in fine motor control. *Exp Neurol.* 1997; 146(1):159-170.

84. McLennan JE, Nakano K, Tyler HR, Schwab RS. Micrographia in Parkinson's disease. *J Neurol Sci.* 1972;15(2):141-152.

85. Arend W, Van Gemmert A, Teulings HL, Stelmach GE. Parkinsonian patients reduce their stroke size with increased processing demands. *Brain Cogn.* 2001; 47(3):504-512.

86. Longstaff MG, Mahant PR, Stacy MA, Van Gemmert AW, Leis BC, Stelmach GE. Discrete and dynamic scaling of the size of continuous graphic movements of parkinsonian patients and elderly controls. *J Neurol Neurosurg Psychiatry.* 2003; 74(3):299-304.

87. Giladi N, McDermott MP, Fahn S, Przedborski S, Jankovic J, Stern M et al. Freezing of gait in PD: prospective assessment in the DATATOP cohort. *Neurology.* 2001;56(12):1712-1721.

88. Arend WA, Van Gemmert AWA, Tuelings HL, Stelmach GE. The influence of mental and motor load on handwriting movements in Parkinsonian patients. *Acta Psychologia.* 1998;100:161-175.

89. Oliveira RM, Gurd JM, Nixon P, Marshall JC, Passingham RE. Micrographia in Parkinson's disease: the effect of providing external cues. *J Neurol Neurosurg Psychiatry.* 1997;63(4):429-433.

90. Teulings HL, Stelmach GE. Control of stroke size, peak acceleration, and stroke duration in Parkinsonian handwriting. *Human Movement Science.* 1991;10:315-334.

91. Trail M, Fox C, Ramig LO, Sapir S, Howard J, Lai EC. Speech treatment for Parkinson's disease. *NeuroRehabilitation.* 2005;20(3):205-221.

92. Farley BG, Koshland GF. Training BIG to move faster: the application of the speed-amplitude relation as a rehabilitation strategy for people with Parkinson's disease. *Exp Brain Res.* 2005;167(3):462-467.

93. Preminger F, Weiss PL, Weintraub N. Predicting occupational performance: handwriting versus keyboarding. *Am J Occup Ther.* 2004;58(2):193-201.

94. Beck H, Shulman LM, Dusaj R, Anderson KE, Weiner WJ. Computer skills in patients with movement disorders. *Parkinsonism Relat Disord.* 2005;11(7):421-426.

95. Rodnitzky R. The Parkinsonisms: identifying what is not Parkinson's disease. *The Neurologist.* 1999;5(6):300-312.

96. Dewey RB. Clinical features of Parkinson's disease. In: Adler CH, Ahlskog JE, eds. *Parkinson's Disease and Movement Disorders: Diagnosis and Treatment Guidelines for the Practicing Physician.* Totowa, NJ: Humana Press; 2000:71-84.

97. Berardelli A, Rothwell JC, Thompson P Deal. Pathophysiology of bradykinesia in Parkinson's disease. *Brain.* 2001;124:2131-2146.

98. Edwards S. *Neurological Physiotherapy.* 2nd ed. London: Churchill Livingston, 2006.

99. Marjama-Lyons JM, Koller WC. Parkinson's disease. Update in diagnosis and symptom management. *Geriatrics.* 2001;56(8):24-30, 33.

100. Fahn S. Description of Parkinson's disease as a clinical syndrome. *Ann N Y Acad Sci.* 2003;991:1-14.

101. Klockgether T. Parkinson's disease: clinical aspects. *Cell Tissue Res.* 2004; 318(1):115-120.

102. Bernatzky G, Bernatzky P, Hesse HP, Staffen W, Ladurner G. Stimulating music increases motor coordination in patients afflicted with Morbus Parkinson. *Neurosci Lett.* 2004;361(1-3):4-8.

103. Pacchetti C, Aglieri R, Mancini F, Martignoni E, Nappi G. Active music therapy and Parkinson's disease: methods. *Funct Neurol.* 1998;13(1):57-67.

104. Hi, M, Trombly CA, Tickle-Degnen L, Wagenaar RC. Effect of one single auditory cue on movement kinematics in patients with Parkinson's disease. *Am J Phys Med Rehabil.* 2004;83(7):530-536.

105. Schettino LF, Rajaraman V, Jack D, Adamovich SV, Sage J, Poizner H. Deficits in the evolution of hand pre-shaping in Parkinson's disease. *Neuropsychologia.* 2004;42(1):82-94.

106. Lim I, van Wegen E, de Goede C, Deutekom M, Nieuwboer A, Willems A et al. Effects of external rhythmical cueing on gait in patients with Parkinson's disease: a systematic review. *Clin Rehabil.* 2005;19(7):695-713.

107. Suteerawattananon M, Morris GS, Etnyre BR, Jankovic J, Protas EJ. Effects of visual and auditory cues on gait in individuals with Parkinson's disease. *J Neurol Sci.* 2004;219(1-2):63-69.

108. Morris ME, Iansek R, Matyas TA, Summers JJ. Stride length regulation in Parkinson's disease. Normalization strategies and underlying mechanisms. *Brain.* 1996;119(Pt 2):551-568.

109. Melnick NE. Basal ganglia disorders: metabolic, hereditary, and genetic. In: Umphred D, ed. *Neurological Rehabilitation.* St. Louis: Mosby; 2001:669-682.

110. Turnbull GI. The role of physical therapy intervention. In: Turnbull GI, ed. *Physical Therapy Management of Parkinson's Disease.* New York: Churchill Livingstone; 1992:91-111.

111. O'shea S, Morris ME, Iansek R. Dual task interference during gait in people with Parkinson disease: effects of motor versus cognitive secondary tasks. *Phys Ther.* 2002;82(9):888-897.

112. Bond JM, Morris M. Goal-directed secondary motor tasks: their effects on gait in subjects with Parkinson disease. *Arch Phys Med Rehabil.* 2000;81(1):110-116.

113. Schwab RS, Chafetz ME, Walker S. Control of two simultaneous voluntary motor acts in normals and in parkinsonism. *AMA Arch Neurol Psychiatry.* 1954; 72(5):591-598.

114. Rochester L, Hetherington V, Jones D, Nieuwboer A, Willems AM, Kwakkel G et al. Attending to the task: interference effects of functional tasks on walking in Parkinson's disease and the roles of cognition, depression, fatigue, and balance. *Arch Phys Med Rehabil.* 2004;85(10):1578-1585.

115. Rochester L, Hetherington V, Jones D, Nieuwboer A, Willems AM, Kwakkel G et al. The effect of external rhythmic cues (auditory and visual) on walking during a functional task in homes of people with Parkinson's disease. *Arch Phys Med Rehabil.* 2005;86(5):999-1006.

116. Wu T, Hallett M. A functional MRI study of automatic movements in patients with Parkinson's disease. *Brain*. 2005;128(Pt 10):2250-2259.

117. Fama R, Sullivan EV. Motor sequencing in Parkinson's disease: relationship to executive function and motor rigidity. *Cortex*. 2002;38(5):753-767.

118. Benecke R, Rothwell JC, Dick JP, Day BL, Marsden CD. Disturbance of sequential movements in patients with Parkinson's disease. *Brain*. 1987;110 (Pt 2):361-379.

119. Jennings PJ. Evidence of incomplete motor programming in Parkinson's disease. *J Mot Behav*. 1995;27(4):310-324.

120. Roy EA, Saint-Cyr J, Taylor A, Lang A. Movement sequencing disorders in Parkinson's disease. *Int J Neurosci*. 1993;73(3-4):183-194.

121. Samuel M, Ceballos-Baumann AO, Blin J, Uema T, Boecker H, Passingham RE et al. Evidence for lateral premotor and parietal overactivity in Parkinson's disease during sequential and bimanual movements. A PET study. *Brain*. 1997; 120(Pt 6):963-976.

122. Cahn DA, Sullivan EV, Shear PK, Pfefferbaum A, Heit G, Silverberg G. Differential contributions of cognitive and motor component processes to physical and instrumental activities of daily living in Parkinson's disease. *Arch Clin Neuropsychol*. 1998;13(7):575-583.

123. Smiley-Oyen AL, Worringham CJ, Cross CL. Practice effects in three-dimensional sequential rapid aiming in Parkinson's disease. *Mov Disord*. 2002; 17(6):1196-1204.

124. Curtis CL, Bassile CC, Cote LJ, Gentile AM. Effects of exercise on the motor control of individuals with Parkinson's disease: case studies. *Neurology Report*. 2001;25(1):2-11.

125. Yekutiel MP. Patients' fall records as an aid in designing and assessing therapy in Parkinsonism. *Disabil Rehabil*. 1993;15(4):189-193.

126. Agostino R, Curra A, Giovannelli M, Modugno N, Manfredi M, Berardelli A. Impairment of individual finger movements in Parkinson's disease. *Mov Disord*. 2003;18(5):560-565.

127. Georgiou N, Bradshaw JL, Sheppard D, Chiu E, Iansek R, Phillips J et al. Motor sequencing problems in Parkinson's disease, Huntington's disease, and Tourette's Syndrome 2: Recent findings involving the provision of advanced information. In: Piek JP, ed. *Motor Behavior and Human Skill: A Multidisciplinary Approach*. Champaign, IL: Human Kinetics; 1998:319-328.

128. McCollum G, Leen TK. Form and exploration of mechanical stability limits in erect stance. *J Mot Behav*. 1989;21(3):225-244.

129. Schenkman M. Treatment and management of a patient with Parkinson's disease. In: Partridge C, ed. *Neurological Physiotherapy: Bases of Evidence for Practice*. London: Whurr Publishers Ltd; 2002:2-11.

130. Kamsma YPT, Brouwer WH, Lakke JP. Training compensational strategies for impaired gross motor skills in Parkinson's disease. *Physiotherapy*. 1995;11:209-229.

131. Henneberg A. Additional therapies in Parkinson's disease patients: useful tools for the improvement of the quality of life or senseless loss of resources? *J Neurol*. 1998;245 Suppl 1:S23-S27.

132. Knott M, Voss DE. *Proprioceptive Neuromuscular Facilitation*. 2nd ed. New York: Harper & Row, 1968.

133. Bobath B. *Adult Hemiplegia: Evaluation and Treatment*. 3rd ed. London: William Heinemann Medical Books, 1990.

134. Gibberd FB, Page NG, Spencer KM, Kinnear E, Hawksworth JB. Controlled trial of physiotherapy and occupational therapy for Parkinson's disease. *Br Med J*. (Clin Res Ed) 1981;282(6271):1196.

135. Miyasaki JM, Martin W, Suchowersky O, Weiner WJ, Lang AE. Practice parameter: initiation of treatment for Parkinson's disease: an evidence-based review: report of the Quality Standards Subcommittee of the American Academy of Neurology. *Neurology*. 2002;58(1):11-17.

136. Fellows SJ, Noth J, Schwarz M. Precision grip and Parkinson's disease. *Brain*. 1998;121(Pt 9):1771-1784.

137. Ashour R, Tintner R, Jankovic J. Striatal deformities of the hand and foot in Parkinson's disease. *Lancet Neurol*. 2005;4(7):423-431.

138. Aydog E, Eksioglu E, Cakci A, Yilmaz O. Hand deformity in Parkinson's disease: case report. *Rheumatol Int*. 2005;25(7):548-549.

139. Kyriakides T, Hewer RL. Hand contractures in Parkinson's disease. *J Neurol Neurosurg Psychiatry*. 1988;51(9):1221-1223.

140. Wagner MB, Kerr G. Mobility. In: Bonder BR, Wanger MB, eds. *Functional Performance in Older Adults*. Philadelphia: F.A. Davis Company; 2002:61-84.

141. Dural A, Atay MB, Akbostanci C, Kucukdeveci A. Impairment, disability, and life satisfaction in Parkinson's disease. *Disabil Rehabil*. 2003;25(7):318-323.

142. Riley D, Lang AE, Blair RD, Birnbaum A, Reid B. Frozen shoulder and other shoulder disturbances in Parkinson's disease. *J Neurol Neurosurg Psychiatry*. 1989;52(1):63-66.

143. Schenkman M, Cutson TM, Kuchibhatla M, Chandler J, Pieper CF, Ray L et al. Exercise to improve spinal flexibility and function for people with Parkinson's disease: a randomized, controlled trial. *J Am Geriatr Soc*. 1998;46(10):1207-1216.

144. Trail M, Pati A, Callendar M. *Managing Neck Weakness in Clients with ALS*. Brochure 1995. Houston, TX, The Methodist Hospital Foundation.

145. Trail M. Managing neck weakness in clients with neuromuscular disease. *OT Practice*. 1997;2(5):53-55.

146. Zesiewicz TA, Cimino CR, Malek AR, Gardner N, Leaverton PL, Dunne PB et al. Driving safety in Parkinson's disease. *Neurology*. 2002;59(11):1787-1788.

147. Grace J, Amick MM, D'Abreu A, Festa EK, Heindel WC, Ott BR. Neuropsychological deficits associated with driving performance in Parkinson's and Alzheimer's disease. *J Int Neuropsychol Soc*. 2005;11(6):766-775.

148. Wood JM, Worringham C, Kerr G, Mallon K, Silburn P. Quantitative assessment of driving performance in Parkinson's disease. *J Neurol Neurosurg Psychiatry*. 2005;76(2):176-180.

149. Stolwyk RJ, Triggs TJ, Charlton JL, Iansek R, Bradshaw JL. Impact of internal versus external cueing on driving performance in people with Parkinson's disease. *Mov Disord*. 2005;20(7):846-857.

150. Homann CN, Suppan K, Homann B, Crevenna R, Ivanic G, Ruzicka E. Driving in Parkinson's disease—a health hazard? *J Neurol*. 2003;250(12):1439-1446.

151. Uc EY, Rizzo M, Anderson SW, Qian S, Rodnitzky RL, Dawson JD. Visual dysfunction in Parkinson disease without dementia. *Neurology*. 2005; 65(12):1907-1913.

152. Eliott SJ, Velde BP. Integration of occupation for individuals affected by Parkinson's disease. *Phys Occup Ther Geriatr*. 2005;24(1):61-80.

153. Jackson PL, Lafleur MF, Malouin F, Richards CL, Doyon J. Functional cerebral reorganization following motor sequence learning through mental practice with motor imagery. *Neuroimage*. 2003;20(2):1171-1180.

154. Yaguez L, Nagel D, Hoffman H, Canavan AG, Wist E, Homberg V. A mental route to motor learning: improving trajectorial kinematics through imagery training. *Behav Brain Res*. 1998;90(1):95-106.

155. Jackson PL, Lafleur MF, Malouin F, Richards C, Doyon J. Potential role of mental practice using motor imagery in neurologic rehabilitation. *Arch Phys Med Rehabil*. 2001;82(8):1133-1141.

156. Fansler CL, Poff CL, Shepard KF. Effects of mental practice on balance in elderly women. *Phys Ther*. 1985;65(9):1332-1338.

157. Yue G, Cole KJ. Strength increases from the motor program: comparison of training with maximal voluntary and imagined muscle contractions. *J Neurophysiol*. 1992;67(5):1114-1123.

158. White A, Hardy L. Use of different imagery perspectives on the learning and performance of different motor skills. *Br J Psychol*. 1995;86(Pt 2):169-180.

159. Janssen JJ, Sheikh AA. Enhancing athletic performance through imagery: an overview. In: Sheikh AA, Korn ER, eds. *Imagery in Sports and Physical Performance*. Amityville, NY: Baywood Publishing Company; 1994:1-22.

160. Dominey P, Decety J, Broussolle E, Chazot G, Jeannerod M. Motor imagery of a lateralized sequential task is asymmetrically slowed in hemi-Parkinson's patients. *Neuropsychologia*. 1995;33(6):727-741.

161. Yaguez L, Canavan AG, Lange HW, Homberg V. Motor learning by imagery is differentially affected in Parkinson's and Huntington's diseases. *Behav Brain Res*. 1999;102(1-2):115-127.

162. Tamir R, Dickstein R, Huberman M. Combination of mental practice and physiotherapy in group treatment of patients with Parkinson's disease. *Mov Disord*. 2006;21(suppl 13):S133-S134. Abstract.

163. Malouin F, Richards CL, Desrosiers J, Doyon J. Bilateral slowing of mentally simulated actions after stroke. *Neuroreport*. 2004;15(8):1349-1353.

164. Suinn RM. Visualization in sports. In: Sheikh AA, Korn ER, eds. *Imagery in Sports and Physical Performance*. Amityville, NY: Baywood Publishing Company; 1994:23-41.

165. Fell NT, Wrisberg CA. Mental rehearsal as a complementary treatment in geriatric rehabilitation. *Phys Occup Ther Geriat*. 2001;18(4):106-111.

166. Korn ER. Mental imagery in enhancing performance: theory and practical exercises. In: Sheikh AA, Korn ER, eds. *Imagery in Sports and Physical Performance*. Amityville, NY: Baywood Publishing; 1994:201-239.

167. Hall CR, Pongrac J. *Movement Imagery Questionnaire*. London, Ontario: The University of Western Ontario, Faculty of Physical Education, 1983.

168. Jackson PL, Doyon J, Richards CL, Malouin F. The efficacy of combined physical and mental practice in the learning of a foot-sequence task after stroke: a case report. *Neurorehabil Neural Repair*. 2004;18(2):106-111.

169. Warner L, McNeill ME. Mental imagery and its potential for physical therapy. *Phys Ther*. 1988;68(4):516-521.

170. Murray J. Sports Psychology: The Essence of Imagery in Tennis. 1995. Available at: http://www.selfhelpmagazine.com/articles/sports/tennis.html. Accessed February 1, 2006.

171. Poole JL. Self-care strategies for people with movement disorders. In: Christiansen CH, Matuska KL, eds. *Ways of Living: Adaptive Strategies for Special Needs*. Bethesda, MD: American Occupational Therapy Association; 2004:257-270.

172. Kielhofner G. Dimensions of doing. In: Kielhofner G, ed. *Model of Human Occupation*. Baltimore, MD: Lippincott Williams & Wilkins; 2002:114-124.

173. Christiansen CH. Functional evaluation and management of self care and other activities of daily living. In: DeLisa J, Gans B, eds. *Rehabilitation Medicine: Principles and Practice.* Philadelphia: Lippincott Williams & Wilkins; 2004:975-1003.

174. Cumming RG, Thomas M, Szonyi G, Salkeld G, O'Neill E, Westbury C et al. Home visits by an occupational therapist for assessment and modification of environmental hazards: a randomized trial of falls prevention. *J Am Geriatr Soc.* 1999;47(12):1397-1402.

175. Wood BH, Bilclough JA, Bowron A, Walker RW. Incidence and prediction of falls in Parkinson's disease: a prospective multidisciplinary study. *J Neurol Neurosurg Psychiatry.* 2002;72(6):721-725.

176. Bloem BR, Grimbergen YA, Cramer M, Willemsen M, Zwinderman AH. Prospective assessment of falls in Parkinson's disease. *J Neurol.* 2001; 248(11):950-958.

177. Grimbergen YA, Munneke M, Bloem BR. Falls in Parkinson's disease. *Curr Opin Neurol.* 2004;17(4):405-415.

178. Barnes KJ. Modification of the physical environment. In: Christiansen C, Baum C., eds. *Occupational Therapy: Overcoming Human Performance Deficits.* Thorofare, NJ: SLACK Incorporated; 1991:701-747.

179. Beattie A, Caird FI. The occupational therapist and the patient with Parkinson's disease. *Br Med J.* 1980;280(6228):1354-1355.

180. Clarke CE, Zobkiw RM, Gullaksen E. Quality of life and care in Parkinson's disease. *Br J Clin Pract.* 1995;49(6):288-293.

181. Clauson M. Everyday use of assistive technology devices by persons with Parkinson's disease. Unpublished professional paper. Texas Woman's University, School of Occupational Therapy, Houston, TX, 1994.

182. Alves G, Wentzel-Larsen T, Larsen JP. Is fatigue an independent and persistent symptom in patients with Parkinson disease? *Neurology.* 2004;63(10):1908-1911.

183. Cianci H, Cloete L, Gardner J, Trail M, Wichmann R. *Activities of Daily Living: Practical Pointers for Parkinson Disease.* Miami: National Parkinson Foundation; 2005.

184. Relf D. Horticulture: a therapeutic tool. *J Rehabil.* 1973;39(1):27-29.

185. VandenDolder RP, Bendzick MA, Larson JM. Horticulture therapy in treatment of Parkinson's Disease. *Mov Disord.* 2006;21(Suppl 1): S143.

186. Relf D. Gardening in raised beds and containers for older gardners and individuals with physical disabilities. Available at http://www.hort.vt.edu. Accessed May 3, 2006.

187. Gardening with people with disabilities. Available at http://www.foodshare.net. Accessed May 3, 2006.

188. Thrive: using gardening to change lives. Available at: http://www.thrive.org.uk. Accessed February 1, 2006.

189. Carryingongardening. Available at: http.www.carryongardening.org.uk. Accessed February 1, 2006.

190. Human issues in horticulture. Available at: http://www.hort.vt.edu. Accessed May 3, 2006.

191. American horticulture therapy association (AHTA). Available at: http:www.ahta.org. Accessed February 1, 2006.

192. *A Kitchen Training Program.* Boserup E, Ed. Cowan MK, trans. Baltimore, MD: American Occupational Therapy Association, 1985.

193. Klinger JL. *Meal Preparation and Training.* Thorofare, NJ: SLACK Incorporated; 1997.

194. Wolf SL, Kutner NG, Green RC, McNeely E. The Atlanta FICSIT study: two exercise interventions to reduce frailty in elders. *J Am Geriatr Soc.* 1993; 41(3):329-332.

195. Wolf SL, Sattin RW, Kutner M, O'Grady M, Greenspan AI, Gregor RJ. Intense tai chi exercise training and fall occurrences in older, transitionally frail adults: a randomized, controlled trial. *J Am Geriatr Soc.* 2003;51(12):1693-1701.

196. Wolf SL, Sattin RW, O'Grady M, Freret N, Ricci L, Greenspan AI et al. A study design to investigate the effect of intense Tai Chi in reducing falls among older adults transitioning to frailty. *Control Clin Trials.* 2001;22(6):689-704.

197. Wolf SL, Coogler C, Xu T. Exploring the basis for Tai Chi Chuan as a therapeutic exercise approach. *Arch Phys Med Rehabil.* 1997;78(8):886-892.

198. Marjama-Lyons J, Smith L, Mylar B, Nelson J, Holliday G, Seracino D. Tai Chi and reduced rate of falling in Parkinson's disease: a single-blinded pilot study. *Mov Disord.* 2000;17[S5], S70.

199. Venglar M. Case report: Tai Chi and Parkinsonism. *Physiother Res Int.* 2005; 10(2):116-121.

200. Chen H, Zhang SM, Schwarzschild MA, Hernan MA, Ascherio A. Physical activity and the risk of Parkinson disease. *Neurology.* 2005;64(4):664-669.

201. Larson EB, Wang L, Bowen JD, McCormick WC, Teri L, Crane P et al. Exercise is associated with reduced risk for incident dementia among persons 65 years of age and older. *Ann Intern Med.* 2006;144(2):73-81.

202. Yaffe K, Barnes D, Nevitt M, Lui LY, Covinsky K. A prospective study of physical activity and cognitive decline in elderly women: women who walk. *Arch Intern Med.* 2001;161(14):1703-1708.

203. Verghese J, Lipton RB, Katz MJ, Hall CB, Derby CA, Kuslansky G et al. Leisure activities and the risk of dementia in the elderly. *N Engl J Med.* 2003; 348(25):2508-2516.

204. Schooler C, Mulatu MS. The reciprocal effects of leisure time activities and intellectual functioning in older people: a longitudinal analysis. *Psychol Aging.* 2001;16(3):466-482.

205. Wang JY, Zhou DH, Li J, Zhang M, Deng J, Tang M et al. Leisure activity and risk of cognitive impairment: the Chongqing aging study. *Neurology.* 2006; 66(6):911-913.
206. Fogel J, Carlson MC. Soap operas and talk shows on television are associated with poorer cognition in older women. *South Med J.* 2006;99(3):226-233.
207. Lindstrom HA, Fritsch T, Petot G, Smyth KA, Chen CH, Debanne SM et al. The relationships between television viewing in midlife and the development of Alzheimer's disease in a case-control study. *Brain Cogn.* 2005;58(2):157-165.
208. World Health Organization. The Heidelberg Guidelines for Promoting Physical Activity among Older Persons. 1996. Geneva, Ageing and Health Programme, Division of Health Promotion, Education and Communication.
209. American Heart Association. Available at: http://www.americanheart.org. Accessed February 8, 2006.
210. Dipietro L. Physical activity in aging: changes in patterns and their relationship to health and function. *J Gerontol A Biol Sci Med Sci.* 2001;56(2):13-22.
211. Grajczyk A, Zollner O. How older people watch television. Telemetric data on the TV use in Germany in 1996. *Gerontology.* 1998;44(3):176-181.
212. Meara J, Mitchelmore E, Hobson P. Use of the GDS-15 geriatric depression scale as a screening instrument for depressive symptomatology in patients with Parkinson's disease and their carers in the community. *Age Ageing.* 1999; 28(1):35-38.
213. Riley KP. Depression. In: Bonder RR, Wagner MB, eds. *Functional Performance in Older Adults.* Philadelphia: FA Davis Company; 2001:306-315.
214. Lomax CL, Brown RG, Howard RJ. Measuring disability in patients with neurodegenerative disease using the 'Yesterday Interview'. *Int J Geriatr Psychiatry.* 2004;19(11):1058-1064.
215. Karlsen KH, Tandberg E, Arsland D, Larsen JP. Health related quality of life in Parkinson's disease: a prospective longitudinal study. *J Neurol Neurosurg Psychiatry.* 2000;69(5):584-589.
216. Verghese J, LeValley A, Derby C, Kuslansky G, Katz M, Hall C et al. Leisure activities and the risk of amnestic mild cognitive impairment in the elderly. *Neurology.* 2006;66(6):821-827.
217. Beard JG, Ragheb MG. Measuring leisure satisfaction. *J Leisure Res.* 1980; 12:20-33.
218. Gregory MD. Occupational behavior and life satisfaction among retirees. *Am J Occup Ther.* 1983;37(8):548-553.
219. Taylor HL, Jacobs DR, Jr., Schucker B, Knudsen J, Leon AS, DeBacker G. A questionnaire for the assessment of leisure time physical activities. *J Chronic Dis.* 1978;31(12):741-755.
220. Bundy AC. Leisure. In: Bonder BR, Wagner MB, eds. *Functional Performance in Older Adults.* Philadelphia: FA Davis, 2001:196-217.
221. Decker JA. *Making the Moments Count: Leisure Activities for Caregiving Relationships.* Baltimore, MD: Johns Hopkins University Press, 1997.
222. Gerber LH, Furst GP. Scoring methods and application of the activity record (ACTRE) for patients with musculoskeletal disorders. *Arthritis Care Res.* 1992; 5(3):151-156.
223. Smith NR, Kielhofner G, Watts JH. The relationships between volition, activity pattern, and life satisfaction in the elderly. *Am J Occup Ther.* 1986;40(4):278-283.
224. Moss MS, Lawton MP. Time budgets of older people: a window on four lifestyles. *J Gerontol.* 1982;37(1):115-123.
225. Lyons M, Orozovic N, Davis J, Newman J. Doing-being-becoming: occupational experiences of persons with life-threatening illnesses. *Am J Occup Ther.* 2002; 56(3):285-295.

Developing an Occupational Therapy Home Program for Patients With Parkinson's Disease

Nancy Lowenstein, MS, OTR, BCPR;
Linda Tickle-Degnen, PhD, OTR/L, FAOTA

Introduction

Quality of life research has shown that people with Parkinson's disease (PD) experience distress associated with feelings of lack of control and mastery, public shame, and social isolation.[1-5] Due to disease processes, the natural flow of daily activity as it was once lived is compromised for the person with PD. Concurrent problems in motor, emotional, and cognitive function (although self-awareness and reality orientation are generally intact) often compound the ability to cope with losses, manage the disease, and find solutions for maintaining competent participation in valued personal, family, work, and community activities. Yet people with PD are similar to aging individuals with other chronic diseases in that they value a life in which they are able to maintain relationships with friends, meaningful time use, and positive emotion.[6] Psychosocial adaptation to PD has been found to be more related to participation in valued daily activities than to the severity of the disease.[7,8] Individuals who maintain the quality of these activities, regardless of disease severity, are less depressed and experience more well-being than those who do not maintain their participation. As a result, an effective occupational therapy intervention program must target directly the maintenance and restoration of participation in valued daily activities as a primary means toward improving quality of life in this population.

In individuals with PD, as well as across various clinical populations, a specificity of training effect has been demonstrated.[9] Performance improves most on tasks that are the most directly trained. For example, if self-care strategies need improvement then self-care strategies must be practiced directly. An effective occupational therapy program must engage the patient in tasks and activities that the patient must actually do in real life (eg, buttoning one's own clothing, or learning to negotiate mobility around one's own kitchen), as opposed to simulated tasks or tasks that are presumed, without strong empirical support, to influence components of real-life activities (eg, stacking cones to develop grasp-and-release ability for meal preparation).

Related to this specificity of training effect, it has been found that learning how to perform an activity of daily living (ADL) in the actual context in which that activity is usually performed is superior to learning in an environment and context in which the activity is not normally performed.[10-12] The most natural context for learning daily life activities is in one's own home and community. Although individual intervention in the home is helpful, group intervention is also beneficial because of the facilitative effect of social support and group influence on regular engagement in self-management activities.[13] As a result, the most beneficial occupational therapy intervention occurs both individually in the patient's home and surrounding community, as well as in a group context, such as in a clinic or a regularly scheduled group in the community.

The purpose of this chapter is to describe occupational therapy home intervention that occurs as part of a rehabilitation program for PD, the effectiveness of which is currently being tested in a randomized controlled trial.[14] The first author is the occupational therapist who works with an intervention team that also involves a physical therapist, a speech and language pathologist, as well as a neurological medical team that monitors optimal medication for all research participants. The second author is a co-investigator involved in planning, implementing, and analyzing the results of the trial. We focus here on one element of the 6-week rehabilitation program: occupational therapy intervention in the home that occurs weekly while the patient also experiences a twice weekly group rehabilitation session in a university clinic. The specific objective of this home intervention, as well as the overall interdisciplinary rehabilitation program, is the improvement of quality of life through a self-management approach to maintaining and restoring participation in valued daily activities in the home and community.

Self-Management Rehabilitation: Research Evidence

Although PD is a chronic, degenerative disease with no known cure, its negative effects on health and quality of life can be controlled and the progression slowed down through a self-management model of illness management combined with optimal medical intervention.[15-17] Self-management rehabilitation involves teaching skills to patients and caregivers that are needed to develop healthy habits and assume an active role in carrying out health care regimens and managing health-related quality of life problems as they arise in daily life.[18,19] Using a client-centered approach, quality of life problems are identified in collaboration with the patient, family, and team members. Evidence-based rehabilitation is directed at setting realistic goals and developing action plans in the context of patient and family preferences, resources, real life needs and capabilities. There is active clinic, home, and community contact to identify potential problems, and check and reinforce progress in implementing action plans.

Evidence suggests that a self-management approach to PD is effective. Montgomery et al[16] found that an individualized patient education program for people with PD slowed the progression of the disease, reduced neurological symptoms, and reduced side effects of medicine compared to a control group. The success of the program appeared to relate to the consistent monitoring of patient symptoms with responsive feedback to both patient and physician, as well as the concrete and individualized suggestions for exercise and other self-management behaviors in the home. Lorig et al[15] found that a 7-week patient education program that targeted the development of self-management skills, including maintaining adequate exercise, among older adults with a variety of chronic illnesses (eg, stroke or arthritis) resulted in significantly improved health behaviors, health status, quality of life, and health service utilization compared to a control condition. Ellis et al,[9] in a cross-national randomized trial, found a 6-week clinical exercise program for PD to effectively improve mobility in the home and community.

Individuals with PD have attributes that prepare them to benefit from self-management rehabilitation. First, they typically have a history of normal functioning in adult life, with developed skills and preferences, and they identify continued and competent involvement in daily life activities and roles as central to their quality of life.[6-8] As a result they bring experience and focused self-knowledge and preferences to their health encounters that enable them to collaborate in goal setting and intervention planning and implementation. Second, they are able to effectively learn new tasks and improve performance through the focused practice of tasks. There are documented statistically and clinically significant practice effects for ADL, such as mobility and self-care[20,21] as well as body functions such as those related to movement[22,23] and voice production.[24] Quantitative research syntheses[20,21] demonstrate that the magnitude of the effect of rehabilitation training on the functioning of patients with PD is equivalent to other findings that demonstrate that older community-residing adults benefit from well-designed rehabilitation interventions.[25]

An effective self-management program capitalizes on these areas of intact functioning in PD, and simultaneously addresses areas of disease-related disability. People with PD learn tasks most efficiently and effectively when the strategies of performing the tasks compensate for disabilities in motor and cognitive initiation and sequencing. These disabilities arise from basal ganglia dysfunction and its effect on prefrontal cortex function.[26,29] For example, evidence is building that people with PD can consciously compensate to a degree for movement impairment, such as akinesia and bradykinesia, by directing their attention consciously to external performance, timing, and sequencing cues[28,29] and, consequently, reduce their dependency on impaired basal ganglia functioning to perform actions. A home program can capitalize on these findings by allowing the individual to practice timing and sequencing strategies during normal daily activities in the home and the community.

THE THEORETICAL BASIS OF A SELF-MANAGEMENT OCCUPATIONAL THERAPY HOME PROGRAM

Figures 10-1 and 10-2 depict elements of self-management occupational therapy that are derived from three theoretical and evidence-based perspectives of health behavior and performance: the theory of planned behavior[30,31] the social cognitive theory of self-regulation,[32] and a person-environment-task model.[33,34] Each of these perspectives strengthens a home intervention approach that targets training in the self-management of PD. The theory of planned behavior contributes elements shown in Figure 10-1 that are related to attitudes and social norms as they influence a person's intentions and goal-

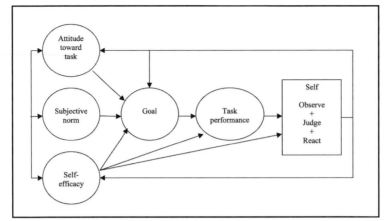

Figure 10-1. Model for self-management rehabilitation that incorporates aspects of theories. Adapted from Ajzen (1991) and Bandura (1991).

Figure 10-2. Task performance as a function of personal abilities, environmental factors, and task parameters.

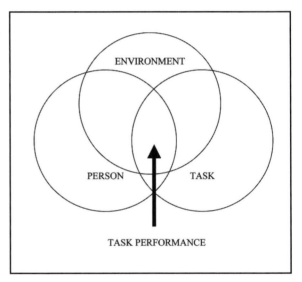

directed behavior. The social cognitive theory of self-regulation contributes elements shown in Figure 10-1 that are related to promoting the patient's self-efficacy and self-regulation of goal-directed behavior during daily task performance. The person-environment-task model identifies elements shown in Figure 10-2 that the patient monitors during task performance and learns to adapt in order to successfully achieve important home and community goals.

Together, the elements shown in these figures guide the occupational therapist in planning home interventions that address: 1) patient preferences and attitudes with respect to forming healthy living goals, 2) patient skills in monitoring and regulating ones' thoughts, feelings, and behavior during occupational tasks, and 3) patient skills for assessing and adapting oneself, the environment, and the occupational task on a daily basis in order to maintain habits that support achievement of goals. The following sections provide descriptions of each element in the figures.

Task Performance

The key element of the model in Figure 10-1 and the focus of intervention in occupational therapy is a task performance. Occupational therapists intervene to facilitate successful performance of tasks related to ADLs (including exercise and medication management); instrumental activities of daily living (IADLs); community participation; and vocational, social, and leisure involvement. What is determined to be a successful performance varies according to the patient and is derived through a collaborative process with the patient, family members, the occupational therapist, and other health care team members. Success may be indicated by patient independence, confidence, or satisfaction in the task performance and the effect of that task performance on overall daily living.

Motivation to Perform a Task

The elements in Figure 10-1 to the left of the task performance element are factors that contribute to the motivation for performing the task. There is a strong and growing body of research that demonstrates that successful outcomes are more likely if both therapist and patient agree on the goal and method of intervention.[35,36] Successful task performance and outcomes are less likely if an intervention goal and task are incongruent with: 1) the patient's own attitude toward a task targeted for intervention; 2) the subjective norm, ie, what the patient perceives to be family's, friends' and others' attitudes toward this task; and 3) the patient's self-efficacy, ie, the belief about control over one's level of functioning during the task.

The paths of the model from attitude toward task and subjective norm to establishment of a goal that then leads to task performance are drawn and modified from Ajzen's[30] theory of planned behavior. An attitude toward a task is a function of beliefs about the outcomes of a task performance as well as an evaluation of those outcomes. For example, a patient may believe that brushing her teeth will make her appearance more socially acceptable and will enable her to maintain strong teeth to support her ability to eat. This belief is conducive to forming a goal of brushing one's teeth regularly. However, favorable beliefs about task outcomes are only one aspect of an attitude that is conducive to forming a goal to perform a task. The patient must also value these outcomes. If the patient does not value a socially acceptable appearance or an ability to eat, her attitude toward the task of teeth brushing will not be conducive to her performing that task.

Ajzen[30] has argued that the subjective norm is also influential in the formation of an intention to perform a behavior or task. The patient's own social support network can be quite influential if the patient believes that individuals in that network approve or disapprove of the patient performing the task, and the patient also wants to comply with those individuals. If the patient believes that others approve of the task performance, but the patient does not care about complying with what others want the patient to do, then the subjective norm will not be supportive to the patient performing the task. For example, the patient will be more likely to set a goal of regular teeth brushing if she believes that valued family and friends think that she should brush her teeth, and the patient wants to comply with their wishes.

A third element that contributes to the motivation to perform a task is the patient's feelings of efficacy related to task performance. The paths of the model from self-efficacy to goal, task performance, and self-observation, judgment and reaction to a task performance are drawn and modified from Bandura's[32] social cognitive theory of self-regulation. Whereas Ajzen's[30] theory primarily contributes elements to the model that are important for planning a task performance, Bandura's[32] theory contributes elements that affect and are affected by the actual task performance, specifically as related to self-efficacy. A patient's self-efficacy with respect to a task performance is a personal belief about one's capability of exercising control over one's level of functioning during the task.[30,31] Patients who believe they can control their level of functioning during the task are more likely to set a goal of doing the task, and, then, while performing the task, monitoring their performance to adjust subsequent beliefs about control. If patients feel little control over personal functioning during the task, they are less likely to want to do the task in the first place. For example, a patient who feels that she can control the quality and efficiency of her teeth brushing is more likely to set a goal of regular teeth brushing than a patient who feels little control over the quality and efficiency of the task performance.

The occupational therapist can maximize the motivation for task performance in the home by first assessing patient attitudes toward tasks that are important for self-management of PD, subjective norms around these tasks, and self-efficacy beliefs related to the tasks. The therapist works collaboratively with the patient to identify tasks that lead to self-management outcomes, and are valued by the patient, supported by the patient's caregivers, and perceived by the patient, realistically, to be within the patient's capacity.[18] Meta-analytic evidence[37] suggests that adult neurological populations in particular are more likely to put effort into task performance and show high quality motor performance in tasks that are perceived by the patients to be purposeful and meaningful as opposed to tasks perceived as non-purposeful or meaningless. The occupational therapist not only seeks to identify self-management goals that are important to the patient, but also educates the patient about which goals are essential for self-management. In this manner, they collaboratively construct a task performance goal. Once a goal is established, the therapist and patient work toward performing the task successfully.

Observing, Judging, and Reacting to Task Performance

Bandura[32] theorized that self-regulation occurs through three sub-functions: self-observation, judgmental processes, and self-reaction to actual task performances in context. These sub-functions are depicted together in the box to the right of the task performance element in Figure 10-1. Self-observation is the process of attending to one's own performance by noting what occurs, how it occurs, and when it occurs during the performance. Judgmental processes include comparing the observed performance against one's own and others' standards of performance. Self-reaction is the process of evaluating positively or negatively one's performance in comparison to these standards and deciding what to do next, eg, to reward or punish oneself. This entire self-monitoring and self-reacting process influences the patient's self-efficacy for future task performance attempts, as well as the attitudes toward the tasks and new goals for task performance. An individual's observations, judgments, and reactions can have a favorable or unfavorable effect on future task performance.

The occupational therapist's role is to teach the patient how to carefully observe his or her own behavior in the context of the task, how to judge it against personal and normative standards, and how to react to the performance realistically and productively. Although Bandura's view of self-reaction is primarily related to affective reactions, in our self-management program we have incorporated an additional type of reaction related to deciding what to do next. That reaction is a response to the question: "Can I change something about myself, the task, or the environment to improve my task performance in the future?" We use the person-environment-task model of task analysis that is shown in Figure 10-2 and is commonly used by occupational therapists to describe occupational performance.[33,34] The model recognizes that task performance is a function of personal abilities (physical, emotional, and cognitive), environmental factors (physical and social), and occupational task parameters (strategies, steps, and methods of performing the task). Each of these elements contributes equally to task performance, and changing any one or all of the elements can modify this performance. For example, the occupational therapist works with a patient who has a goal of brushing her teeth regularly to observe her own skills of brushing teeth and monitoring its regularity, to note elements in the environment that support or hinder her performance, and to identify different means of performing the teeth brushing task that may be simpler to repeat on a regular basis.

SELF-MANAGEMENT OCCUPATIONAL THERAPY IN THE HOME

Successful home programs need to be individually tailored to the patient and his or her environment. It has been this author's experience that health care providers often tell individuals with chronic diseases that rehabilitation is not going to be effective and therefore they are not frequently referred. Additionally, Beatty et al[38] found that individuals with chronic diseases had difficulty accessing rehabilitation services due mostly to insurance barriers. Insurance companies do not want to pay for "maintenance" therapy, and often those with chronic diseases are put into this category by insurance companies. Therefore, individuals have often either given up an occupation or activity, or have made slow adaptations as their skills have diminished or changed. The goal of a home program should be to encourage the patient to identify his or her strengths and deficits, to teach adaptations and compensatory techniques, to allow for practice of a skill in the context in which it will be performed, and to teach the patient methods to solve problems as they arise.

Evaluation

All occupational therapy intervention should start with a thorough client-centered assessment that includes an occupational history as well as an assessment of contextual factors and patient factors.[39] Using client-centered assessments before component based ones will assist the clinician and patient in goal collaboration. It is also important to discuss the different environments that the patient usually functions within (work and community settings) and for the occupational therapist to understand the barriers that these other contexts pose. Essential to a self-management model is to assist the patient in identifying the problems at the participation, activity, and patient factor levels. Excellent tools for assessment at the participation level are the Canadian Occupational Performance Measure, 4th edition (COPM),[40] the Occupational Performance History Interview II (OPHI-II) Version 2.1,[41] and Occupational Self Assessment (OSA) Version 2.2.[42] The COPM and the OPHI-II are semi-structured interviews and the OSA is a patient self-assessment. These tools assist the therapist in obtaining information regarding the patient's self-perception of his or her abilities in the areas of self-care, productivity, and leisure. The value of these tools, versus a component based occupational therapy evaluation, is that by using these assessments, the occupational therapist allows the patient to identify his or her goals and priorities. In this way, the patient, not the occupational therapist, has control of the intervention process. One non-OT assessment for the participation level is the Parkinson's Disease Quality of Life Questionnaire-39 Item Version (PDQ-39).[5,43] An assessment at the activity level would be the Unified Parkinson's Disease Rating Scale (UPSRS).[44] For assessment at the patient factors level, there are various component-based assessments for perceptual, cognitive, and motor skills.

In home care, the focuses of occupational therapy intervention for patients with PD are the areas of functional mobility in and around different environments: bathing, dressing, handwriting, and computer access. Occupational therapists are also skilled at addressing issues around transfers and mobility pertaining to chairs, beds, and cars—all activities that individuals with PD may have difficulty performing. Additionally, the present authors believe that the role of OT is to assist a patient in developing habits and routines that encourage healthy behaviors, such as exercise routines, energy conservation techniques, medication routines, and organizing the patient's environment to maximize his or her independence.

Intervention

Using the Person Environment Occupation Model,[33,34] one of the goals of a home self-management program for individuals with PD is to educate patients in monitoring their own performance of the task, as well as adjust their performance by asking the question: "Can I change something about myself, the task, or the environment in order to improve performance?" Occupational therapists bring the unique ability to analyze tasks, activities, and occupations in the contexts in which they are commonly performed and make adjustments in order to achieve optimal performance. This skill is the focus of occupational therapy intervention in the home for individuals with PD. After learning the skills of activity analysis, the patients are able to adjust their performance as their condition varies on a daily, monthly, or yearly basis. An example of this might be the individual who is able to make a cup of tea or coffee easily when at the "peak" of his or her medication, but when the medication effects are wearing off, and the patient is more rigid or slower in his or her movements, may need to make adjustments such as using a microwave to heat the water, or a covered mug to carry it. It is the authors' experience that patients with PD are best served by learning skills to adapt to different situations, rather than one adaptation that might not be useful as their condition changes daily, monthly, or yearly. This is not to say that occupational therapists do not also address compensatory skills for self-care, productivity, and leisure activities, but embedded into each teaching session should be instruction on how to problem solve as the patient's condition changes.

For the occupational therapist, it is important to have an understanding of the particular issues that individuals with PD face. These include their medication "on" and "off" times,[45,46] use of cognitive methods (such as consciously thinking about the movement),[28,29] and practice of an activity in the context in which it is frequently performed in order to improve performance.[37,47] All interventions must be individually tailored for each patient's unique needs and goals. Including significant others in the practice of tasks can assist the patient in accurately monitoring his or her performance by allowing external feedback and cueing during the performance. Additionally, by including significant others in the intervention, the occupational therapist can educate these individuals in correct ways to provide cueing and feedback. For instance, family members may be providing too much assistance during an ADL task. When they are taught to provide correct verbal cueing, the patient may be able to function more independently. Additionally, performing tasks in the context in which they are usually completed is key to improving performance for individuals with PD.[37,47]

In learning to monitor their performance, it may be useful for patients to keep a log or chart of medication peaks and lows, of falls, or of how long it takes to do an activity during different times of the day. These charts are easy to create (Figure 10-3) and are most effective when they require checks or simple abbreviations, as micrographia is frequently a problem for individuals with PD.[46] The authors have found videotaping to be a useful tool in giving visual feedback to patients. Individuals with PD often develop a "stooped"

Time	Symptom	Medication	Activity	Comments

Figure 10-3. Sample log for client to record.

posture or festinating gait, yet when told to stand straight or to take bigger strides they are unable to properly compensate because they feel they are going to fall backward. However, when they view their posture or gait on video, this visual feedback can help to show the correct posture or gait. For instance, when individuals see that they are stooped forward during walking, and can also see and feel what they look like while straight, they are better able to incorporate this proprioceptive feedback into their actual walking.

Environmental modifications are an important intervention for individuals with PD. This involves not just making sure that grab bars are installed in the bathroom, but also that visual cues are used throughout the home to assist in walking.[48] Visual cues, such as lines on the floor or looking at a spot on the wall, during walking can act as cues for stride length or prevent freezing in doorways.[26,49] The occupational therapist can help patients identify effective visual and sensory strategies to use around their home and in the community. For instance, an individual who is having difficulty walking down a hallway to go to the bathroom and frequently freezing in the doorway to the bathroom can be taught to look at a spot directly in front of him or her and walk toward this. While walking in the grocery store or mall, an individual can be taught to visualize the lines on the floor tiles and step over them or to pick a spot at the end of the aisle and walk toward that spot.

Ergonomics is another area for the occupational therapist to consider in the home. Micrographia, a frequent symptom, can pose a significant issue in the lives of individuals with PD. Many patients may already be using a computer or limiting their writing to only important tasks, such as bill paying or check writing. By assessing the ergonomic set-up of the individual's computer station and ensuring that the arms are fully supported, that the keyboard and mouse are in the best positions, and by teaching them to use the built-in accessibility features in Mac and PC computers, their computer use can improve tremendously. Tremors[46] are a frequent problem reported by patients that interfere with both computer use and handwriting. Fortunately, there are built-in features on all computers for tremors. These features, known as filter keys, filter out repeated key strokes and sticky keys to assist with one-handed typing. These can be found under the accessibility features of both PC and Mac computers. In this same accessibility area, there are ways to change the screen display for visual issues, as well as the cursor options and blink rate. Mouse click speed sensitivity can be altered and the mouse can be changed from right-handed to left-handed use. Furthermore, there are many assistive technology adaptations that are available, and a referral to an assistive technology consultant may be appropriate for the patient. One adaptation that may be useful for individuals with PD is the Assistive Mouse Adapter, available from Montrose Secam Limited (Iver, Bucks, England), a British electronics company. This mouse was developed specifically for individuals with tremors and is able to filter out the shaking of the cursor caused by tremors (http://domino.watson.ibm.com/comm/pr.nsf/pages/news.20050314_mouseadapter.html).

Functional mobility is another key area to address in the home.[50] For individuals with PD, this may include bed mobility (rolling in bed, getting in and out of bed), and getting on and off of furniture, especially soft chairs, couches, recliners, and rocking chairs. Getting in and out of cars may also be an area to assess for intervention. Teaching the patient to assess the factors that may be causing the mobility problem is as important as teaching the correct technique. For instance, patients might determine they need to strengthen their quads and improve their trunk flexibility to assist in the mechanics needed for rising from a soft chair, or they may determine that they need to sit in only in hard chairs with armrests. By using proper techniques (slide to the front of the chair, place feet underneath their knees, rock forward a few times to gain momentum, and push up on armrests), they are able to get up independently. Lastly, they may determine that at certain times of the day, they cannot sit in chairs that are difficult to rise from.

As mentioned earlier, in the authors' practice we have noted that tremor may be a significant issue for individuals with PD. Tremor at rest may create feelings of embarrassment and lead to social isolation. Strategies to cope with tremor may include putting hands in pockets when standing still or holding a small object in one hand and moving it from one hand to another.

Case Study

Mr. R is a 68-year-old male with a 10-year history of PD. He lives at home with his wife in a two-story home. There is a garage that leads to the house with four steps into the kitchen. On the first floor are the kitchen, living room, dining room, family room, and half bath. The second floor has three bedrooms, one being the master bed/bath combination. One of the bedrooms was converted to a home office, with a computer desk, computer, chair, and horizontal file cabinets. Mr. R is retired from his job as an accountant. He presented upon home evaluation with the following COPM issues (Table 10-1). Bed Mobility: His bed was very high, with a new mattress, and a heavy comforter. When looking at the Person Environment Occupation model and bed mobility, Mr. R decided that he did not need to change anything about himself, however by changing from a heavy comforter to an electric blanket, his bed mobility would be improved. By doing vocal and oral motor exercises, he noticed that he was not being asked to repeat himself as often. Setting up a regular exercise space in his house and changing his attitude toward exercise (this attitude change was reinforced by improvements in mobility that he was experiencing through regular exercise) allowed him to engage in regular exercise again. Mr. R began a regular walking program with the occupational therapist and kept a chart of his time and distance. He also walked after he had taken his medications. When Mr. R was discharged from occupational therapy, he had developed a regular exercise routine of walking and doing stretches and strengthening and flexibility exercises that he had learned with the occupational therapist during his sessions. Additionally, he took it upon himself to find a place to walk in the winter, and decided that he could return to assistant coaching a high school junior varsity basketball team. Prior to OT treatment being initiated, he had assumed he could not coach, as his voice could not be heard and he would not be able to move along the sidelines. Upon discharge, Mr. R's endurance had improved significantly so that he was walking a mile a day. He reported increased flexibility in his trunk movements, less stiffness when off medication, and more energy for work and leisure.

TABLE 10-1

COPM for Case Study

COPM Problem	Change Self	Change Activity/ Strategy	Change Environment
Bed mobility	Trunk rotation exercises	Satin sheets or satin PJs	Purchase electric blanket
Soft voice	Vocal exercises	Phone amplifier	
Improve walking	Leg exercises	Walk with someone or with metronome	Walk on smooth surfaces Set up outside walking route
Exercise more	Change attitude toward exercise	Break exercise up into smaller time periods (stretch during commercial breaks)	Set up exercise area in home
Freezes when walking in open spaces	Do heavy work when meds at peak	Look at point in distance and walk toward that	Wear Walkman or iPod while walking and listen to songs at correct walking speed

CONCLUSION

The key to home intervention for individuals with PD is to collaboratively identify the patient's goals, to teach problem-solving skills, and to practice the task in the context in which it is performed. Because PD is chronic and progressive, it is important to teach patients the skills needed to manage their disease on a daily basis, as well as throughout the weeks, months, and years. Patients may need to be referred to occupational therapy several times over the course of the disease to assist with problem solving in new contexts or to learn and practice skills as their condition changes. It is imperative that the therapist educate patients about the recurring needs for occupational therapy that may occur over the course of time so they feel empowered to ask for referrals from their physician, as needed.

ACKNOWLEDGMENT

This chapter was supported in part by Grant Number NAG21152 (PI, Robert Wagenaar; Co-I, Tickle-Degnen) from the National Institute of Aging of the National Institutes of Health (NIH). Its contents are solely the responsibility of the author and do not necessarily represent the official views of NIH.

REFERENCES

1. Brod M, Mendelsohn GA, Roberts B. Patients' experiences of Parkinson's disease. *J Gerontol B Psychol Sci Soc Sci.* 1998;53(B):213-222.
2. Koplas PA, Gans HB, Wisely MP, Kuchibhatla M, Cutson TM, Gold DT et al. Quality of life and Parkinson's disease. *J Gerontol A Biol Sci Med Sci.* 1999;54(A):M197-M202.
3. Lyons KD, Tickle-Degnen L. The dramaturgical challenges of Parkinson's disease. *Occup Ther J Res.* 2003;23(1):27-34.
4. Nijhof G. Parkinson's disease as a problem of shame in public appearance. *Sociol Health Illness.* 1995;17(2):193-205.
5. Peto V, Jenkinson C, Fitzpatrick R, Greenhall R. The development and validation of a short measure of functioning and well being for individuals with Parkinson's disease. *Qual Life Res.* 1995;4(3):241-248.
6. Lawton MP. Quality of life in chronic illness. *Gerontology.* 1999;45(4):181-183.
7. Herrmann M, Freyholdt U, Fuchs G, Wallesch CW. Coping with chronic neurological impairment: a contrastive analysis of Parkinson's disease and stroke. *Disabil Rehabil.* 1997;19(1):6-12.
8. Livneh H, Antonak RF. Review of research on psychosocial adaptation to neuromuscular disorders: I. Cerebral Palsy, Muscular Dystrophy, and Parkinson's Disease. *J of Soc Behav and Personality.* 1994;9(5):201-230.
9. Ellis T, de Goede C, Feldman RG, Wolters EC, Kwakkel G, Wagenaar RC. Efficacy of a physical therapy program in patients with Parkinson's disease: a randomized controlled trial. *Arch Phys Med Rehabil.* 2005;86(4):626-632.
10. Gilbertson L, Langhorne P, Walker A, Allen A, Murray GD. Domiciliary occupational therapy for patients with stroke discharged from hospital: randomized controlled trial. *BMJ.* 2000;320(7235):603-606.
11. Matteliano M, Mann W, Tomita M. Comparison of home based older patients who received occupational therapy with patients not receiving occupational therapy. *Phys Occup Ther Geriatrics.* 2000;21(1):22-33.
12. Von Koch L, Wottrich AW, Homquist LW. Rehabilitation in the home versus the hospital: the importance of context. *Dis Rehab.* 1998;20(10):367-372.
13. Carron AV, Hausenblas HA, Mack D. Social influence and exercise: a meta-analysis. *J Sport Exer Psychol.* 1996;18(4):1-16.
14. Tickle-Degnen L, Ellis T, Wagenarr RC. Evidence-based rehabilitation for the self-management of Parkinson's disease. Platform presentation. American Occupational Therapy Association 85th Annual Conference, May 12–15, 2005, Long Beach, CA. 2005.
15. Lorig KR, Sobel DS, Stewart AL, Brown BW, Bandura A, Ritter P et al. Evidence suggesting that a chronic disease self-management program can improve health status while reducing hospitalization: a randomized trial. *Med Care.* 1999;37(1):5-14.
16. Montgomery EB, Lieberman A, Singh G, Fries JF. Patient education and health promotion can be effective in Parkinson's disease: a randomized controlled trial. *Am J Med.* 1994;97(5):429-435.
17. Von Korff M, Gruman J, Schaefer J, Curry SJ, Wagner EH. Collaborative management of chronic illness. *Ann Intern Med.* 1997;127(12):1097-1102.
18. Lyons KD. Self-management of Parkinson's disease: guidelines for program development and evaluation. *Phys Occup Ther Geriatrics.* 2003;21(3):17-31.
19. Neufeld P, Kniepmann K. Wellness and self-management programs for persons with chronic disabling conditions. *OT Practice.* 2003;8(13):17-21.
20. de Goede CJ, Keus SH, Kwakkel G, Wagenaar RC. The effects of physical therapy in Parkinson's disease: a research synthesis. *Arch Phys Med Rehabil.* 2001;82(4):509-515.
21. Murphy S, Tickle-Degnen L. The effectiveness of occupational therapy-related treatments for persons with Parkinson's disease: a meta-analytic review. *Am J Occup Ther.* 2001;55(4):385-392.
22. Behrman AL, Cauraugh JH, Light KE. Practice as an intervention to improve speeded motor performance and motor learning in Parkinson's disease. *J Neurol Sci.* 1991;174(2):127-136.
23. Ma HI, Trombly CA, Wagenaar RC, Tickle-Degnen L. Effect of one single auditory cue on movement kinematics in patients with Parkinson's disease. *Am J Phys Med Rehabil.* 2004;83(5):530-536.
24. De Angelis EC, Mourao LF, Ferraz HB, Behlau MS, Pontes PA, Andrade LA. Effect of voice rehabilitation on oral communication of Parkinson's disease patients. *Acta Neurol Scand.* 1997;96(4):199-205.
25. Clark F, Azen SP, Zemke R, Jackson J, Carlson M, Mandel D et al. Occupational therapy for independent-living older adults. A randomized controlled trial. *JAMA.* 1997; 278(16):1321-1326.
26. Morris ME, Iansek R. Characteristics of motor disturbance in Parkinson's disease and strategies for movement rehabilitation. *Human Mvt Sci.* 1996;15(5):649-669.
27. Zalla T, Sirigu A, Pillon B, Dubois B, Grafman J, Agid Y. Deficit in evaluating pre-determined sequences of script events in patients with Parkinson's disease. *Cortex.* 1998; 34(4):621-628.
28. Marchese R, Diverio M, Zucchi F, Lentino C, Abbruzzese G. The role of sensory cues in the rehabilitation of parkinsonian patients: a comparison of two physical therapy protocols. *Mov Disord.* 2000;15(5):879-883.

29. Montgomery EB, Jr. Rehabilitative approaches to Parkinson's disease. *Parkinsonism Relat Disord.* 2004;10 Suppl 1:S43-S47.

30. Ajzen I. The theory of planned behavior. *Organiz Behav Human Decision Processes.* 1991;50(2):179-211.

31. Ajzen I. Perceived behavioral control, self-efficacy, locus of control, and the theory of planned behavior. *J Appl Soc Psychol.* 2002;32(4):665-683.

32. Bandura A. Social cognitive theory of self-regulation. *Organiz Behav Human Decision Processes.* 1991;50:248-287.

33. Fisher AG. Uniting practice and theory in an occupational framework. 1998 Eleanor Clarke Slagle Lecture. *Am J Occup Ther.* 1998;52(7):509-521.

34. Law M, Cooper B, Strong S, Stewart D, Rigby P, Letts L. The Person-Environment-Occupation Model: A transactive approach to occupational performance. *Can J Occup Ther.* 1996;63(1):9-23.

35. Law M. Does client-centered practice make a difference. In: Law M, ed. *Client-Centered Occupational Therapy.* Thorofare, NJ: SLACK Incorporated; 1998:19-27.

36. Martin DJ, Garske JP, Davis MK. Relation of the therapeutic alliance with outcome and other variables: a meta-analytic review. *J Consult Clin Psychol.* 2000;68(3):438-450.

37. Lin K, Wu C, Tickle-Degnen L, Coster W. Enhancing occupational performance through occupationally embedded exercise: a meta-analytic review. *Occup Ther J Res.* 1997; 17(1):25-47.

38. Beatty PW, Hagglund KJ, Neri MT, Dhont KR, Clark MJ, Hilton SA. Access to health care services among people with chronic or disabling conditions: patterns and predictors. *Arch Phys Med Rehabil.* 2003;84(10):1417-1425.

39. Occupational therapy practice framework: domain and process. *Am J Occup Ther.* 2002; 56(6):609-639.

40. Law M, Baptiste S, Carswell A, McColl M, Polatajko H, Pollock N. *Canadian Occupational Performance Measure.* 4th ed. Ottawa: CAOT Publications, 2005.

41. Kielhofner G, Forsyth K, de las Heras CG, Hayashi MJ, Raymond L. Observational assessments. In: Kielhofner G, ed. *Model of Human Occupation.* Baltimore, MD: Lippincott Williams & Wilkins; 2002:191-212.

42. Henry AD, Baron KB, Mouradian L, Curtin C. Reliability and validity of the self-assessment of occupational functioning. *Am J Occup Ther.* 1999;53(5):482-488.

43. Peto V, Jenkinson C, Fitzpatrick R. PDQ-39: a review of the development, validation and application of a Parkinson's disease quality of life questionnaire and its associated measures. *J Neurol.* 1998;245 Suppl 1:S10-S14.

44. Fahn S, Elton R. Unified Parkinson's Disease Rating Scale. In: Fahn S, Elton R, and Members of the UPDRS Development Committee (Jankovic J.) *Recent Developments in Parkinson's Disease.* New York: MacMillan; 1987: 153-163.

45. Samil A, Nutt JG, Ransom BR. Parkinson's disease. *Lancet.* 2004;363(9423):1783-1793.

46. Nutt JG, Wooten GF. Clinical practice. Diagnosis and initial management of Parkinson's disease. *N Engl J Med.* 2005;353(10):1021-1027.

47. Trombly CA, Wu CY. Effect of rehabilitation tasks on organization of movement after stroke. *Am J Occup Ther.* 1999;53(4):333-344.

48. Bagley S, Kelly TN. The effects of visual cues on the gait of independently mobile Parkinson's disease patients. *Physiotherapy.* 1991;77:415-420.

49. Jiang Y, Norman KE. Effects of visual and auditory cues on gait initiation in people with Parkinson's disease. *Cl Rehab.* 2006;20(1):36-45.

50. Morris ME. Movement disorders in people with Parkinson disease: a model for physical therapy. *Phys Ther.* 2000;80(6):578-597.

Voice and Speech Disorders in Parkinson's Disease and Their Treatment

Cynthia M. Fox, PhD, CCC-SLP; Lorraine Olson Ramig, PhD, CCC-SLP;
Shimon Sapir, PhD, CCC-SLP; Angela Halpern, MS, CCC-SLP;
Jill Cable, MS, CCC-SLP; Leslie A. Mahler, PhD, CCC-SLP;
Becky G. Farley, PhD, PT

Introduction

Oral communication is vital in education, employment, social functioning, and self-expression. Nearly 300 million children and adults worldwide have a neurological disorder that may impair their ability to communicate orally. The prevalence of disordered communication is particularly high (89%) in the nearly 7 million people worldwide with Parkinson's disease (PD); however, only 3% to 4% receive speech treatment.[1-3] Soft voice, monotone, breathiness, hoarse voice quality, and imprecise articulation,[3-6] together with lessened facial expression (masked facies),[7-8] contribute to limitations in communication in the vast majority of people with PD. Consequently, they are "less likely to participate in conversations" or have "confidence in communication" as compared to healthy aging adults.[9] In addition, dysphagia (disordered swallowing), which may be associated with life-threatening pneumonia, has been reported in as many as 95% of patients[10] (see Chapter 12 for detailed discussion on swallowing disorders in PD). Despite optimal medical management,[11-13] most people with PD have significant speech deficits that negatively impact their quality of life.[14] Affected individuals become disabled or retire early, are forced to give up activities they enjoy, incur substantial medical costs, and have increased mortality.[15] PD costs the United States $5.6 billion annually in direct health-related expenses, disability-related costs, and lost productivity.[16] With PD predicted to increase four-fold by 2040,[17] the potential negative impact of disordered communication in this population is clear.

Successful treatment of speech disorders in people with progressive neurological diseases such as PD can be challenging.[18-22] Although medical treatments, including neuropharmacological as well as neurosurgical methods, may be effective in improving limb symptoms, their impact on speech production remains unclear.[23-29] In addition, previous speech treatment approaches for people with PD, focusing on articulation and rate and delivered in non-intensive regimes, have limited efficacy data and limited evidence of long-term success. Recently, however, a speech treatment approach called LSVT®-LOUD (Lee Silverman Voice Treatment), which emphasizes increasing amplitude of motor output by training vocal loudness and self-monitoring of vocal loudness, has generated the first Level I efficacy data for successfully treating voice and speech disorders in this population.[30-32] Research has documented perceptual, acoustic, aerodynamic, and physiologic improvements in speech and voice and, most recently, using positron emission tomography (PET), neural reorganization in parallel with demonstrated treatment efficacy.[33-37] This established efficacy has offered a unique opportunity to explore and define key elements for successful speech treatment in PD (eg, treatment target, mode of delivery), which has implications not only for speech therapy but other areas of rehabilitation (eg, physical therapy and occupational therapy) as well. This chapter will: 1) review speech and voice characteristics associated with PD; 2) discuss medical, surgical, and behavioral speech treatment approaches for PD; 3) summarize data from LSVT-LOUD and describe components of the LSVT-LOUD speech treatment approach; and 4) highlight ongoing and future research directions in speech rehabilitation for PD.

SPEECH AND VOICE CHARACTERISTICS IN PARKINSON'S DISEASE

Disorders of laryngeal, respiratory, and articulator function have been documented across a number of perceptual, acoustic, and physiological studies in people with PD.[38-44] Although the neural mechanisms underlying these voice and speech disorders are unclear,[45-50] they have traditionally been attributed to the motor signs of the disease (rigidity, bradykinesia, hypokinesia, and tremor). In particular, inadequate muscle activation, the pathophysiologic mechanism underlying bradykinesia/hypokinesia in PD,[51-53] has been implicated as a cause of many speech-system disorders. An additional explanation for the speech and voice impairment is a deficit in the sensory processing related to speech.[35,54-55] Collectively, the hypothesized features underlying the speech disorder in patients with PD[56] include: 1) reduced amplitude of neural drive to the muscles of the speech mechanism that may result in a "soft voice that is monotone,"[57-59] 2) a problem in sensory perception of effort that prevents a person with PD from accurately monitoring his or her vocal motor output that results in,[58,60] 3) the individual's difficulty in independently generating (internal cueing/scaling) the right amount of effort to produce adequate vocal loudness.[61-62] This section will review characteristics of speech and voice impairment in PD patients, including laryngeal and respiratory disorders, articulatory disorders, and deficits in sensory processing related to speech.

Laryngeal and Respiratory Disorders

Darley et al[63] described perceptual characteristics of speech and voice in patients with PD. They identified reduced loudness, monopitch, monoloudness, reduced stress, breathy, hoarse voice quality, imprecise articulation, and short rushes of speech as the classic features of speech and voice in people with PD. Collectively, these speech symptoms are called *hypokinetic dysarthria*.[63] Logemann and colleagues[3] conducted a study of 200 people with PD to examine vocal-tract control and to quantify and describe features of the disorder. Eighty-nine percent of the people with PD in the study presented with laryngeal disorders, comprising breathiness, hoarseness, roughness, and tremulousness. Ho et al[2] studied 200 PD patients and found that voice problems were first to occur, with other speech problems (prosody, articulation, and fluency) gradually appearing later and accompanying more severe motor signs. Sapir and colleagues[36] studied 42 people with PD who sought treatment for their speech problems. Eighty-six percent had an abnormal voice, and this problem tended to occur early in the disease course. Later, with symptom progression, prosodic, fluency, and articulation abnormalities occurred. Furthermore, Aronson[19] and Stewart et al[64] have also observed that voice disorders might occur very early in the disease process.

Acoustic descriptions of voice characteristics of people with PD have also been documented. Vocal sound pressure level (SPL) has been measured. Early studies varied in reporting a reduction in vocal SPL in these people.[65-70] However, Fox and Ramig[9] more recently compared 29 people with PD with an age- and gender-matched control group and found that vocal SPL was 2 to 4 decibels (at 30 cm) lower across a number of speech tasks in people with PD. A 2- to 4-decibel change is equal to a 40% perceptual change in loudness.[9] Furthermore, Ho and colleagues[71] found voice intensity of patients with PD to decay much faster than that observed in a healthy comparison group during various speech tasks.

Results related to fundamental frequency (acoustic correlate of pitch) in the speech of people with PD have consistently reported a reduced frequency.[65-67,69-70,72] Fundamental frequency variability has been reported to be consistently lower in PD patients as compared to healthy aging people.[66-67,69] These findings support the perceptual characteristics of monopitch or monotonous speech typically observed in this patient population.[4-5,73]

Disordered laryngeal function has been documented through a number of imaging studies of the vocal folds (videoendoscopic studies). Hansen et al[74] reported vocal fold bowing (lack of medial vocal fold closure) in 30 out of 32 people with PD. Blumin and colleagues[75] used videostroboscopy and fiberoptic endoscopic techniques, as well as a voice handicap index (VHI) questionnaire, to assess laryngeal function in 15 people with severe PD. They reported 13 (87%) patients had significant vocal fold bowing, and 14 (93%) had a significant self-reported voice handicap. Smith and colleagues[37] documented that 12 of 21 patients with PD in their study demonstrated a form of glottal incompetence (bowing, anterior or posterior chink) on flexible fiberoptic views. Perez et al[76] studied 29 people with PD and observed 50% of them demonstrated difficulties with phase closure of the vocal folds, 46% demonstrated an asymmetrical vibratory pattern, and 55% had laryngeal tremor (vertical laryngeal tremor being the most common).

The mechanisms underlying laryngeal disorders in people with PD have been investigated with electromyographic (EMG) techniques. EMG studies of speech in PD demonstrate either a reduction of neural drive to the laryngeal muscles[38] or abnormally elevated muscle activity[40-42,77-79] and poor reciprocal suppression of laryngeal and respiratory muscles.[80] Hirose and Joshita[81] studied data from the thyroarytenoid (TA) muscles in an individual with parkinsonism who had limited vocal fold movement. They observed no reduction in the number of motor unit discharges and no pathological discharge patterns (such as polyphasic or high amplitude voltages). They reported loss of reciprocal suppression of the TA during inspiration and interpreted this as evidence of deterioration in the reciprocal adjustment of the antagonist muscles associated with rigidity. This finding is consistent with deficits in sensory gating characteristics of PD.[82] Gallena and colleagues[77] used TA EMG and nasoendoscopy to compare laryngeal physiology during speech of people with PD on versus off levodopa, and of people without PD. Significant differences were found between patients and non-patients in the on and off conditions: some patients were observed to have higher levels of laryngeal muscle activation, more vocal fold bowing and greater impairment in voice onset and offset control when they were off levodopa than when they were on levodopa, and in comparison to the healthy controls. Luschei et al[83] studied single motor unit activity in the TA muscle in people with PD and suggested the firing rate of the TA motor units was decreased in males with PD in the study. The investigation reported that this finding as well as those in past studies suggest that PD affects rate and variability in motor unit firing in the laryngeal musculature. Baker et al[38] found that absolute TA amplitudes during a known loudness level task in people with PD were lowest for the group of patients with PD when compared to young normal adults and normal aging adults. Relative TA amplitudes were also decreased in both the aging and PD groups when compared to the young normal adults. The authors concluded that reduced levels of TA muscle activity may contribute to the reduced vocal loudness that is observed in people with PD and aging populations. The reduction in TA activity may also reflect sensory gating anomalies and is contrary to the notion of laryngeal muscle rigidity as the cause of hypophonia in PD.

A number of studies have documented evidence of disordered respiratory function in patients with PD. Researchers reported reduced vital capacity,[84-86] a reduction in the total amount of air expended during maximum phonation tasks,[87] reduced intraoral air pressure during consonant/vowel productions,[88-89] and abnormal airflow patterns.[80,90] The origin of these respiratory abnormalities may be related to variations in airflow resistance resulting from abnormal movements of the vocal folds and supralaryngeal area[80] or abnormal chest wall movements and respiratory muscle activation patterns.[47,89,91]

Articulatory Disorders

In addition to voice abnormalities, disorders in speech articulation have also been documented. Imprecise consonants have been observed in people with PD.[3,73,84] Logemann et al[3,73] reported articulation problems in 45% of the 200 unmedicated PD patients they studied. Ho and colleagues[2] have also documented that nearly half of 200 people with PD they studied had articulatory or fluency problems. Sapir et al[92] found abnormal articulation in 50% of 42 medically treated patients with PD. Disordered rate of speech has also been reported in some people with PD. While rapid rates, or short rushes of speech, have been described in 6% to 13% of people with PD,[66-67,74,93-94] Canter[66] found slower than normal rates. *Palilalia* or stuttering-like speech dysfluencies have been observed in some PD patients.[4,92]

Acoustic correlates of disordered articulation have been studied and include problems with timing of vocal onsets and offsets (voicing during normally voiceless closure intervals of voiceless stops), and spirantization (presence of fricative-like, aperiodic noise during stop closures).[45,95-96] In another study,[97] dysarthric speakers with PD showed longer voice onset times (VOTs) than normal. Such abnormal VOTs may reflect a problem with movement initiation,[97] which may be related to deficits in internal cueing, timing, and/or sensory gating.[45,92] McRae and colleagues[98] studied acoustic and perceptual consequences of articulatory rate changes in the speech of patients with PD and the speech of age-matched healthy controls. They reported that the PD group exhibited smaller measures of acoustic working space and more severe perceptual estimates of speech articulation than the control speakers. The reduction in working vowel space is indicative of reduced motility of the articulators, consistent with hypokinetic articulation characteristics of speech in PD. Flint and colleagues[99] compared the speech of patients with PD to that of people with major depression and healthy controls. Both major depression and PD groups had significantly shortened VOT and decreased F2 transition compared to controls, suggesting reduced range of articulatory movements.

Kinematic analysis of jaw movements in people with PD has also documented disordered articulatory movements.[100-105] Researchers consistently report that people with

PD show a significant reduction in the size and peak velocity of jaw movements during speech when compared to healthy people with normal speech.[97,103,106] The reduction in range of movement has been attributed to rigidity of the articulatory muscles;[107-108] however, this may be related to a problem with sensorimotor perception and/or scaling of speech and non-speech movements.[2,45,54-55,109]

EMG studies of the lip and jaw muscles in people with and without PD have provided some evidence for increased levels of tonic resting and background activity,[40-42,78-79] as well as for loss of reciprocity between agonist and antagonist muscle groups.[40-41,78,105,110] These findings are consistent with evidence for abnormal sensorimotor gating in the orofacial and limb systems, which are presumably related to basal ganglia dysfunction.[82,111-112] Whether or not these abnormal sensorimotor findings are indicative of excess stiffness or rigidity in the speech musculature is not clear.[100,103-104,111]

The presence and severity of speech impairment in people with PD is related, in many cases, to the speech task being performed. Caligiuri[101] used kinematic analyses of lip displacement amplitude, peak instantaneous velocity, and movement time to assess the effects of rate of speech on articulatory function in patients with PD. He found that lip movements became hypokinetic when the rate increased to 5 to 7 syllable/sec, which is the typical rate of conversational speech, but not at a slower rate. Kempler and Van Lancker[113] found that the speech of a dysarthric individual with PD was much less intelligible during spontaneous speech than during the production of the same utterances in other modes, such as repetition, reading, or singing. Rosen and colleagues[114] studied decline in vocal intensity in PD patients and matched controls across different tasks (eg, vowel prolongation, syllable repetition, sentences). They found that the PD speakers had no significant difference in intensity decline from the healthy speakers in vowel prolongation. However, vocal intensity of speakers with PD declined more rapidly than that of controls in syllable repetition tasks. Bunton and Kientz[115] examined the impact of a concurrent motor task on speech intelligibility in people with PD. They reported that the dual task condition resulted in speech of lesser intelligibility than speaking alone, and speech during the concurrent motor task was more representative of conversational speech when the subjects with PD were unaware they were being recorded. In summary, measures of speech in people with PD are affected by the task demands, with more automatic and/or challenging ("real life") speech tasks unmasking deficits in speech articulation and intelligibility.

Sensory Observations

Although the speech problems associated with PD are considered to be related to the motor dysfunctions of the disease, sensory problems in these people have been recognized for years.[58,112,116] Numerous investigators documented sensorimotor deficits in the orofacial system[82,111-112,116-117] and abnormal auditory, temporal, and perceptual processing of voice and speech,[45,54-55,82,109,112,118-119] and they have been implicated as important etiologic factors in speech and voice abnormalities secondary to PD.[56] Behavioral evidence from limb and speech motor systems for sensory processing disorders in PD includes errors on tasks of kinesthesia;[120-122] difficulties with orofacial perception, including decreased jaw proprioception, tactile localization on tongue, gums, and teeth, and targeted and tracking head movements to perioral stimulation;[82] problems utilizing proprioceptive information for normal movement;[82,121] and abnormal higher order processing of afferent information as demonstrated by abnormal reflex and voluntary motor responses to proprioceptive input.[123] Overall, the basal ganglia may be an area in the brain where sensory information related to movement is filtered[82] in that it "gates out" sensory information when it is not relevant for a motor action, or when it is overly familiar. Thus, one aspect of PD might include complex deficits in the utilization of specific sensory inputs to organize and guide movements.

Problems in sensory perception of effort have been identified as an important focus of successful speech and voice treatment.[124] Specifically, it is often observed that soft-speaking people with PD report that their voices are not reduced in loudness, but rather, their spouse "needs a hearing aid."[9,125] When these same people are asked to speak in a louder voice, they often comment, "I feel like I am shouting," despite the fact that listeners judge the louder voice to be within normal range. If PD patients hear a tape recording of themselves using increased loudness, they can easily recognize that their voice sounds within normal limits, despite the fact they feel they are talking too loud. This suggests that the breakdown may be in online feedback (auditory and proprioceptive) and/or feed-forward while speaking.

Some insights into the sensory deficits affecting speech and voice in people with PD have been provided by Ho and colleagues.[55,109] One study examined the regulation of speech loudness to increased levels of background noise and instantaneous auditory feedback in soft-speaking people with PD and age- and gender-matched controls. The people in the control group automatically adjusted the loudness of their voice while reading aloud and during conversation by decreasing their loudness when presented with increasing levels of instantaneous auditory feedback and increasing their loudness with more background noise. The patients with PD demonstrated an abnormal pattern of speech loudness modulation and failed to increase or decrease loudness in response to the auditory feedback and background noise in the same manner as people in the control group. When given explicit auditory cues to increase loudness, the people with PD were able to increase their speech loudness. These findings further suggest a problem with online or autophonic scaling of loudness in people with PD that can be overridden, in the short term, with explicit external cueing. The difference in voice loudness regulation with explicit versus implicit cues is extremely important, as it suggests that the hypophonia in PD patients is at least partially related to a deficit in internal (implicit) cueing, and that this deficit can be compensated for by external cueing. It also indicates that the hypophonia is not necessarily related to peripheral deficits such as muscle rigidity.

In relation to explicit versus implicit cueing, a number of studies have evaluated the impact of stimulated (say that twice as loud; explicit cue) versus treated loudness (sixteen 60-minute sessions of individual LSVT-LOUD therapy; trained implicit cue). Across a series of stimulated vocal loudness studies, changes in respiratory and articulatory changes as well as improved fundamental frequency (F0) and F0 variability have been documented in non-disordered speakers.[126] In speakers with PD, stimulated loudness has resulted in improved or maintained levels of motor stability[127] and increased activity with reduced variability in EMG studies of laryngeal and articulatory muscles.[128] Others studies have reported that stimulating vocal loudness in healthy people augments the acoustic variable of F0 declination and final-word lengthening.[129] In a recent study comparing vowel space in stimulated and treated loudness, Will and colleagues[130] documented significant acoustic differences in vowel space accompanying increased loudness only in the treated condition in patients with PD (not the stimulated condition). These findings are consistent with Tjaden and Wilding,[131] who did not find an impact of stimulated loudness on acoustic measures of co-articulation in PD. Further support for the difference between stimulated and trained loudness comes from the work of Liotti et al,[33] who documented changes in brain activation in five subjects with PD following training in LSVT-LOUD for 1 month. These neural changes were not observed pre-treatment with brief experimenter-cued increases in loudness (ie, stimulated loudness). Taken together, these findings suggest that while stimulating loudness or providing the explicit cue does impact speech production,[132] lasting changes in speech-motor coordination and reorganization appear to require intensive training.

Problems with self-perception of vocal loudness may also be related to motor-to-sensory cortical gating mechanisms. Studies have demonstrated self-initiated, speech-induced inhibitory influences on neuronal activity in the auditory cortex, via feed-forward efferent mechanisms.[133] Dysfunction of such feed-forward mechanisms has been documented in people with schizophrenia, and has been linked to inner speech and auditory hallucinations.[134] Studies by Liotti and colleagues[135] using PET and evoked response potentials (ERPs) have demonstrated the presence of abnormal (excessive) auditory cortex activity during speech in people with PD, suggesting abnormal collateral gating of auditory neurons. This abnormality has been shown to be partially reversed (reflected in a reduction in excessive auditory activity) in response to intensive voice treatment (LSVT-LOUD) and in parallel with improvement in voice and speech function and dopaminergic activity in the striatofrontal network. Importantly, the motor-to-sensory gating mechanisms are not specific to the vocal and auditory systems, and can involve other sensory systems relevant to speech, such as the somatosensory system and its striatocortical connections.[136]

In an additional study of neural functioning post-LSVT-LOUD, the mechanism of strategy shift was further probed by using transcranial magnetic simulation (TMS) with PET, a novel technique of task-independent connectivity mapping.[137] The behavioral and imaging findings confirm that speech treatment in PD hypophonia results in short-term changes in the speech motor network. These data indicate that LSVT-LOUD facilitates a strategy shift during task by recruiting right hemisphere speech motor areas, as well as recruiting right hemispheric multimodal sensory integration and auditory areas. A significant finding was the appearance post-LSVT-LOUD of activity in right Brodmann area (BA) 21/22 and superior temporal sulcus (STS), both in activation and correlation maps. This was interpreted as a possible mechanism of action for improved monitoring of paralinguistic features of speech following LSVT-LOUD (clinically referred to as *auditory recalibration*). One additional study examined sensory (auditory) feedback control on speech in a single subject with PD using behavioral perturbations of both amplitude (loudness) and pitch (frequency) during voicing tasks pre/post LSVT-LOUD.[138] Pre-LSVT-LOUD, the subject with PD demonstrated a lack of vocal response to perturbations in amplitude and pitch feedback while sustaining the vowel "ah," consistent with impaired audio-vocal gating. Post-LSVT-LOUD, behavioral responses (as measured by audio recordings) to perturbations in speech feedback revealed that this individual developed a faster, more automatic response to amplitude perturbations as a result of LSVT-LOUD training. Thus, preliminary data suggest that patients with PD may have altered cortical responses to pitch and amplitude perturbations, which are modified immediately post-LSVT-LOUD training. Further research into the nature of this apparent impaired audio-vocal gating and its role in speech disorders is needed.

To summarize, the hypophonia in people with PD might be related to deficits in internal (implicit) cueing, abnormal scaling or regulation of the gain of movement amplitude, abnormal gating of the somatosensory cortex, abnormal gating of the auditory cortex via feed-forward mechanisms, abnormal perception of one's own voice, or a combination of these. Future research on the role of sensory problems in the speech and voice characteristics of parkinsonian speech is necessary.[56]

Summary of Parkinson's Related Speech Dysfunction

Perceptual, acoustic, physiological, and sensory processing data have documented varying degrees of dysfunction in different aspects of speech in people with PD. The most common perceptual speech characteristics are reduced loudness, monopitch, hoarse voice, and imprecise articulation. Acoustic studies of speech of those with PD appear to parallel perceptual studies and have shown evidence of reduced vocal SPL, reduced vocal

SPL range, reduced fundamental frequency range, and abnormal articulatory acoustics, such as spirantization. Physiological studies of articulatory muscles have revealed reduced amplitude and speed of movements from a kinematic analysis, EMG activity, and abnormal vocal fold closure patterns. Finally, sensory studies have revealed sensorimotor deficits that include errors on tasks of kinesthesia; difficulties with orofacial perception, including decreased jaw proprioception, tactile localization on tongue, gums and teeth; and targeted and tracking head movements to perioral stimulation. The neurophysiological mechanisms underlying speech and voice disorders in PD are still poorly understood at this time, particularly in regard to deficits in sensory processing.

TREATMENT FOR SPEECH AND VOICE DISORDERS

Management of speech and voice disorders in people with PD has been challenging for both medical and rehabilitation practitioners. This has been due, in part, to the lack of precise understanding of the neuropathology of speech and voice disorders in PD. Current treatments for speech and voice disorders in people with PD consist of medical therapies including pharmacological treatments and surgical procedures, behavioral speech therapy, or a combination thereof.[139-140] Medical therapies alone are not as effective for treating speech symptoms as they are for limb motor symptoms. Thus, speech symptoms are often grouped with other axial symptoms (eg, balance, gait, posture) that are also considered less responsive to traditional medical therapies. At this time, a combination of medical therapy (eg, optimal medication) with behavioral speech therapy appears to offer the greatest improvement for speech dysfunction.[140] There are a number of recent papers that have reviewed the literature related to speech treatment in PD, including pharmacological, surgical, and behavioral interventions for this population.[140-143] This chapter will highlight key findings from those recent reviews to help guide clinician choices for recommendations for speech treatment and set the stage for future work in the area of speech treatment and PD.

Pharmacological Treatments

Several studies assessed the effects of levodopa and dopamine agonists on voice and speech functions in PD. Gallena and colleagues[144] reported positive effects of administering levodopa in some of the six people with early PD who had not started anti-Parkinson's medications (de novo). De Letter and colleagues[145] assessed the effects of levodopa on speech intelligibility in 10 patients with PD and reported significant improvement in speech intelligibility with levodopa on, compared to off, medication. Goberman and colleagues[146] examined the acoustic-phonatory characteristics of speech in nine people with PD and fluctuating motor symptoms before and after taking levodopa. They found that differences in speech between on and off medication were small, although in some people phonation clearly improved. Although these and other studies[147-149] have documented improvements in some aspects of speech and voice with levodopa, many other studies, reviewed elsewhere,[140,141,150] have failed to find significant improvement in voice and speech functions with levodopa or dopamine agonists. These negative findings question the role dopamine plays in hypokinetic dysarthria, and raise the possibility that other non-dopaminergic or special dopaminergic mechanisms may play an important etiologic role. Indeed, clonazepam (dosage 0.25 to 0.5 mg/d), a non-dopaminergic agent, has been reported to significantly improve speech in 10 of 11 people with PD and hypokinetic dysarthria.[151] At this time, it appears that pharmacological treatment alone is not sufficient for managing the symptoms of hypokinetic dysarthria in people with PD.

Surgical Treatments

Recently, much attention has been paid to the effects of neurosurgery, in particular Deep Brain Stimulation (DBS) procedures, on speech and voice of people with PD. Pahwa and colleagues,[152] in a 5-year follow-up study of unilateral or bilateral thalamic DBS (DBS-THAL) in 38 individuals with essential tremor (ET) or PD, found that 75% of the individuals with PD treated with bilateral DBS-THAL developed dysarthria as a side-effect of the surgery. Rodriguez-Oroz and colleagues[153] describe a multicenter, 1-year and 3- to 4-year follow-up study of a large cohort of patients with severe PD. Forty-nine patients were treated with bilateral DBS of the subthalamic nucleus (DBS-STN) and 20 with bilateral DBS of the globus pallidus (DBS-GPi). The authors reported negative effects associated with DBS, to include: decline in cognition, difficulties with speech, gait disorders, instability, and depression. These negative effects were more common in the STN group. Krack and colleagues,[154] in a 5-year follow-up prospective study of bilateral DBS of the STN in 49 individuals with advanced PD, reported that from 1 to 5 years post-surgery, speech, along with akinesia, postural stability, and freezing of gait, were worse on medication. The authors do make the point, however, that this decline is consistent with what would naturally be seen in PD. The authors also state that off medication, the only motor function not to improve from baseline was speech.

Several studies examined specific aspects of voice, speech, and related orofacial and respiratory-laryngeal functions associated with DBS treatment of PD. Santens and colleagues[155] studied lateralized effects of DBS-STN on various aspects of speech in individuals with PD. They reported significant differences between left and right stimulation. Unlike right-sided stimulation, left-sided stimulation resulted in a negative effect on articulation, prosody, and intelligibility. With bilateral stimulation, no significant differences in speech characteristics were observed between on and off stimulation. Wang and colleagues[156] also studied the effects of unilateral DBS-STN on respiratory/phonatory systems of speech production in 6 individuals with PD. Speech data were collected at baseline in the medication-off state, and at 3 months post-DBS off medication with stimulation-on, and with stimulation-off. Stimulation-on improved Unified Parkinson's Disease Rating Scale (UPDRS-III) motor section scores in all patients (non-speech tasks were rated). The authors note that for both right and left STN, stimulation-on resulted in mildly better intensity and duration than stimulation-off during sustained phonation. However, a noticeable increase was only seen with stimulation in the right STN. In comparison, vowel duration and vocal intensity demonstrated a significant decline (from baseline) in three patients who received left DBS-STN. Wang and colleagues attributed the latter findings to micro lesions of the probable dominant hemisphere for speech for the right-handed individuals in this study.

Some studies indicate improvement in voice and speech functions associated with DBS. Gentil and colleagues[157] assessed the effects of bilateral DBS-STN on hypokinetic dysarthria in patients with PD. Through acoustic analysis and force measurements of the articulatory organs, they noted that DBS-STN reduced reaction and movement time of the articulatory organs, increased maximal strength and precision of these organs, and improved respiratory and phonatory functions. In a previous study, Gentil and colleagues[158] compared the effects of bilateral DBS-STN versus DBS-Vim on oral control in 14 individuals with PD. They used force transducers to sample ramp-and-hold force contractions generated by the upper lip, lower lip, and tongue at 1- and 2-newton target force levels, as well as maximal force. After an overnight withdrawal from pharmacological medication, the patients were evaluated under two conditions: during bilateral DBS and one hour after DBS was turned off. With STN stimulation, dynamic and static control of the articulatory organs improved greatly, whereas with Vim stimulation it worsened. In another study of 26 patients with

PD treated with bilateral DBS-STN, Gentil and colleagues,[159] using acoustic analysis of voice, found that, compared to off-stimulation, on-stimulation resulted in shorter duration of sentences, words and pauses, increased duration of sustained vowels, increased variability in voice F0 in sentences, and increased stability of voice F0 while sustaining vowels. There was no difference in vocal intensity between the on- and off-stimulation conditions. In still another study, Pinto and colleagues[160] assessed the impact of bilateral DBS-STN on forces of the tongue, upper lip, and lower lip. Twenty-six individuals with PD were evaluated before and after DBS surgery. They reported that with stimulation on, there was improvement in motor examination scores of the UPDRS. In addition, during an articulatory force task, reaction time, maximal voluntary force, movement time, imprecision of the peak force, and the hold phase were improved. They also reported that these beneficial effects of DBS on articulatory forces continued through the different times of post-surgical follow-up (3 months, 1 to 2 years, 3 to 5 years). The authors report, however, that dysarthria (assessed by the UPDRS) was worsein patient subgroups with a 1- to 2-year and 3- to 5-year post-surgical follow-up, as compared to a 3-month follow-up subgroup. The incongruence between improved articulatory forces and deterioration in dysarthria is puzzling, although it may be accounted for by the notion that dysarthria in PD is related to high-level sensorimotor functions rather than to peripheral motor deficits. Also, the force task may have inadvertently provided external cueing, which induced optimal performance, whereas conversational speech was without such cueing, thus showing poor performance.

Dromey and colleagues[161] studied the effects of bilateral DBS-STN on acoustic measures of voice in seven individuals with PD. Acoustic recordings of voice were made before surgery in the medication-off and medication-on conditions and after surgery in the medication-off and medication-on conditions with and without electrical stimulation. Six months following surgery, statistically significant increases in variability of fundamental frequency and sound pressure level were reported in the medication/stimulation on condition. The authors note, however, that these results may not be observed as a functional change in speech. Rousseaux and colleagues[162] studied the effects of bilateral DBS-STN on speech parameters and intelligibility in seven dysarthric patients with PD. Speech was evaluated in six conditions: before and 3 months after surgery, stimulation turned off or on, and with and without medication. Overall, performance level on the UPDRS-III improved significantly with DBS post-implantation lip movements showed some positive effects, and mild improvement was observed in the voice. The authors state that articulation did not show change; however, they do say that a slight reduction in intelligibility was observed in the on-stimulation condition, especially in the on-drug condition. Large variability was noted between individual patients, with negative effects on intelligibility demonstrated in a few patients; mostly those who exhibited dysarthria pre-surgery.

Saint-Cyr and colleagues[163] studied neuropsychological consequences of chronic bilateral DBS-STN in 11 individuals with advanced PD (age = 67 +/− 8 years, verbal IQ = 114 +/− 12). They were evaluated in their best "on state" with tests assessing frontostriatal functions at pre-surgery, and at 3 to 6 months and 9 to 12 months (n = 10) post-surgery. Saint-Cyr and colleagues noted that at 3 to 6 months post-surgery, there were significant declines in working memory, speed of mental processing, bimanual motor speed and coordination, set switching, phonemic fluency, long-term consolidation of verbal material, and the encoding of visuospatial material. These declines were more consistently observed in the individuals who were 69 and older (n = 6). At 9 to 12 months postoperative, only learning based on multiple trials had recovered and tasks reliant on the integrity of frontostriatal circuitry either did not recover or gradually worsened over time. Based on these findings, Saint-Cyr and colleagues concluded that bilateral DBS-STN can have a negative impact on various aspects of frontal executive functioning, especially in patients 69 years and older.

The overall picture that emerges from these studies indicates marked improvement with DBS in primary motor deficits (rigidity, akinesia, bradykinesia, tremor), especially off-medication, and improvement in dyskinesia with medication. In terms of the speech motor system, improvements were documented during non-speech task, with minimal therapeutic or adverse effects on voice and speech functions, and in some individuals, deterioration in executive functions. Although the follow-up studies suggest deterioration in speech and cognition following DBS, it is not clear to what extent this deterioration is due to the DBS surgery, to the spread of electrical current from DBS, and to the natural degenerative progression of the disease. In addition, Tornqvist and colleagues note that amplitude and frequency settings can have a large impact on speech intelligibility.[165]

Effects of Transcranial/Subdural Stimulation on Speech

Dias and colleagues[166] studied the effects of repetitive transcranial magnetic stimulation (rTMS) on vocal function in 30 people with PD. They examined two different sets of rTMS parameters: active or sham 15 Hz rTMS of the left dorsolateral prefrontal cortex (LDLPFC) and active 5 Hz rTMS of the primary motor cortex (M1)-mouth area. Acoustic and perceptual analysis of voice and voice-related quality of life (V-RQOL) were employed using a blind rater. Stimulation of the M1-mouth induced a significant improvement of the voice F0 and intensity. Stimulation of the LDLPFC resulted in mood amelioration and subjective improvement of the V-RQOL, but not in objective measures of voice F0 and intensity.

Pagni and colleagues[167] studied the effects of extradural motor cortex stimulation in three patients with PD. They found that unilateral stimulation relieved, partially or dramatically, tremor, akinesia, standing, anteropulsion, gait, dysphagia, speech, and swallowing, as well as levodopa-induced symptoms such as dyskinesia and psychiatric complications. They also found that the results of the stimulation did not fade away and that drug dosage was reduced by 50%.

Thus, these two studies suggest that transcortical/transdural stimulation of the motor cortex may have therapeutic effects on voice, speech, and swallowing, in addition to the positive effects on other motor and cognitive functions. Additional studies are needed to corroborate these preliminary observations.

Current data reveal that pharmacological and neurosurgical approaches alone do not improve speech and voice consistently and significantly.[139,141] However, due to the heterogeneity of published studies, it can be difficult to make conclusive statements regarding the effects of neurosurgical approaches.[168] Future studies, with more controlled variables, are needed to better understand the impact of these neurosurgical procedures on voice and speech. In addition, an important consideration will be to include detailed voice and speech assessments. Behavioral speech therapy should be considered as an adjunct for improving speech and voice even for optimally medicated PD patients and for those who have undergone neurosurgical procedures. Stewart and colleagues[169] acknowledge the need for a team approach to treatment including behavioral speech therapy to optimize the benefits of surgery.

Behavioral Speech and Voice Therapy for PD

For many years, speech and voice disorders in people with PD were considered resistant to traditional behavioral speech therapy.[18-21,170] Although changes in speech may be achieved in the treatment room, the challenge of carryover and long-term maintenance has been encountered consistently over a wide range of speech therapies that have been applied to this population.[93] These approaches have included training in control of speech rate, prosody, loudness, articulation, and respiration.[171] Speech therapy with assistive instruments, such as delayed auditory feedback (DAF), voice amplification devices, and pacing boards have also shown limited long-term success.[93,172-173] Reviews of evidence-based practice for behavioral speech therapy for individuals with PD have recently been reported in the literature[142] and will be summarized here, including: *Movement Disorders* review,[142] Cochrane review,[174,175] and Academy of Neurologic Communication Disorders and Sciences (ANCDS) review.[143]

The Evidence Based Medical Review for the Treatments of Parkinson's Disease sponsored by the Movement Disorder Society published a review of speech therapy for PD in 2002.[142] This review stated that there were a varied number of speech therapies reported in the literature, but very few clinical trials. This report critiqued four Level-I randomized controlled studies with the following inclusion criteria: randomized controlled studies, treatments with a duration of at least 2 weeks, a minimum of 10 patients with idiopathic PD, and objective assessments of speech functioning before and after the speech therapy protocol.[124,176-179] The quality of these Level 1 studies was measured according to CONSORT guidelines. Summary findings from this review concluded that there was insufficient evidence to conclude on the efficacy of speech therapy. The authors recommended that future clinical research should include larger, randomized, prospective, and controlled studies. In addition, the use of functional neural imaging studies to examine people with PD pre- and post-speech therapy to determine the functional and anatomic changes related to speech treatment was suggested.[142] Furthermore, the authors proposed that behavioral speech therapies should be intensive and focus on loudness or prosody based on the evidence reviewed.[176-177,179]

Since the publication of the Movement Disorders review, other Level 1 studies for speech therapy in PD have been published. One study by Ramig and colleagues[180] was independently reviewed by the primary author of the section responsible for speech therapy and it was concluded to be of high quality Level I evidence (Goetz, personal communication, 2003).

Deane and colleagues in the Cochrane review[174,175] also examined behavioral speech therapy studies. These authors included only randomized controlled studies and analyzed quality of the studies based on CONSORT guidelines. In two publications, the results of studies comparing speech therapy to a placebo or no intervention and studies comparing two forms of speech therapy were analyzed;[177,178] in the second publication, two randomized controlled trials comparing two different forms of speech therapy were analyzed.[34,179] Again, the authors concluded there was insufficient evidence to support or refute the efficacy of one form of speech therapy over another. Both of the Cochrane review publications were based on studies published before February 2001. Currently, an update of information from the Cochrane review for speech therapy and PD is taking place. The updated Cochrane review will include and analyze randomized controlled studies that have been published or are in progress from 2001 to the present. In 2006, the National Institute for Clinical Excellence in the United Kingdom published new guidelines for the diagnosis and management of Parkinson's disease in which it was recommended that speech and language therapy should be available for people with PD, including speech therapy programs such as LSVT-LOUD.[181]

Members of the ANCDS reviewed the evidence for behavioral management of respiratory and phonatory dysfunction from dysarthria including studies of speech therapy for people with PD.[143] These authors did not limit the review to randomized controlled trials; rather, they included case, single subject, and group designs. The strength of evidence was based on the following factors: type of study (eg, case, single subject, group), primary focus of treatment (eg, biofeedback, LSVT-LOUD), number of people, medical diagnosis, replicability, psychometric adequacy (eg, reliability), evidence for control, measures of impairment, measures of activity or participation, and study conclusions. For speech therapy related to PD, this review included 3 studies of biofeedback devices totaling 39 people; 5 studies with devices (eg, delayed auditory feedback) totaling 16 people; 14 studies of LSVT-LOUD totaling ~90 people, and 3 miscellaneous studies of group treatment. For a table outlining details of these studies, see Yorkston et al.[143]

Conclusions from the review reported that LSVT-LOUD has the greatest number of outcome measures associated with any speech treatment examined. Furthermore, the authors summarized that for the most part outcomes were positive and can be interpreted with confidence.[143] Recommendations for future research for biofeedback, devices, and group treatment approaches included having a larger number of people in studies, well-controlled replicable and reliable studies of well-defined populations, and control or comparison group studies (randomized controlled studies). Recommendations for future research in LSVT-LOUD included additional documentation of long-term maintenance effects, large multi-site effectiveness studies (clinical trials), alternative modes of administration (eg, different dosages of intensity), and further study of treated patients with PD to better define predictors of success or failure with the treatment.

INTENSIVE VOICE TREATMENT FOR PD

Over the past 15 years, research on LSVT-LOUD has focused on improving speech and voice in people with PD and has generated the first Level I evidence for efficacious speech treatment in PD.[31,180,182] LSVT-LOUD trains amplitude (vocal loudness) as a single motor control parameter, thereby targeting inadequate muscle activation, the pathophysiologic mechanism underlying bradykinesia/hypokinesia in PD.[51-53] LSVT-LOUD incorporates: 1) enhancing the voice source (consistent with improving the carrier in the classic engineering concept of signal transmission),[183] 2) using vocal loudness as a trigger for distributed system-wide effects across the speech production system, and 3) recalibrating sensorimotor processes so people with PD integrate improved speech into functional communication. Unlike other forms of speech treatment, LSVT-LOUD requires intensive, high effort exercise combined with a simple, redundant and salient treatment target to transfer loudness into functional daily living. Elements of logic for this approach were drawn from work in engineering, speech intelligibility, motor speech development, motor disorders, neurology, and speech treatment.[52,132,184-189] Furthermore, the standardized protocol for LSVT-LOUD adheres to many of the fundamental principles of exercise and motor training that have been shown to promote neural plasticity and brain reorganization in animal models of PD[190] and human stroke-related hemiparesis.[191] The unique combination of targeting vocal loudness in a training mode that is high effort and intensive may be essential elements in why LSVT-LOUD has been so successful.

Summary of Research Data From LSVT-LOUD

Initial research compared LSVT-LOUD to a respiratory treatment (RESP) where both treatments were matched for mode of delivery (eg, intensive, high effort, homework, positive reinforcement).[33,176,180,182] These studies documented that in people with PD, the combined approach of treating vocal fold adduction and respiratory drive (LSVT-LOUD) generated the greatest and most lasting positive (statistically significant) impact on vocal sound pressure level (SPL). Data from this work documented a range of laryngeal and respiratory changes accompanying post-treatment increases in SPL.[34,36,128,192-193] These findings were consistent with perceptual data demonstrating improved loudness and voice quality.[194] Overall, data suggest that those with PD increased vocal SPL and improved speech production using phonatory mechanisms associated with vocal SPL

Figure 11-1. LSVT-LOUD is designed to improve the phonatory source and scale up amplitude across the speech mechanism with the global variable "LOUD." Increases in loudness can trigger increases in respiratory volumes, vocal fold adduction, articulatory valving, and vocal tract opening. These factors may all contribute to improved speech intelligibility with the simple target of "LOUD."

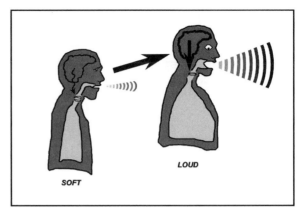

control in the non-disordered larynx.[195] There was no evidence of vocal hyperfunction post-treatment; to the contrary, LSVT-LOUD has been shown to reduce laryngeal hyperfunction[196] and improve voice quality.[194] In addition, distributed effects across the speech production system following LSVT-LOUD were documented. These effects extended beyond voice[36] to include improved articulation,[197-198] facial expression,[199] and preliminary data supporting improved swallowing efficiency in individuals with mild swallowing impairments.[200]

The impact of LSVT-LOUD on articulation in an individual with PD was first identified by Dromey and colleagues[197] when they reported post-treatment improvements in articulation reflected in measures of transition duration, rate, and extent. More recently, a comparison of articulatory acoustics in PD (treated and untreated) and a healthy control group were examined.[198] Data documented articulatory acoustics measures improved significantly (formant frequency 2 (F2) of /u/ and the ratio of F2 of /u/ and F2 of /i/ (F2i/u)) in the subjects who received LSVT-LOUD and were significantly correlated with perceptual improvements in vowel ratings. The impact of treatment on facial expression was compared in a preliminary study across subjects who received LSVT-LOUD versus RESP treatment where subjects who received LSVT-LOUD were rated significantly more expressive post-treatment, compared with RESP treatment.[199] Preliminary assessment of the impact of LSVT-LOUD on swallowing used standardized radiographic studies to define any changes that may have resulted post-treatment. Results indicated a 51% reduction in the number of overall swallow disorders after LSVT-LOUD on several bolus types.[200] The nature of the swallow disorders that resolved with LSVT-LOUD were oral tongue and tongue base disorders, indicating that the effect of treatment extended to orofacial musculature from the focus of the treatment on respiratory/laryngeal function.

Targeting Vocal Loudness in PD—Is There Something Special About LOUD?

Collectively, these findings suggest that training amplitude (vocal loudness) stimulates generalized neural motor activation across the speech production system (Figure 11-1). These speech system–wide effects are consistent with the concept of global parameters.[201-204] The neurological bases of such global motor effects are not known; however, McClean and Tasko[205] reported evidence for neural coupling of orofacial muscles to neural systems of laryngeal and respiratory control in human studies. These authors suggested that a potential source of this observed neural coupling may be from efferent drive from a common brain region to motoneurons innervating orofacial, laryngeal, and respiratory muscles. Neural coupling may explain, in part, the potential spread of effects from stimulation of increased vocal effort and loudness (respiratory and laryngeal systems) to orofacial muscles. Similar findings have been reported in the limb motor system where a focus on training increased amplitude (large, axial body movements) resulted in improvements in balance and posture, as well as more distal functioning (eg, reaching).[206]

Another explanation for the distributed and lasting impact of LSVT-LOUD is that it involves and stimulates phylogenetically old neural systems, especially the emotive brain, which is an important part of the survival mechanism. Speech production is a learned, highly practiced motor behavior, with many of its movements regulated in a quasiautomatic fashion[207-208]; loudness scaling is a task that both animals and humans engage in all their lives.[55,109,209-212] Thus, the regulation of vocal loudness for speech may involve a phylogenetically old system that has been adapted, through learning, for speech audibility and intelligibility purposes. In humans, lesions to different parts of the central nervous system, especially the limbic system (LS), the anterior cingulate cortex (ACC), the paramedian thalamic nuclei, and the basal ganglia, produce hypophonia, hypoprosodia, and hypokinetic articulatory movements.[54,109,213-215] Studies in animals suggest that the LS, ACC, thalamus, and basal ganglia are involved in emotive and other survival-related vocalizations[216]; they also suggest that these neural structures are involved, directly or indirectly, in the readiness to vocalize and the intensity of vocalization.[209,217-222]

Brain changes induced by LSVT-LOUD as measured with PET imaging[33] reflect improvements in the basal ganglia, LS, prefrontal cortex, and right hemisphere functions. As indicated earlier, these neural systems are involved in vocalization, loudness regulation, and vocal learning, which collectively can account for the significant and long-term effects of LSVT-LOUD on speech in people with PD and other neurological disorders. Perspectives such as these may help explain why LSVT-LOUD improves voice and speech production in PD, as compared to less successful treatments that have focused on rate or articulation, which involve primarily cortical, phylogenetically newer neural centers.

Role of Mode of Treatment Delivery in Successful Speech Outcomes

Another consideration in the interpretation of positive outcomes following LSVT-LOUD is that, unlike other forms of speech treatment, LSVT-LOUD has been delivered in high effort (effort expended by clients) and intensive mode (frequency and duration of treatment sessions: 16 individual 60-minute treatment sessions in 1 month). This intensive mode of delivery has not been a part of previous speech treatment approaches focused on articulation or rate. Although principles such as intensity of motor training have long been accepted in terms of behavioral recovery and improved function, only recently has the neurobiological phenomenon underlying such principles been stringently validated for the positive effects on central nervous system functioning.[223-225] For example, it was previously thought that the adult brain had limited capacity to "heal itself;" however, there is now increasing evidence to the contrary[223-225] and the adaptive capacity of the nervous system, known as neural plasticity, has begun to be quantified. Fundamental principles of exercise and motor training that contribute to neural plasticity and brain reorganization in animal models of PD[190] and human stroke-related hemiparesis[191] have been identified (Table 11-1). The translation of these principles of neural plasticity to therapeutic approaches for patients with PD is an area of great research interest. Although LSVT-LOUD was developed long before these data were widely published, today we recognize that the mode of delivery of LSVT-LOUD is consistent with principles of motor learning,[226] and more recently, these principles are believed to promote neural plastic-

TABLE 11-1

Translation of Some of the Proposed Principles Underlying Neural Plasticity (Column 1) to Proposed Deficits in Parkinson's Disease (Column 2) and the Corresponding Rationale and Task in LSVT-LOUD (Column 3)

Intensity[190,241-242]		
Principle Intensive practice is important for maximal plasticity. Intensity can be increased via frequency, repetitions, force/resistance, effort, and accuracy. Intensity increases activation of corticostriatal terminals inducing synaptic plasticity in the striatum.	**Deficit specific to PD** Intensive, high effort training can be difficult in PD due to sensory deficits, force control, fatigue, depression, and progressive loss of cardiac sympathetic innervation.	**LSVT-LOUD** Train intensively 1 hour/day, 4 days/week, for 4 weeks; multiple repetitions (15 or more); increase resistance, amplitude (within healthy range) effort, accuracy; and daily homework exercises. Train maximum perceived effort.
Use It or Lose It/ Use It and Improve It[224,243-244]		
Principle Spared, but compromised DA neurons highly vulnerable to bouts of inactivity/activity. Inactivity may accelerate deficits. Post-exercise intervention, there may be a minimum use requirement to maintain positive effects.	**Deficit specific to PD** Deficits are subtle—not "red flag" to seek speech therapy. Getting early PD to recognize need for exercise and then convincing them to continually exercise is challenging. Decreased physical activity may be a catalyst in degenerative process.	**LSVT-LOUD** Educate people with PD on subtle deficits and improve motor function that directly impacts real life. Retrain a new way of speaking in everyday life (LOUD), thus, normal activity offers continuous exercise.
Saliency[33,56,245-246]		
Principle Practicing rewarding tasks (success/emotionally salient) activates basal ganglia circuitry. Rewards are associated with phasic modulation of DA levels critical to induction of striatal plasticity and learning/relearning in PD.	**Deficit specific to PD** People with early PD may experience lack of awareness of subtle motor deficits, depression, loss of motivation and a feeling of "helplessness." Thus, they feel they do not need, or would not benefit from, speech therapy.	**LSVT-LOUD** We train salient familiar movements (core patterns) of speech promoting success. We provide homework tasks that reinforce success of LOUD in emotionally salient social interactions. We provide extensive positive feedback.

continued

TABLE 11-1, CONTINUED
Translation of Some of the Proposed Principles Underlying Neural Plasticity (Column 1) to Proposed Deficits in Parkinson's Disease (Column 2) and the Corresponding Rationale and Task in LSVT-LOUD (Column 3)

Complexity[33,247-250]		
Principle Complex movements or environmental enrichment have been shown to promote greater structural plasticity (spine density, protein expression/synapse number) in adjacent and remote interconnected regions than simple movements.	**Deficit specific to PD** As basal ganglia pathology progresses, there is a loss in automaticity requiring greater conscious attention to task. When required to perform dual tasks, insufficient attentional resources results in the decrement in one or both of the concurrent tasks.	**LSVT-LOUD** Train complexity of movement with single patient focus (LOUD) to multiple motor tasks. Retrain automaticity of amplitude (LOUD) in familiar movements. Progress complexity over 4 weeks by varying contexts, adding dual cognitive/motor loads, and increasing duration and difficulty of speech tasks (progress from words to conversation).
Timing Matters[243,251-254]		
Principle Early exercise has the potential to: rescue DA neurons, prevent chronic disuse, promote system-wide plasticity, and halt disease progression—particularly to the asymptomatic side.	**Deficit specific to PD** People with early PD have subtle physical underactivity (small movements/soft voice). This may be coupled with a lack of awareness or self-correction, leading to further inactivity.	**LSVT-LOUD** Train people with early PD when they may not have deficits in all systems (laryngeal and orofacial). Train strategies to raise awareness/avoid neglect and increase muscle activation for normal effort/amplitude required for within normal limits vocal loudness.

ity.[224] This mode of delivery may be one key component underlying positive outcomes following LSVT-LOUD in people with PD.

Fundamentals of LSVT-LOUD

The LSVT-LOUD approach centers on a specific therapeutic target: increasing vocal loudness (increasing amplitude of movement). This key target acts as a "trigger" to increase effort and coordination across the speech production system. The LSVT-LOUD is a standardized therapeutic protocol that includes three daily tasks (sustained vowel "ah," high/low "ah," functional phrases), which take up the first half of the treatment session, and a speech hierarchy (words/phrases, sentences, reading, conversation) that takes up the second half of the session.[124] The key treatment fundamentals are:

1. *Single focus: Amplitude.* LSVT-LOUD has a single focus on increasing amplitude of motor output by training vocal loudness. Even for subjects who have multiple speech difficulties (eg, soft, hoarse voice with mumbled speech), only training vocal loudness (amplitude) is targeted. In this manner, the focus for treatment remains simple and redundant for the subject (LOUD). Data document other aspects of speech (eg, hoarseness, intelligibility) will improve over time with the single focus on vocal loudness.

2. *High effort/Intensive treatment.* LSVT-LOUD requires high effort physical exercise of the speech motor system. Therapists push subjects with PD to complete multiple repetitions of each task (minimum of 15) at a patient-perceived effort level of 8 or more (scale 1 to 10, with 10 being the most effort). LSVT-LOUD is delivered 4 days a week for 4 weeks (1-hour sessions).

3. *Sensory calibration.* LSVT-LOUD teaches subjects with PD that what feels too loud is actually within normal limits. There is behavioral evidence from limb and speech motor systems for sensory processing disorders in PD as summarized earlier. These deficits are a barrier in carryover of treatment effects outside of the therapy room because normal vocal loudness "feels" too loud. By directly addressing this sensory mismatch, LSVT-LOUD teaches people with PD to recalibrate their perception of normal loudness so that by the end of 1 month of therapy, they spontaneously speak with improved loudness.

4. *Shaping optimal voice quality.* LSVT-LOUD is designed to train LOUD speech that is healthy (ie, no unwanted strain or excessive vocal fold closure). People with PD are never taught to speak too loud. Therapists will shape the voice quality through use of modeling ("do what I do") or tactile/visual cues. In this manner, there is minimal cognitive loading with extensive instructions or explanations.

5. *Carryover/homework.* Due to sensorimotor challenges that accompany PD, carryover of treatment effects from the therapy room out into the real world can be difficult. Carryover exercises are daily assignments to use LOUD speaking in real-life situations. The difficulty of the carryover assignment matches the level of the hierarchy where the person is working (eg, words, sentences, reading, conversation). People with PD are made accountable for completing carryover tasks so that they are forced to use LOUD in the "real world." This helps people with PD realize that what feels like exaggerated speaking is accepted as normal loudness by others.

6. *Maintenance.* The goal of LSVT-LOUD is to teach subjects with PD a new way of speaking in everyday life. This use of vocal loudness in everyday speaking provides continuous exercise. In addition, people with PD are taught to establish a routine of daily LSVT-LOUD exercises so that they can and will continue to practice once the individual therapy is completed.

Although LSVT-LOUD is effective for most patients with PD, there are challenges that can diminish treatment outcomes with LSVT-LOUD, including people who have severe depression, moderate to severe dementia, atypical parkinsonism (eg, multiple-system atrophy, progressive supranuclear palsy), or people who have had neurosurgery for their PD (eg, DBS). These people are more challenging to treat during therapy due to factors such as difficulty putting forth maximum effort, more difficulty staying on task, easily confused, or on/off drug effects.[56,227] Many times, the ultimate treatment outcomes are adjusted for those patients with advanced PD or those who have had surgical intervention. Instead of striving for self-generated improved loudness in daily conversation, the end treatment goal may be self-generated loudness in 10 functional phrases and cued loudness during conversational speech. Although treatment outcomes are adjusted in these patients, they can, and do, make significant gains in communication abilities that are important to both the person with PD and his or her family members.

LSVT-LOUD Applied to Other Motor Systems

Recently principles of LSVT-LOUD were applied to limb movement in people with PD (LSVT-BIG) and have been documented to be effective in the short term.[206] Specifically, training increased amplitude of limb and body movement (Bigness) in PD patients has documented improvements in amplitude (trunk rotation/gait) that generalized to improved speed (upper/lower limbs), balance, and quality of life.[206] In addition, people were able to maintain these improvements when challenged with a dual task.

The extension of this work to a novel integrated treatment program that simultaneously targets speech and limb motor disorders in people with PD has been proposed. Results from pilot work have been completed in 11 people with PD: 9, Stage I (3 de novo) and 2, Stage II. Data revealed all subjects increased vocal SPL (loudness) during sustained vowels and reading (average 10 db SPL increase across both tasks) and increased stride length/velocity during gait (average of 9 cm).[228-230] The gains in vocal SPL and gait stride length were comparable to previously published data from independently training LSVT-LOUD (range 8 to 13 dB SPL)[33,180] or LSVT-BIG (range 9 to 30 cm).[206] These changes in speech and gait function had a positive impact of 28% on disease severity (UPDRS-motor section) and 27% on quality of life (PDQ-summary score). These data document that individuals with early PD (unilateral Stage I) are able to improve beyond baseline levels. These subjects reported continuing the use of BIG and LOUD strategies in daily living. One subject commented, "In my normal everyday life, I just exaggerate my movements. I keep things BIG when I reach for things, or when I bend or when I walk; and when I talk, I keep my voice strong." There is a great need to simplify rehabilitation approaches for patients with PD due to the progressive nature of the disorder, cognitive challenges that make motor learning difficult, and logistical and financial burdens that intensive speech and physical therapies present. A whole body, amplitude-based treatment program that simultaneously delivers speech and physical therapy may be one possible solution.

Technology-Assisted Treatment Delivery

It is recognized that there are practical challenges of delivering speech treatment intensively (4 individual sessions a week for 4 weeks). In fact, any treatment regime (speech, physical, or occupational therapy) that is consistent with plasticity promoting principles and incorporates elements such as intensity and multiple repetitions, will require going beyond the one-to-one (patient to clinician) classic paradigm of treatment delivery. There are not enough therapists to deliver this efficacious dosage of treatment to all the people with PD in need—a need which will only increase dramatically in the coming years with the aging of the Baby Boomer population. The use of group therapy is not an option as it does not enable the efficacious requirement of each person working to his or her maximum effort levels for the entire 1-hour treatment session. Furthermore, continued exercise following the conclusion of speech treatment and tune-up sessions are needed as the disease progresses.

Advances in computer and Web-based technology offer potentially powerful solutions to the problems of treatment accessibility, efficacious dosage delivery, and long-term maintenance in rehabilitation. For example, a program for upper limb motor deficits following stroke has been developed for delivery of constraint induced therapy—a program that requires intensive motor training (eg, 6 hours/day for 2 weeks). This computerized system, called AutoCITE, was documented to result in comparable outcomes to live delivery of the therapy.[231] Computer technology has also been developed for delivery of an intensive speech treatment (LSVT-LOUD) and is discussed next.

Halpern et al[232-233] reported on the use of a personal digital assistant (PDA) as an assistive device for delivering LSVT-LOUD to patients with PD. This PDA, named the LSVT-LOUD Companion (LSVT-LOUDC), was designed to meet the challenges of treatment accessibility and frequency that they often encounter. The LSVT-LOUDC is specially programmed to collect data and provide feedback as it guides patients through the LSVT-LOUD exercises, enabling them to participate in therapy sessions at home. Fifteen people with PD participated in this study, during which nine voice treatment sessions were completed with a speech therapist and seven sessions were completed independently at home utilizing the LSVT-LOUDC. Acoustic data collected in a sound-treated booth before and after the 16 treatment sessions demonstrated that following treatment, the people with PD made significant gains in vocal loudness across a variety of voice and speech tasks. These results were similar to previously published data on 16 face-to-face sessions both immediately post-treatment and at 6-month follow-up.[232-233] These pilot findings support feasibility of the LSVT-LOUDC and support further development of technology-based approaches to enhance treatment accessibility.

An evolution of the LSVT-LOUDC has been the development of an LSVT-LOUD virtual speech therapist (LSVT-LOUDVT). This is a perceptive animated character, modeled after expert LSVT-LOUD speech therapists, that delivers LSVT-LOUD in a computer-based program. This work builds on the well-established foundation of experimental efficacy data[33,176,180,182] and state-of-the-art learning tools, incorporating intelligent animated agents.[234-235,238-240] A prototype of the LSVT-LOUDVT has been developed and clinical testing has begun. In addition, research into effectiveness of delivering intensive speech therapy via Telehealth systems or other Web-enabled speech therapy systems will continue to enhance accessibility to the intensive sensorimotor training important for successful speech outcomes.

Conclusion

Voice and speech disorders occur in the majority of people with PD, and significantly hinder communication, physical and psychological well-being, and overall quality of life. Although all aspects of speech production may be affected, disordered voice is one of the most common problems. Previous forms of treatment for the disorder of speech and voice in PD patients have had modest or inconsistent effects, with minimal long-term maintenance of therapeutic gains. The LSVT-LOUD, an intensive treatment program that addresses increased vocal loudness and improved sensory perception of vocal effort and loudness, has been extensively documented to be a successful approach in the short and long term. LSVT-LOUD has been shown to produce favorable effects on articulation, swallowing, and facial expression in people with PD, although these findings are based on preliminary efficacy data. The success of LSVT-LOUD may be related to the uniquely pervasive impact of training vocal loudness across the entire speech production mechanism, the intensive mode of delivery that is consistent with neural plasticity promoting principles, or some combination of the two. Improvement in voice, speech, and swallowing functions in the context of a degenerative disease may prove, in future research, to be indicative of neural plasticity, as preliminary brain studies post-LSVT-LOUD already suggest. The principles of LSVT-LOUD have been applied to the limb motor system, with preliminary data suggesting a positive impact. The possibility of a hybrid treatment approach that simultaneously delivers speech and physical therapy, with a common treatment target of increased amplitude (BIG and LOUD) is an intriguing area of ongoing research. The use of computer technology to deliver LSVT-LOUD offers promise for increasing access to this treatment for all people with PD in need. Although the degenerative course of PD cannot be altered at this time, improving oral communication is an important component in developing the highest levels of functioning and independence for patients with PD. There are many exciting avenues of ongoing and future speech research that will clarify our understanding of the underlying mechanism of speech disorders in PD and impact development of rehabilitation strategies over the next decade.

Case Study

The following case study serves as an example of how a patient with PD and a moderate voice and speech severity level may respond to LSVT-LOUD. This patient attended 1-hour individual treatment sessions 4 days a week for 4 weeks. He completed a total of 16 sessions within 1 month.

Medical History

Mr. Smith, a 49-year-old male with idiopathic Parkinson's disease, stage II (Hoehn and Yahr[255]), had been diagnosed approximately 2 years prior to his enrollment in the LSVT-LOUD program. He received a score of 13.0 on the UPDRS Motor Exam section indicating mild motor disability. His initial symptoms included a foot flap and flexing of the left arm. Parkinson's medications were Sinemet CR and Eldepryl. He did not experience dyskinesias or "on/off" symptoms. He reported a tremor in the fourth finger of his left hand.

Medical history did not include any other significant health problems.

Mr. Smith was employed full-time as a family physician and was president of the local American Parkinson Disease Association (APDA).

Voice and Speech Symptoms

At the time of enrollment in the LSVT-LOUD, Mr. Smith complained of reduced loudness, vocal fatigue, hoarseness, monotonicity, and mumbling. The speech language pathologist rated his overall voice and speech impairment as moderate and described his perceptual voice and speech characteristics to include reduced loudness, monotonicity, and slurring.

A motor speech examination revealed the structures and functions of the speech mechanism to be within normal limits. Mr. Smith reported inconsistent difficulty swallowing liquids and solids. He was referred to a local hospital for a dysphagia assessment. His hearing was within normal limits bilaterally.

Pre-Treatment Laryngeal Exam

A pre-treatment laryngeal exam with videolaryngostroboscopy revealed a mild degree of incomplete vocal fold closure and mild false fold and anterior to posterior supraglottic hyperadduction.

Neuropsychological Testing

Neuropsychological testing revealed cognitive functioning to be within normal limits. Psychosocial testing did not reveal depression (Beck Depression Inventory) or emotional distress as a result of his PD. However, Mr. Smith reported that due to the PD, he had reduced the amount of work done at home and was pursuing social entertainment less frequently.

Objective Experimental and Perceptual Results

Mr. Smith's pre-treatment maximum duration of sustained vowel phonation was within normal limits, but dramatically improved immediately post-treatment (from approximately 24 to 38 seconds). With increased vocal effort training in therapy, both duration and loudness increased, yet Mr. Smith did not develop abusive or hyperfunctional vocal behaviors. In fact, his false fold and anterior to posterior supraglottic hyperfunctioning were eliminated post-treatment. This is attributed to improved vocal fold adduction and less need for compensatory behaviors.

From pre- to immediately post-treatment, Mr. Smith's vocal SPL increased in all tasks. Increases in vocal SPL during maximum duration of sustained vowel phonation averaged 21 dB SPL (decibels of sound pressure level). Reading vocal SPL increased 12 dB SPL and vocal SPL during conversational monologue increased 6 dB. Mr. Smith's increases in Standard Semitone Deviation (STSD) document improvement in pitch variability, suggesting greater vocal intonation from pre- to immediately post-treatment.

Articulatory acoustic analyses were also carried out on the speech of this patient. Immediately post-treatment results revealed improvements on articulatory acoustic measures such as frication duration, rise time, and the vowel duration to whole word duration ratio.[188] Therefore, even though articulation was not targeted during treatment, these results suggest generalization of vocal effort to articulation.

Mr. Smith's (P) pre-, immediately post-treatment perceptual ratings documented improvements in monotonicity (ie, improvement of: Patient ratings (P) = 26%, Spouse Ratings (S) = 49%) and hoarseness (ie, improvement of: P = 26%, S = 18%) as the most improved perceptual variables from pre- to immediately post-treatment. Mr. Smith rated his intelligibility reduced from pre- to immediately post-treatment. This phenomenon frequently occurs because many patients are unaware of the extent of their voice and speech disorder prior to treatment. Treatment tends to increase their awareness and as a result patients may rate themselves as worse post-treatment, when in fact, they have improved. Immediately post-treatment, Mr. Smith reported that he was no longer experiencing vocal fatigue at the end of the day.

At 6 months and 1 year post-treatment, Mr. Smith remained at or above pre-treatment baseline levels and immediately post-treatment levels on all objective experimental and perceptual measures except for the variable STSD in conversational monologue.

Post-Treatment Laryngeal Exam

Mr. Smith's immediately post-treatment videolaryngostroboscopy exam revealed complete vocal fold closure and no supraglottic hyperfunctioning. At 6 months and 1 year post-treatment, the exam revealed continued complete vocal fold closure.

Treatment Observations

Although Mr. Smith was aware of his voice problems pre-treatment, he did not believe individuals were having trouble hearing or understanding him. He thought his hoarseness was related to upper respiratory infections. Therefore, because he was a physician, he treated himself with antibiotics for several months. Mr. Smith believed he was compensating for the reduced loudness and hoarseness by speaking less frequently. He stated that his voice problems had forced him to leave a medical clinic job because he believed he could not "vocally compete" with the other physicians when requesting assistance from the nurses.

Mr. Smith easily learned the LSVT-LOUD techniques. Performance on his daily variables and hierarchical speech loudness drills continued to improve as the weeks progressed. However, despite the implementation of many calibration tasks (ie, retraining sensory perception of adequate vocal loudness), successful calibration was challenging. Mr. Smith was taken to a local deli and asked to order using his "loud, strong" voice. Sitting at an outside cafe table conversing while the traffic whizzed by helped convince Mr. Smith that the LSVT-LOUD techniques were working. His audiotaped reading from a children's book using his "loud, strong" voice was played for his coworkers (ie, nurses and office staff). He was surprised to hear they did not believe that it was his voice. His wife told him that after treatment she heard the "rich, resonant" voice that had attracted her to him 25 years ago. Mr. Smith willingly practiced, attempted to use the LSVT-LOUD techniques in social situations, and received positive reinforcement. However, it was not until the fourth week of treatment that he started to become convinced that using increased vocal effort and loudness were improving his communication skills.

In his immediately post-treatment videotaped voice recording session, Mr. Smith discussed his difficulty with calibration. He reported the realization that there were "probably" individuals who had not heard or understood him prior to treatment, but that he still worried about being "too loud." At 1 year post-treatment, he stated during his videotaped voice recording session that his learning extended beyond the 16 sessions. As he received more and more positive feedback from family and friends about his voice, he realized that increased vocal effort in order to speak louder was necessary.

Summary

Mr. Smith is an example of the importance of and need for calibration. Even for someone who willingly practiced outside of treatment and easily mastered the "THINK LOUD" technique, it was difficult for him to realize that he needed to use the loud voice. Fortunately, his family and friends provided the necessary feedback to aid his calibration.

REFERENCES

1. Hartelius L, Svensson P. Speech and swallowing symptoms associated with Parkinson's disease and multiple sclerosis: a survey. *Folia Phoniatrica Logo Pedica*. 1994;46:9-17.
2. Ho A, Iansek R, Marigliani C, Bradshaw JL, Gates S. Speech impairment in a large sample of people with Parkinson's disease. *Behavl Neurol*. 1998;11:131-137.
3. Logemann J, Fisher H, Boshes B, Blonsky E. Frequency and concurrence of vocal tract dysfunctions in the speech of a large sample of Parkinson patients. *J Speech Hearing Dis*. 1978;43:47-57.
4. Darley FL, Aronson AE, Brown JR. Clusters of deviant speech dimensions in the dysarthrias. *J Speech Hearing Res*. 1969a;12:462–469.
5. Darley FL, Aronson A, Brown J. Differential diagnostic patterns of dysarthria. *J Speech Hearing Res*. 1969b;12:246-269.
6. Scott S, Caird FL. Speech therapy for Parkinson's disease. *BMJ*. 1981;283:1088.
7. Pitcairn TK, Clemie S, Gray JM, Pentland B. Non-verbal cues in the self-presentation of parkinsonian patients. *Br J Clin Psychol*. 1990a;29:177-184.
8. Pitcairn TK, Clemie S, Gray JM, Pentland B. Non-verbal cues in the self-presentation of parkinsonian patients. *Br J Clin Psychol*. 1990b;25:85-92.
9. Fox C, Ramig L. Sound pressure level and self-perception of speech and voice in men and women who have idiopathic Parkinson disease. *Am J Speech Language Pathol*. 1997;2:29-42.
10. Logemann J, Blonsky R, Boshes B. Dysphagia in parkinsonism. *JAMA*. 1975;231:69-70.
11. Koller WC, Tse W. Unmet medical needs in Parkinson's disease. *Neurology*. 2004;62(Suppl 1):S1-8.

12. Krack P, Batir A, Van Blercom N, Chabardes S, Fraix V, Ardouin C, Koudsie A, Limousin PD, Benazzouz A, LeBas JF, Benabid AL, Pollak P. Five-year follow-up of bilateral stimulation of the subthalamic nucleus in advanced Parkinson's disease. *N Engl J Med*. 2003;349(20):1925-1934.

13. Olanow CW, Jankovic J. Neuroprotective therapy in Parkinson's disease and motor complications: a search for a pathogenesis-targeted, disease-modifying strategy. *Mov Disord*. 2005;20(Suppl 11):S3-10.

14. Sapir S, Ramig LO, Countryman S, Fox C. Voice, speech, and swallowing disorders. In: Factor S, Weiner W, eds. *Parkinson's Disease: Diagnosis and Clinical Management* (2nd ed.). New York, Demos Medical Publishing; 2007:75-86.

15. Wermuth L, Stenager EN, Stenager E, Boldsen J. Mortality in patients with Parkinson's disease. *Acta Neurol Scand*. 1995;92:55-58.

16. Bryson HM, Milne RJ, Chrisp P. Selegiline: an appraisal of the basis of its pharmacoeconomic and quality-of-life benefits in Parkinson's disease. *Pharmacoeconomics*. 1992;2:118-36.

17. Tompkins P, Herman L. How many people in the U.S. have PD? Parkinson's Information Exchange, July, 1998. Available at http://www.parkinsons-information-exchange-network-online.com/parkmail3a/1998c/msg00789.html.

18. Allan CM. Treatment of non-fluent speech resulting from neurological disease: treatment of dysarthria. *Br J Disord Comm*. 1970;5:3-5.

19. Aronson AE. *Clinical Voice Disorders*. New York: Thieme-Stratton, 1990.

20. Greene, HCL. *The Voice and Its Disorders*. London: Pitman Medical, 1980.

21. Sarno MT. Speech impairment in Parkinson's disease. *Arch Phys Med Rehabil*. 1968:269–275.

22. Weiner WJ, Lang AE. *Movement Disorders: A Comprehensive Survey*. Mount Kisco, NY: Futura; 1989.

23. Baker K, Ramig LO, Johnson A, Freed C. Preliminary speech and voice analysis following fetal dopamine transplants in 5 individuals with Parkinson disease. *J Speech Hearing Res*. 1997;40:615-626.

24. Ghika J, Ghika-Schmid F, Fankhauser H, et al. Bilateral contemporaneous posteroventral pallidotomy for the treatment of Parkinson's disease: neuropsychological and neurological side effects. Report of four cases and review of the literature. *J Neurosurg*. 1999;2:313-321.

25. Kompoliti K, Wang QE, Goetz CG, Leurgans S, Raman R. Effects of central dopaminergic stimulation by apomorphine on speech in Parkinson's disease. *Neurology*. 2000;54:458-462.

26. Larson K, Ramig LO, Scherer RC. Acoustic and glottographic voice analysis during drug-related fluctuations in Parkinson's disease. *J Med Speech Language Pathol*. 1994;2:211-226.

27. Rigrodsky S, Morrison EB. Speech changes in parkinsonism during L-dopa therapy: preliminary findings. *J Am Geriatr Soc*. 1970;18:142-151.

28. Wang E, Kompoliti K, Jiang J, Goetz CG, An instrumental analysis of laryngeal responses to apomorphine stimulation in Parkinson disease. *J Med Speech Lang Pathol*. 2002;8:175-186.

29. Wolfe VI, Farvin JS, Bacon M, Waldrop W. Speech changes in Parkinson's disease during treatment with L-dopa. *J Comm Disord*. 1975; 8(3):271–279.

30. Ramig LO, Sapir S., Countryman S, Pawlas AA, O'Brien C, Hoehn M, Thompson LL. Intensive voice treatment (LSVT) for patients with Parkinson's disease: a 2 year follow up. *J Neurol Neurosurg Psychiatry*. 2001a;71:493-498.

31. Ramig LO, Sapir S, Fox C, Countryman S. Changes in vocal loudness following intensive voice treatment (LSVT) in individuals with Parkinson's disease: a comparison with untreated patients and normal age-matched controls. *Mov Disord*. 2001b;16:79-83.

32. Goetz C. Personal communication. 2003.

33. Liotti M, Ramig LO, Vogel D, New P, Cook CI, Ingham RJ, Ingham JC, Fox PT. Hypophonia in Parkinson's disease. Neural correlates of voice treatment revealed by PET. *Neurology*. 2003;60:432-440.

34. Ramig L, Countryman S, Thompson L, Horii Y. Comparison of two forms of intensive speech treatment for Parkinson disease. *J Speech Hearing Res*. 1995;38:1232-1251.

35. Ramig LO, Dromey C. Aerodynamic mechanisms underlying treatment-related changes in SPL in patients with Parkinson disease. *J Speech Hearing Res*. 1996;39:798-807.

36. Sapir S, Ramig LO, Hoyt P, Countryman S, O'Brien C, Hoehn M. Speech loudness and quality 12 months after intensive voice treatment (LSVT) for Parkinson's disease: a comparison with an alternative speech treatment. *Folia Phoniatr Logo*. 2002;54:296-303.

37. Smith M, Ramig LO, Dromey C, Perez K, Samandari R. Intensive voice treatment in Parkinson's disease: laryngostroboscopic findings. *J Voice*. 1995; 9:453-459.

38. Baker K, Ramig LO, Luschei E, Smith M. Thyroarytenoid muscle activity associated with hypophonia in Parkinson disease and aging. *Neurology*. 1998;6:1592-1598.

39. Beukelman DR. *Recent Advances in Clinical Dysarthria*. Boston: College-Hill Press; 1989.

40. Leanderson R, Meyerson BA, Persson A. Effect of L dopa on speech in parkinsonism: an EMG study of labial articulatory function. *J Neurol Psychiatry*. 1971;43:679-681.

41. Leanderson R, Meyerson BA, Persson, A. Lip muscle function in parkinsonian dysarthria. *Acta Otolaryngol*. 1972;74:350-357.

42. Moore CA, Scudder, RR. Coordination of jaw muscle activity in parkinsonian movement: description and response to traditional treatment. In: Yorkston KM, Beukelman DR, eds. *Recent Advances in Clinical Dysarthria*. Boston: College-Hill Press, 1989.

43. Yorkston KM. Treatment efficacy: dysarthria. *J Speech Hearing Res*. 1996;39:S46-S57.

44. Yorkston KM, Miller RM, Strand EA. *Management of Speech and Swallowing in Degenerative Diseases*. Communication Skill Builders, 1997.

45. Ackermann H, Ziegler W. Articulatory deficits in parkinsonian dysarthria: an acoustic analysis. *J Neurol Neurosurg Psychiatry*. 1991;54:1093-1098.

46. Ackermann H, Konczak J, Hertrich I. The temporal control of repetitive articulatory movements in Parkinson's disease. *Brain Lang*. 1997;56:312-319.

47. Estenne M, Hubert M, Troyer AD. Respiratory muscle involvement in Parkinson's disease. *N Engl J Med*. 1984;311:1516.

48. Hanson WR, Metter EJ. DAF speech rate modification in Parkinson's disease: a report of two cases. In: Berry WR, eds. *Clinical Dysarthria*. San Diego, CA: College-Hill Press; 1983.

49. Hoodin RB, Gilbert HR. Nasal airflows in Parkinsonian speakers. *J Comm Disord*. 1989a;22:169-180.

50. Hoodin RB, Gilbert HR. Parkinsonian dysarthria: an aerodynamic and perceptual description of velopharyngeal closure for speech. *Folia Phoniatr*. 1989b;41:249-258.

51. Farley BG, Sherman S, Koshland GF. Shoulder muscle activity in Parkinson's disease during multijoint arm movements across a range of speeds. *Exp Brain Res*. 2004;154:160-175.

52. Hallett M, Khoshbin S. A physiological mechanism of bradykinesia. *Brain*. 1980;103:301-314.

53. Pfann KD, Buchman AS, Comella CL, Corcos DM. (2001). Control of movement distance in Parkinson's disease. *Mov Disord*. 2001;16:1048-1065.

54. Ho AK, Iansek R, Bradshaw JL. Regulations of parkinsonian speech volume: the effect of interlocuter distance, *J Neurol Neurosurg Psychiatry*. 1999;67:199-202.

55. Ho AK, Bradshaw JL, Iansek T. Volume perception in parkinsonian speech. *Mov Disord*. 2000;15:1125-1131.

56. Fox CM, Morrison CE, Ramig LO, Sapir S. Current perspectives on the Lee Silverman Voice Treatment (LSVT) for people with idiopathic Parkinson's disease. *Am J Speech Lang Pathol*. 2002;11:111-123.

57. Albin RL, Young AB, Penny JB. The functional anatomy of basal ganglia disorders. *Trends Neuroscience*. 1989;12:366-375.

58. Barbeau A, Sourkes TL, Murphy CF. Les catecholamines de la maladie de Parkinson's. In: Ajuria Guerra J, ed. *Monoamines et Systeme Nerveux Central*. Geneve: George; 1962.

59. Penny JB, Young AB. Speculations on the functional anatomy of basal ganglia disorders. *Annu Rev Neurosci*. 1983;6:73-94.

60. Berardelli A, Dick JP, Rothwell JC, Day BL, Marsden CD. Scaling of the size of the first agonist EMG burst during rapid wrist movements in patients with Parkinson's disease. *J Neurol Neurosurg Psychiatry*. 1986;49(11):1273-1279.

61. Demirci M, Grill, McShane, Hallet, M. Impairment of kinesthesia in Parkinson's disease. *Neurology*. 1995;45:A218.

62. Stelmach GE. Basal ganglia impairment and force control. In: Requin J, Stelmach GE, eds. *Tutorial in Motor Neuroscience*. Netherlands: Kluwer Academic Publishers, 1991.

63. Darley FL, Aronson AE, Brown JR. *Motor Speech Disorders*. Philadelphia: W.B. Saunders, 1975.

64. Stewart C, Winfield L, Hunt A, Bressman SB, Fahn S, Blitzer A, Brin MF. Speech dysfunction in early Parkinson's disease. *Mov Disord*. 1995;10:562-565.

65. Canter GJ. Speech characteristics of patients with Parkinson's disease: I. Intensity, pitch and duration. *J Speech Hearing Disord*. 1963; 28:221-229.

66. Canter GJ. Speech characteristics of patients with Parkinson's disease: III. Articulation, diadochokinesis and overall speech adequacy. *J Speech Hearing Disorders*. 1965a;30:217-224.

67. Canter GJ. Speech characteristics of patients with Parkinson's disease: II. Physiological support for speech. *J Speech Hearing Disorders*. 1965b;30:44-49.

68. Ludlow CL, Bassich CJ, Relationships between perceptual ratings and acoustic measures of hypokinetic speech. In: McNeil MR, Rosenbek JC, Aronson AE, eds. *Dysarthria of Speech: Physiology-Acoustics-Linguistics-Management*. San Diego, CA: College-Hill Press; 1983.

69. Ludlow CL, Bassich, CJ. Relationships between perceptual ratings and acoustic measures of hypokinetic speech. In: McNeil MR, Rosenbek JC, Aronson AE, eds. *The Dysarthrias: Physiology, Acoustics, Perception, Management*. San Diego: College-Hill Press, 1984.

70. Metter EJ, Hanson WR. Clinical and acoustical variability in hypokinetic dysarthria. *J Comm Disord*. 1986;19:347-366.

71. Ho AK, Iansek R, Bradshaw JL. Motor instability in parkinsonian speech intensity. *Neuropsychiatry, Neuropsychology and Behavl Neurology*. 2001;14:109-116.

72. Fraile V, Cohen H. Prosody in Parkinson's disease: relations between duration, amplitude and fundamental frequency range. Paper presented at the International Neuropsychological Society 23rd Annual Meeting, Seattle, WA, 1995.

73. Logemann J, Boshes B, Fisher, H. The steps in the degeneration of speech and voice control in Parkinson's disease. In: Siegfried J, ed. *Parkinson's Disease: Rigidity, Akinesia, Behavior*. Vienna: Hans Huber; 1973.

74. Hansen DG, Gerratt BR, Ward PH. Cinegraphic observations of laryngeal function in Parkinson's disease. *Laryngoscope*. 1984;94:348-353.

75. Blumin JH, Pcolinsky DE, Atkins JP. Laryngeal findings in advanced Parkinson's disease. *Ann Otol Rhinol Laryngol*. 2004;113:253-258.

76. Perez K, Ramig LO, Smith M, Dromey C. The Parkinson larynx: tremor and videostroboscopic findings. *J Voice*. 1996;10:354-361.

77. Gallena S., Smith PJ, Zeffiro T, Ludlow CL. Effects of levodopa on laryngeal muscle activity for voice onset and offset in Parkinson disease. *J Speech Lang Hear Res*. 2001;44:1284-1299.

78. Hunker CJ, Abbs JH. Physiological analyses of parkinsonian tremors in the orofacial system. In: McNeil MR, Rosenbek JC, Aronson AE, eds. *The Dysarthrias: Physiology, Acoustics, Perception, Management*. San Diego, CA: College-Hill Press; 1984.

79. Netsell R, Daniel B, Celesia GG. Acceleration and weakness in parkinsonian dysarthria. *J Speech Hearing Disord*. 1975;40:170-178.

80. Vincken WG, Gauthier SG, Dollfuss RE, Hanson RE, Parauay CM, Cosio MG. Involvement of upper-airway muscles in extrapyramidal disorders, a cause of airflow limitation. *N Engl J Med*. 1984;311:438-442.

81. Hirose H, Joshita Y. Laryngeal behavior in patients with disorders of the central nervous system. In: Hirano M, Kirchner JA, Bless DM, eds. *Neurolaryngology: Recent Advances*. Boston: Little, Brown; 1987.

82. Schneider JS, Diamond SG, Markham CH. Deficits in orofacial sensorimotor function in Parkinson's disease. *Ann Neurol*. 1986;19:275-282.

83. Luschei, ES, Ramig, LO, Baker, KL, Smith ME. Discharge characteristics of laryngeal single motor units during phonation in young and older adults and in persons with Parkinson disease. *J Neurophysiol*. 1999;81:2131-2139.

84. Cramer W. De spaak bij patienten met Parkinsonisme. *Logop Phoniatr*. 1940;22:17-23.

85. De la Torre R, Mier M, Boshes B. Evaluation of respiratory function: Preliminary observations. *Quart Bull Northwestern Univ Med School*. 1960; 34:332-336.

86. Laszewski Z. Role of the department of rehabilitation in preoperative evaluation of parkinsonian patients. *J Am Geriatr Soc*. 1956;4:1280-1284.

87. Mueller PB. Parkinson's disease: motor-speech behavior in a selected group of patients. *Folia Phoniatr*. 1971;23:333-346.

88. Marquardt TP. *Characteristics of Speech in Parkinson's Disease: Electromyographic, Structural Movement and Aerodynamic Measurements*. Seattle: University of Washington, 1973.

89. Solomon NP, Hixon TJ. Speech breathing in Parkinson's disease. *J Speech Hear Res*. 1993;36:294-310.

90. Schiffman PL. A "saw-tooth" pattern in Parkinson's disease. *Chest*. 1985;87:124-126.

91. Murdoch BE, Chenery HJ, Bowler S, Ingram JCL. Respiratory function in Parkinson's subjects exhibiting a perceptible speech deficit: a kinematic and spirometric analysis. *J Speech Hearing Disord*. 1989;54:610-626.

92. Sapir S, Pawlas AA, Ramig LO, Countryman S, O'Brien C, Hoehn M, Thompson L. Voice and speech abnormalities in Parkinson disease: relation to severity of motor impairment, duration of disease, medication, depression, gender, and age. *J Med Speech Lang Pathol*. 2001;9:213-226.

93. Adams SG. Hypokinetic dysarthria in Parkinson's disease. In: McNeil MR, ed. *Clinical Management of Sensorimotor Speech Disorders*. New York: Thieme; 1997.

94. Hammen VL, Yorkston KM, Beukelman DR. Pausal and speech duration characteristics as a function of speaking rate in normal and parkinsonian dysarthric individuals. In: Yorkston KM, Beukelman DR, eds. *Recent Advances in Clinical Dysarthria*. Boston: College-Hill Press, 1989.

95. Uziel A, Bohe M, Cadilhac J, Passouant P. Les troubles de la voix et de la parole dans les syndromes Parkinson'siens. *Folia Phoniatrica*. 1975;27(3):166-176.

96. Weismer G. Articulatory characteristics of parkinsonian dysarthria: segmental and phrase-level timing, spirantization and glottal-supraglottal coordination. In: McNeil M, Rosenbek J, Aronson A, eds. *The Dysarthrias: Physiology, Acoustics, Perception and Management*. San Diego, CA: College-Hill Press; 1984.

97. Forrest K, Weismer G, Turner GS. Kinematic, acoustic, and perceptual analyses of connected speech produced by parkinsonian and normal geriatric adults. *J Acoust Soc Am*. 1989;85:2608-2622.

98. McRae PA, Tjaden K, Schoonings B. Acoustic and perceptual consequences of articulatory rate change in Parkinson disease. *J Speech Lang Hear Res*. 2002;45:35-50.

99. Flint AJ, Black SE, Campbell-Taylor I, Gailey GF, Levinton, C. Abnormal speech articulation, psychomotor retardation, and subcortical dysfunction in major depression. *J Psychiatr Res*. 1993;27:309-319.

100. Caligiuri MP. Labial kinematics during speech in people with Parkinsonian rigidity. *Brain*. 1987;110:1033-1044.

101. Caligiuri MP. The influence of speaking rate on articulatory hypokinesia in Parkinsonian dysarthria. *Brain Lang.* 1989a;36:493-502.

102. Caligiuri MP. Short-term fluctuations in orofacial motor control in Parkinson's disease. In: Yorkson KM, Beukelman DR, eds. *Recent Advances in Clinical Dysarthria.* Boston: College Hill; 1989b.

103. Connor NP, Abbs JH, Cole KJ, Gracco VL. Parkinsonian deficits in serial multiarticulate movements for speech. *Brain.* 1989;112:997-1009.

104. Conner NP, Abbs JH. Task-dependent variations in Parkinsonian motor impairments. *Brain.* 1991;114:321-332.

105. Hirose H, Kiritan S, Ushijima T, Yoshioka H, Sawashima M. Patterns of dysarthric movements in people with Parkinsonism. *Folia Phoniatr.* 1981;33:204-215.

106. Dromey C. Articulatory kinematics in people with Parkinson's disease using different speech treatment approaches, *J Med Speech Lang Pathol.* 2001;8:155-161.

107. Gath I, Yair E. Analysis of vocal tract parameters in Parkinsonian speech. *J Acoust Soc Am.* 1988;84:1628-1634.

108. Rosenfeld D. Parmacologic approaches to speech motor disorders. In: Vogel D, Cannito M eds. *Treating Disordered Speech Motor Control.* Austin: Pro-ed;1991:111-152.

109. Ho AK, Bradshaw JL, Iansek R, Alfredson R. Speech volume regulation in Parkinson's disease: effects of implicit cues and explicit instructions. *Neuropsychologia.* 1999;37:1453-1460.

110. Hirose H. Pathophysiology of motor speech disorders (dysarthria). *Folia Phoniatr* (Basel). 1986;38:61-88.

111. Caligiuri MP, Abbs JH. Response properties of the perioral reflex in Parkinson's disease. *Exp Neurol.* 1987;98:563-572.

112. Schneider JS, Lidsky TI. *Basal Ganglia and Behavior: Sensory Aspects of Motor Functioning.* Toronto: Hans Huber, 1987.

113. Kempler D, Van Lancker D. Effect of speech task on intelligibility in dysarthria: a case study of Parkinson's disease. *Brain Lang.* 2002;80:449-464.

114. Rosen KM, Kent RD, Duffy JR. Task-based profile of vocal intensity decline in Parkinson's disease. *Folia Phiatr Logop.* 2005;57:28-37.

115. Bunton K, Keintz CK. Effects of a concurrent motor task on speech intelligibility for speakers with Parkinson disease. Paper presented at the Biennial Conference on Motor Speech, Austin, TX, March 2006.

116. Koller WC. Sensory symptoms in PD. *Neurology.* 1984;34:957-959.

117. Diamond SG, Schneider JS, Markham CH. Oral sensorimotor defects in people with Parkinson's disease. *Adv Neurol.* 1987;45:335-338.

118. Graber S, Hertrich I, Daum I, Spieker S, Ackermann H. Speech perception deficits in Parkinson's disease: underestimation of time intervals compromises identification of durational phonetic contrasts. *Brain Lang.* 2002;82: 65-74.

119. Solomon,NP, Robin DA, Lorell DM, Rodnitzky RL, Luschei ES. Tongue function testing in Parkinson's disease: indicators of fatigue. In: Till JA, Yorkston KM, Beukelman DR, eds. *Motor Speech Disorders: Advances in Assessment and Treatment.* Baltimore: Paul H. Brookes, 1994.

120. Demirci M, Grill S, McShane L, Hallett M. A mismatch between kinesthetic and visual perception in Parkinson's disease. *Ann Neurol.* 1997;41: 781-788.

121. Jobst EE, Melnick ME, Byl NN, Dowling GA, Aminoff MJ. Sensory perception in Parkinson's disease. *Arch Neurol.* 1997;54:450-454.

122. Klockgether T, Borutta M, Rapp H, Spieder S, Dichgans J. A defect of kinesthesia in Parkinson's disease. *Brain.* 1997;120:460-465.

123. Rickards C, Cody FW. Proprioceptive control of wrist movements in Parkinson's disease. *Brain.* 1997;120:977-990.

124. Ramig LO, Pawlas A, Countryman S. *The Lee Silverman Voice Treatment (LSVT): A Practical Guide to Treating the Voice and Speech Disorders in Parkinson Disease.* Iowa City, IA: National Center for Voice and Speech, 1995b.

125. Marsden CD. The mysterious motor function of the basal ganglia: the Robert Wartenberg lecture. *Neurology.* 1982;32:514-439.

126. Dromey C, Ramig L. The effect of lung volume on selected phonatory and articulatory variables. *J Speech Lang Hear Res.* 1998a;41:491-502.

127. Kleinow J, Smith A, Ramig L. Speech stability in Idiopathic Parkinson disease: effects of rate and loudness manipulations. *J Speech Lang Hear Res.* 2001;44:1041-1051.

128. Ramig L, Sapir S, Baker K, Hinds S, Spielman J, Brisbie A, Stathopoulos E, El-Sharkawi A, Logemann J, Fox C, Johnson A, Borod J, Luschei E, Smith M. The "big picture" on the role of phonation in the treatment of individuals with motor speech disorders: or "What's up with loud?" Paper presented at the TenthBiennial Conference on Motor Speech, San Antonio, TX. (March 2000).

129. Watson PJ, Hughes D. The relationship of vocal loudness manipulation to prosodic Fo and durational variables in healthy adults. *J Speech Lang Hear Res.* 2006;49:636-644.

130. Will L, Spielman J, Ramig L. Stimulated or trained loudness: is there a difference and does it matter? Paper presented at the Conference on Motor Speech Disorders. Austin, March 2006.
131. Tjaden K, Wilding GE. Rate and loudness manipulations in dysarthria: acoustic and perceptual findings. *J Speech Lang Hear Res.* 2004;47:766-783.
132. Schulman R. Articulatory dynamics of loud and normal speech. *J Acoust Soc Am.* 1989;85:295-312.
133. Curio G, Neuloh G, Numminen J, Jousmaki V, Hari R. Speaking modifies voice-evoked activity in the human auditory cortex. *Hum Brain Mapp.* 2000;9:183-191.
134. Ford JM, Mathalon DH. Electrophysiological evidence of corollary discharge dysfunction in schizophrenia during talking and thinking. *J Psychiatr Res.* 2004;38:37-46.
135. Liotti M, Vogel D, Sapir S, Ramig L, New P, Fox P. Abnormal auditory gating in Parkinson's disease before & after LSVT. Paper presented at the Annual Meeting of the American Speech, Language and Hearing Association, Washington DC, November, 2000.
136. Boecker H, Ceballos-Baumann A, Bartenstein P, et al. Sensory processing in Parkinson's and Huntington's disease: investigations with 3D H(2)(15)O-PET. *Brain.* 1999;122:1651-1665.
137. Narayana S, Vogel D, Brown S, Franklin C, Zhang W, Lancaster J, Fox P. Mechanism of action of voice therapy in Parkinson's hypophonia—a PET study. A poster presented at the 11th Annual Meeting of the Organization for Human Brain Mapping. Toronto, Ontario, Canada. 2005
138. Houde J, Nagarajan S, Heinks T, Fox C, Ramig L, Marks W, The effects of voice therapy on feedback control in parkinsonian speech. *Mov Disord.* 2004;19:S403.
139. Schulz GM, Peterson T, Sapienza CM, Greer M, Friedman W. Voice and speech characteristics of persons with Parkinson's disease pre- and post-pallidotomy surgery: preliminary findings. *J Speech Lang Hear Res.* 1999;42:1176-1194.
140. Schultz GM, Grant MK. Effects of speech therapy and pharmacologic and surgical treatments on voice and speech in Parkinson's disease: a review of the literature. *J Commun Disord.* 2000;33:59-88.
141. Pinto S, Ozsancak C, Tripoliti E, Thobois S, Limousin-Dowsey P, Auzou P. Treatments for dysarthria in Parkinson's disease. *Lancet.* 2004;3:547-556.
142. Speech therapy in Parkinson's disease. *Mov Disord.* 2002;17suppl:S163-166.
143. Yorkston KM, Spencer KA, Duffy JR. Behavioral management of respiratory/phonatory dysfunction from dysarthria: a systematic review of the evidence. *J Med Speech Lang Pathol.* 2003;11:xiii-xxxviii.
144. Gallena S, Smith PJ, Zeffiro T, Ludlow CL. Effects of levodopa on laryngeal muscle activity for voice onset and offset in Parkinson disease. *J Speech Lang Hear Res.* 2001;44:1284-1299.
145. De Letter M, Santens P, Van Borsel J. The effects of levodopa on word intelligibility in Parkinson's disease. *J Commun Disord.* 2005;38:187-196.
146. Goberman A, Coelho C, Robb M. Phonatory characteristics of parkinsonian speech before and after morning medication: the ON and OFF states. *J Commun Disord.* 2002;35:217-39
147. Sanabria J, Ruiz PG, Gutierrez R, Marquez F, Escobar P, Gentil M, Cenjor C. The effect of levodopa on vocal function in Parkinson's disease. *Clin Neuropharmacol.* 2001;24:99-102.
148. Cahill LM, Murdoch BE, Theodoros DG, Triggs EJ, Charles BG, Yao AA. Effect of oral levodopa treatment on articulatory function in Parkinson's disease: preliminary results. *Motor Control.* 1998;2:161-172.
149. Jiang J, Lin E, Wang J, Hanson DG. Glottographic measures before and after levodopa treatment in Parkinson's disease. *Laryngoscope.* 1999; 109:1287-1294.
150. Trail M, Fox C, Ramig LO, Sapir S, Howard J, Lai EC. Speech treatment for Parkinson's disease. *NeuroRehabilitation.* 2005;20:205-221.
151. Biary N, Pimental PA, Langenberg PW. A double-blind trial of clonazepan in the treatment of parkinsonian dysarthria. *Neurology.* 1988;38:255-258.
152. Pahwa R, Lyons KE, Wilkinson SB et al. Long-term evaluation of deep brain stimulation of the thalamus. *J Neurosurg.* 2006;104:506-512.
153. Rodriguez-Oroz MC, Obeso JA, Lang AE et al. Bilateral deep brain stimulation in Parkinson's disease: a multicentre study with 4 years follow-up. *Brain.* 2005;128:2240-2249.
154. Krack P, Batir A, Van Blercom N et al. Five-year follow-up of bilateral stimulation of the subthalamic nucleus in advanced Parkinson's disease. *N Engl J Med.* 2003;349:1925-34.
155. Santens P, De Letter M, Van Borsel J et al. Lateralized effects of subthalamic nucleus stimulation on different aspects of speech in Parkinson's disease. *Brain Lang.* 2003;87:253-258.
156. Wang E, Verhagen Metman L, Bakay R, et al. The effect of unilateral electrostimulation of the subthalamic nucleus on respiratory/phonatory subsystems of speech production in Parkinson's disease—a preliminary report. *Clin Linguist Phon.* 2003;17:283-289.
157. Gentil M, Pinto S, Pollak P et al. Effect of bilateral stimulation of the subthalamic nucleus on parkinsonian dysarthria. *Brain Lang.* 2003;85:190-196.
158. Gentil M, Garcia-Ruiz P, Pollak P et al. Effect of bilateral deep-brain stimulation on oral control of patients with parkinsonism. *Eur Neurol.* 2000;44: 147-152.

159. Gentil M, Chauvin P, Pinto S et al. Effect of bilateral stimulation of the subthalamic nucleus on parkinsonian voice. *Brain Lang.* 2001;78:233-240.
160. Pinto S, Gentil M, Fraix V et al. Bilateral subthalamic stimulation effects on oral force control in Parkinson's disease. *J Neurol.* 2003;250:179-187.
161. Dromey C, Kumar R, Lang AE et al. An investigation of the effects of subthalamic nucleus stimulation on acoustic measures of voice. *Mov Disord.* 2000;15:1132-1138.
162. Rousseaux M, Krystkowiak P, Kozlowski O et al. Effects of subthalamic nucleus stimulation on parkinsonian dysarthria and speech intelligibility. *J Neurol.* 2004;251:327-334.
163. Saint-Cyr JA, Trepanier LL, Kumar R et al. Neuropsychological consequences of chronic bilateral stimulation of the subthalamic nucleus in Parkinson's disease. *Brain.* 2000;123:2091-2108.
164. McIntyre CC, Mori S, Sherman DL et al. Electric field and stimulating influence generated by deep brain stimulation of the subthalamic nucleus. *Clin Neurophysiol.* 2004;115:589-595.
165. Tornqvist AL, Schalen L, Rehncrona S. Effects of different electrical parameter settings on the intelligibility of speech in patients with Parkinson's disease treated with subthalamic deep brain stimulation. *Mov Disord.* 2005;20:416-423.
166. Dias AE, Barbosa ER, Coracini K et al. Effects of repetitive transcranial magnetic stimulation on voice and speech in Parkinson's disease. *Acta Neurol Scand.* 2006;113:92-99.
167. Pagni CA, Zeme S, Zenga F. Further experience with extradural motor cortex stimulation for treatment of advanced Parkinson's disease. Report of 3 new cases. *J Neurosurg Sci.* 2003;47:189-193.
168. Boucai L, Cerquetti D, Merello M. Functional surgery for PD treatment: a structured analysis of a decade of published literature. *Br J Neurosurg.* 2004;18:213-222.
169. Stewart M, Desaloms JM, Sanghera, MK. Stimulation of the subthalamic nucleus for the treatment of Parkinson's disease: post operative management, programming and rehabilitation. *J Neurosci Nurs.* 2005;37:108-114.
170. Greene, HCL. *The Voice and Its Disorders.* London: Pitman Medical, 1980.
171. Yaryura-Tobias JA, Diamond B, Merlis S. Verbal communication with L-dopa treatment. *Nature.* 1971;234:224-225.
172. Downie AW, Low JM, Lindsay DD. Speech disorders in parkinsonism: usefulness of delayed auditory feedback in selected cases. *Br J Disord Comm.* 1981a;16:135-139.
173. Helm N. Management of palilalia with a pacing board. *J Speech Hearing Disord.* 1979;44:350-353.
174. Deane KHO, Whurr R, Playford ED, Ben-Shlomo Y, Clarke CE. Speech and language therapy for dysarthria in Parkinson's disease: a comparison of techniques (Cochrane Review). In: *The Cochrane Library.* Chichester, UK: John Wiley & Sons, Ltd., Issue 2, 2004.
175. Deane KHO, Whurr R, Playford ED, Ben-Shlomo Y, Clarke CE. Speech and language therapy versus placebo or no intervention for dysarthria in Parkinson's disease (Cochrane Review), In: *The Cochrane Library.* Chichester, UK: John Wiley & Sons, Ltd, Issue 2, 2004.
176. Ramig LO, Countryman S, O'Brien C, Hoehn M, Thompson L. Intensive speech treatment for patients with Parkinson's disease: short and long term comparison of two techniques. *Neurology.* 1996;47:1496-1504.
177. Johnson J, Pring T. Speech therapy and Parkinson's disease: a review and further data. *Br J Disord Commun.* 1990;125:183-194.
178. Robertson SJ, Thomson F. Speech therapy in Parkinsons disease: a study of the efficacy and long term effects of intensive treatment. *Br J Disord Commun.* 1984;18:213-224.
179. Scott S, Caird FI. Speech therapy for Parkinson's disease. *J Neurol Neurosurg Psychiatry.* 1983;46:140-144.
180. Ramig LO, Sapir S, Countryman S, Pawlas AA, O'Brien C, Hoehn M, Thompson L. Intensive voice treatment (LSVT®) for people with Parkinson's disease: A 2 year follow-up. *J Neurol Neurosurg Psychiatry.* 2001a;71:493-498.
181. NICE, National Collaborating Centre for Chronic Conditions. *Parkinson's Disease: National Clinical Guideline for Diagnosis and Management in Primary and Secondary Care.* London: Royal College of Physicians; 2006.
182. Ramig L, Sapir S, Fox C, Countryman S. Changes in vocal intensity following intensive voice treatment (LSVT®) in people with Parkinson disease: a comparison with untreated people and with normal age-matched controls. *Mov Disord.* 2001b;16:79-83.
183. Titze I. *Vocal Fold Physiology: Frontiers in Basic Science.* San Diego, CA: Singular Publishing Group Inc.; 1993.
184. Albert M, Sparks R, Helm N. Melodic intonation therapy for aphasia. *Arch Neurol.* 1973;29:130-131.
185. Hargrove P, McGarr N. In: Wertz R, ed. *Prosody of Communication Disorders.* San Diego, CA: Singular Publishing Group, 1994.
186. Ling D. *Speech and the Hearing Impaired Child: Theory and Practice.* Washington, DC: The Alexander Graham Bell Association for the Deaf, Inc.; 1976.
187. Munhall K, Ostry D, Parush A. Characteristics of velocity profiles of speech movements. *J Exper Psychology: Human Perception and Performance.* 1986;11:457-474.
188. Picheny M, Durlach N, Braida I. Speaking clearly for the hard of hearing II: acoustic characteristics of clear and conversational speech. *J Speech Hear Res.* 1986;29:434-446.

189. Worringham C, Stelmach G. The contribution of gravitational torques to limb position sense. *Exp Brain Res*. 1985;61:38-42.
190. Fisher B, Petzinger G, Nixon K, Hogg E, Bremmer S, Meshul C, Jakowec M. Exercise-induced behavioral recovery and neuroplasticity in the 1-methyl-4-phenyl-1,2,3,6-tetrahydropyridine-lesioned mouse basal ganglia. *J Neurosci Res*. 2004;77:378-390.
191. Liepert J, Miltner W, Bauder H, Sommer M, Dettmers C, Taub E, Weiller C. Motor cortex plasticity during constraint-induced movement therapy in stroke patients. *Neuroscience Letters*. 1998;250:5-8.
192. Garren K, Brosovic G, Abaza M, Ramig, L. Voice therapy and Parkinson disease: measures of vocal fold adduction. A paper presented at the Voice Symposium. Philadelphia, PA, June, 2000.
193. Huber J, Stathopoulos E, Ramig L, Lancaster S. Respiratory function and variability in individuals with Parkinson disease: pre and post Lee Silverman Voice Treatment (LSVT®). *J Med Speech Lang Pathol*. 2003;11:185-201.
194. Baumgartner C, Sapir S, Ramig L. Voice quality changes following phonatory-respiratory effort Treatment (LSVT) versus respiratory effort treatment for individuals with Parkinson disease. *J Voice*. 2001;15:105-114.
195. Sundberg J, Titze I. Vocal intensity in speakers and singers. *J Acoust Soc Am*. 1992;83:1536-1552.
196. Countryman S, Hicks J, Ramig L, Smith M. Supraglottic hyperfunction in an individual with Parkinson disease: treatment outcome. *Am J Speech Lang Path*. 1996;6:85-94.
197. Dromey C, Ramig L, Johnson A. Phonatory and articulatory changes associated with increased vocal intensity in Parkinson disease: a case study. *J Speech Hear Res*. 1995;38:751-763.
198. Sapir S, Spielman J, Ramig L, Story B, Fox C. Effects of Intensive Voice Treatment (LSVT®) on vowel articulation in dysarthric individuals with idiopathic Parkinson disease: acoustic and perceptual findings. *J Speech Lang Hearing Res*. 2007;50:899-912.
199. Spielman J, Borod J, Ramig L. Effects of Intensive Voice Treatment (LSVT) on facial expressiveness in Parkinson's disease: Preliminary data. *Cogn Behav Neurol*. 2003;16:177-188.
200. El Sharkawi A, Ramig L, Logemann J, Pauloski B, Rademaker A, Smith C, Pawlas A, Baum, S, Werner C. Swallowing and voice effects of Lee Silverman Voice Treatment: a pilot study. *Journal of Neurology, Neuropsychiatry, and Psychiatry*. 2002;72:31-36.
201. Allen G. Segmental timing control in speech production. *Journal of Phonetics*. 1973;1:219-237.
202. Dromey C, Ramig L. The effect of lung volume on selected phonatory and articulatory variables. *J Speech Lang Hear Res*. 1998a;41:491-502.
203. Dromey C, Ramig L. Intentional changes in sound pressure level and rate: their impact on measures of respiration, phonation, and articulation. *J Speech Lang Hear Res*. 1998b;41:1003-1018.
204. Gandour J, Dechongkit S, Ponglorpisit S, Khunadorn F. Speech timing at the sentence level in Thai after unilateral brain damage. *Brain Lang*. 1994;46: 419-438.
205. McClean MD, Tasko SM. Association of orofacial with laryngeal and respiratory motor output during speech. *Exp Brain Res*. 2002;146:481-489.
206. Farley BG, Koshland GF. Training BIG to move faster: the application of the speed-amplitude relation as a rehabilitation strategy for people with Parkinson's disease. *Exp Brain Res*. 2005;11:1-6 (Epub ahead of print)
207. Ackermann H, Wildgruber D, Daum I, Grodd W. Does the cerebellum contribute to cognitive aspects of speech production? A functional magnetic resonance imaging (fMRI) study in humans. *Neuroscience Lett*. 1998;247:187-190.
208. Hirano S, Kojima H, Naito Y, Honjo I, Kamoto Y, Okazawa H, Ishizu K, Yonekura Y, Nagahama Y, Fukuyama H, Konishi J. Cortical speech processing mechanisms while vocalizing visually presented languages. *Neuroreport*. 1996;8: 363-367.
209. Jurgens U, Kirzinger A, von Cramon D. The effects of deep-reaching lesions in the cortical face area on phonation. A combined case report and experimental monkey study. *Cortex*. 1982;18:125-130.
210. Kitchen DM, Cheney DL, Seyfarth RM. Male chacma baboons (Papio hamadryas ursinus) discriminate loud call contests between rivals of different relative ranks. *Anim Cogn*. 2005;8:1-6.
211. Leinonen L, Laakso ML, Carlson S, Linnankoski I. Shared means and meanings in vocal expression of man and macaque. *Logoped Phoniatr Vocol*. 2003;28:53-61.
212. Tecumseh FW. The phonetic potential of nonhuman vocal tracts: comparative cineradiographic observations of vocalizing animals. *Phonetica*. 2000;57:205-218.
213. Jurgens U, von Cramon D. On the role of the anterior cingulate cortex in phonation: a case report. *Brain Lang*. 1982;15:234-248.
214. Meissner I, Sapir S, Kokmen E, Stein SD. The paramedian diencephalic syndrome: a dynamic phenomenon. *Stroke*. 1987;18:380-385.
215. Sapir S, Aronson AE. Clinician reliability in rating voice improvement after laryngeal nerve section for spastic dysphonia. *Laryngoscope*. 1985;95:200-202.
216. Seyfarth RM, Cheney DL. Meaning and emotion in animal vocalizations. *Ann N Y Acad Sci*. 2003;1000:32-55.

217. Davis P, Zhang S, Winkworth A, Bandler R. Neural control of vocalization: respiratory and emotional influences. *J Voice.* 1996;10:23-38.

218. Jurgens U, Zwirner P. The role of the periaqueductal grey in limbic and neocortical vocal fold control. *Neuroreport.* 1996;25:2921-2923.

219. Larson C. The midbrain periaqueductal gray: a brainstem structure involved in vocalization. *J Speech Hear Res.* 1985;28:241-249.

220. Muller-Preuss P, Newnan J, Jurgens U. Anatomical and physiological evidence for a relationship between the 'cingular' vocalization area and the auditory cortex in the squirrel monkey. *Brain Res.* 1980;202:307-315.

221. Ploog, D. Phonation, emotion, cognition, with reference to the brain mechanisms involved. *Ciba Found Symp.* 1979;69:79-98.

222. West RA, Larson CR. Neurons of the anterior mesial cortex related to faciovocal activity in the awake monkey. *J Neurophysiol.* 1995;74:1856-1869.

223. Cotman CW, Berchtold NC. Exercise: a behavioral intervention to enhance brain health and plasticity. *Trends in Neurosci.* 2002;25:295-301.

224. Kleim J, Jones T, Schallert T. Motor enrichment and the induction of plasticity before or after brain injury. *Neurochem Res.* 2003;11:1757-1769.

225. Vaynman S, Gomez-Pinilla F. License to run: exercise impacts functional plasticity in the intact and injured central nervous system by using neurotrophins. *Neurorehabil Neural Repair.* 2005;19:283-295.

226. Schmidt RA, Lee TD. *Motor Control and Learning: A Behavioral Emphasis.* Champaign, IL: Human Kinetic Publishers, 1999.

227. Countryman S, Ramig L, Pawlas A. Speech and voice deficits in Parkinsonian Plus syndromes: Can they be treated? *J Med Speech Lang Path.* 1994;2:211-225.

228. Fox C, Farley B., Ramig L, McFarland. An integrated speech and physical therapy approach for Parkinson disease: training Big and Loud. Paper presented at the Biannual Conference on Motor Speech, Austin, TX. March, 2006.

229. Fox CM, Farley BG. *Learning Big and Loud™: an integrated rehabilitation approach to Parkinson's disease.* Program No. 874.10, 2004 Abstract Viewer and Itinerary Planner. Washington, DC: Society for Neuroscience, Online 2004.

230. Fox CM, Farley BG, Ramig, LO, McFarland D. An integrated rehabilitation approach to Parkinson's disease: learning Big and Loud. *Mov Disord.* 2005;20:S127.

231. Taub E, Lum PS, Hardin P, Mark BW, Uswatte G. AutoCITE: automated delivery of CI therapy with reduced effort by therapists. *Stroke.* 2005;36:1301-1304.

232. Halpern AE, Matos C, Ramig LO, Petska J, Spielman J. LSVTC—A PDA Supported Speech Treatment for Parkinson's disease. A poster presented to the Annual American Speech-Language-Hearing Association Meeting, Philadelphia, PA, 2004.

233. Halpern A, Matos C, Ramig L, Petska J, Spielman J, Bennett J. LSVTC—A PDA supported speech treatment for Parkinson's disease. Presented at the 9th International Congress of Parkinson's Disease and Movement Disorders. New Orleans, LA, 2005.

234. Barker LJ. Computer-assisted vocabulary acquisition: the CSLU Vocabulary Tutor in oral deaf education. *J Deaf Stud Deaf Educ.* 2003;8:187-198.

235. Cole R, Carmell R, Conners P, Macon M, Wouters J, de Villiers J et al. Intelligent animated agents for interactive language training. Proceedings of StiLL: ESCA Workshop On Speech Technology in Language Training. Stockholm, Sweden, 1998.

236. Cole R, Massaro DW, deVilliers J, Rundle B, Shobaki K, Wouters J et al. New tools for interactive speech and language training: using animated conversational agents in the classrooms of profoundly deaf children. In: Proceedings of ESCA/SOCRATES Workshop on Method and Tool Innovations for Speech Science Education, London; 1999.

237. Cole R, VanVuuren S, Pellom B, Hacioglu K, Ma J, Movellan J, Schwartz JS et al. Perceptive animated interfaces: first steps toward a new paradigm for human-computer interaction. Proceedings of the IEEE: Special Issue on Human Computer Multimodal Interface. 2003;91(9):1391-1405.

238. COLIT03 website: http://cslr.colorado.edu/beginweb/reading/reading.html, provides an overview of reading tutors that use animated agent technologies as part of the Colorado Literacy Tutor project.

239. LLOUD03 website: http://cslr.Colorado.edu/beingweb/animated_speech_therapist.html, provides short videos comparing the LSVT virtual therapist to a human therapist.

240. Stone P. Revolutionizing language instruction in oral deaf education. In: Proceedings of the International Conference of Phonetic Sciences, San Francisco, CA, 1999.

241. Robichaud JA, Pfann KD, Vaillancourt DE, Comella CL, Corcos DM. Force control and disease severity in Parkinson's disease. *Mov Disord.* 2005;20:441-450.

242. Pisani A, Centonze D, Bernardi G, Calabresi P. Striatal synaptic plasticity: implications for motor learning and Parkinson's disease. *Mov Disord.* 2005;20(4):395-402.

243. Jones TA, Chu CJ, Grande LA, Gregory AD. Motor skills training enhances lesion-induced structural plasticity in the motor cortex of adult rats. *J Neurosci.* 1999;19(22):10153-10163.
244. Tillerson J, Cohen A, Caudle M, Zigmond M, Schallert T, Miller G. Forced nonuse in unilateral parkinsonian rats exacerbates injury. *J Neurosci.* 2002;22(15):6790-6799.
245. Alexander GE, Crutcher MD. Functional architecture of basal ganglia circuits: neural substrates of parallel processing. *Trends Neurosci.* 1990;13:266-271.
246. Graybiel AM. The basal ganglia and chunking of action repertoires. *Neurobiol Learn Mem.* 1998;70:119-136.
247. Comery TA, Shar R, Greenough WT. Differential rearing alters spine density on medium-sized spiny neurons in the rat corpus striatum: evidence for association of morphological plasticity with early response gene expression. *Neurobiol Learn Mem.* 1995;63:217-219.
248. Kleim JA, Lussnig E, Schwarz ER, Comery TA, Greenough WT. Synaptogenesis and Fos expression in the motor cortex of the adult rat after motor skill learning. *J Neurosci.* 1996;16:4529-4535.
249. Plautz EJ, Milliken GW, Nudo RJ. Effects of repetitive motor training on movement representations in adult squirrel monkeys: role of use versus learning. *Neurobiol Learning Memory.* 2000;74:27-55.
250. Brown RG, Marsden CD. Dual task performance and processing resources in normal subjects and patients with Parkinson's disease. *Brain.* 1991;114:215-231.
251. Brizard M, Carcenac C, Bemelmans A, Feuerstein, Mallet J, Savasta M. Functional reinnervation from remaining DA terminals induced by GDNF lentivirus in a rat model of early Parkinson's disease. *Neurobiol Dis.* 2006;21:90-101.
252. Faherty CJ, Raviie Shepherd K, Herasimtschuk A, Smeyne RJ. Environmental enrichment in adulthood eliminates neuronal death in experimental Parkinsonism. *Mol Brain Res.* 2005;134:170-179.
253. Tillerson J, Cohen A, Philhower J, Miller G, Zigmond M, Schallert T. Forced limb-use effects on the behavioral and neurochemical effects of 6-hydroxydopamine. *J Neurosci.* 2001;21(12):4427-4435.
254. Tillerson JL, Caudle WM, Reveron ME, Miller GW. Exercise induces behavioral recovery and attenuates neurochemical deficits in rodent models of Parkinson's disease. *Neurosci.* 2003;119:899-911.
255. Hoehn M, Yahr M. Parkinsonism: onset, progression and mortality. *Neurology.* 1967;19:427-442.

Parkinson's Disease and Swallowing: Neural Control, Disorders, and Treatment Techniques

Leslie A. Mahler, PhD, CCC-SLP; Michelle R. Ciucci, PhD, CCC-SLP; Lorraine Olson Ramig, PhD, CCC-SLP; Cynthia M. Fox, PhD, CCC-SLP

INTRODUCTION

Dysphagia, or a disorder of swallowing, involves difficulty moving food and liquid safely through the aerodigestive pathway. Dysphagia is common in many neurologic disorders, and it is estimated that as many as 95% of people with Parkinson's disease (PD) have a dysphagia.[1,2] Dysphagia associated with PD has been reported to affect all stages of swallowing (oral, pharyngeal, and esophageal) and is more prevalent in the advanced stages of PD.[3-6] The potential impact of swallowing disorders in PD can include discomfort, difficulty taking oral medications, and an inability to maintain hydration and nutrition.[7] Effective management of dysphagia is important to maintain health and quality of life for people with PD. Synthetic dopamine is the traditional pharmacological agent for management of PD symptoms; however, the effects of dopamine on improving swallowing have not been clearly demonstrated.[1,5,8] Traditional behavioral swallowing treatment techniques have focused on postures, maneuvers, diet modifications, and alternatives to oral feeding to maximize safe and pleasurable oral intake for people with PD. Preliminary data from a neurosurgical intervention has demonstrated improvement of some aspects of swallowing.[9] Finally, a preliminary study of the effect of intensive voice treatment, LSVT®-LOUD, has provided evidence of improved swallowing.[10]

NORMAL SWALLOWING

A normal swallow depends on the rapid transfer of a liquid or food bolus from the oral cavity to the stomach while protecting the airway. Efficient bolus movement requires coordinated neuromuscular contractions and relaxations that create zones of high pressure above the bolus and zones of negative pressure below the bolus. Some of the events that make up the pattern of bolus transfer are under direct neural control and can be changed voluntarily. These include lip movement, tongue movement for mastication, and anterior to posterior oral bolus propulsion. Other aspects of swallowing such as vocal fold closure, laryngeal elevation, pharyngeal peristalsis, and upper esophageal sphincter relaxation are more accurately characterized as being semiautomatic and are controlled by central pattern generators involving brainstem pathways.[11-18]

Oral Stage

The oral stage of the swallow involves bolus preparation (oral preparation phase) and transport of the bolus from the oral cavity to the pharynx (oral transport phase) and includes both voluntary control and more automatic central pattern generators (for mastication).[17] The oral preparation phase of swallowing can be highly variable in duration depending on taste, environment, hunger, motivation, and consciousness for humans.[19] Jaw closing muscles including the temporalis, masseter, and medial pterygoid stabilize the mandible. The suprahyoid and infrahyoid muscles position the hyoid during bolus transport and the extrinsic and intrinsic muscles of the tongue move and propel the bolus posteriorly. Facial and buccal muscles are recruited during the oral stage of swallowing to create an anterior lip seal and prevent food from pocketing laterally between the cheeks and the teeth or under the tongue.

The extrinsic muscles of the tongue, including the genioglossus, hyoglossus, styloglossus, and palatoglossus, pull the tongue in an anterior and superior direction to make contact with the hard palate at the onset of the oral transport phase. This closes the oral cavity anteriorly. Simultaneously, the hyoid bone elevates. Next, the intrinsic muscles of the tongue recruit in an anterior to posterior sequence to change the shape of the tongue and to propel the bolus into and through the pharynx.[20] Coordination of the jaw-closing muscles with the tongue and hyoid bone movement is dependent on sensory feedback involving receptors in the jaw-closing muscles and the suprahyoid and infrahyoid structures.[20] The afferent fibers involved in swallowing are those traveling within a variety of cranial nerves (CN) including the maxillary branch of the trigeminal nerve (V), the glossopharyngeal nerve (IX), and the superior branch of the vagus nerve (X).[19]

Sensory feedback from the oral region is vital to initiate and assist the voluntary portion of the oral phase.[20] The oral cavity and tongue have mechanoreceptors, chemoreceptors, and thermoreceptors that provide sensory information about the bolus size, taste, temperature, and consistency. There is more recruitment of mechanoreceptors when greater stabilization of the mandible is needed.[20] For example, with a bolus that is difficult to chew, the facial nerve (VII) has a specialized sensory branch, the chorda tympani, that mediates taste and motor autonomic fibers from the superior salivatory nucleus of the brainstem that provide moisture to the mouth through submandibular and sublingual glands.[21]

Pharyngeal Stage

The initiation of the pharyngeal swallow varies depending on the consistency of the bolus. For thin liquid consistencies, the swallow is typically initiated when the head of the bolus reaches the point between the anterior faucial arches and the point where the tongue base crosses the lower rim of the mandible. However, the timing of pharyngeal swallow initiation for solid boluses varies. There is a gradual accumulation of a solid bolus on the posterior surface of the tongue and even into the valleculae prior to initiation of the swallow. Therefore, the initiation of a swallow may occur at any time during bolus transport from the anterior faucial arches for liquids to the hypopharynx for solids. The sequence of pharyngeal activity for this stage typically begins with the elevation of the velum, closure of the larynx from an inferior to superior direction beginning with the true vocal folds, anterosuperior movement of the larynx due to contraction of the suprahyoid muscles, superior to inferior constriction of the pharyngeal constrictor muscles, and opening of the upper esophageal sphincter. This sequence is stable; that is, the order of events does not vary. This has been demonstrated using EMG during swallowing in humans in the upright position,[18,22,23] in upright compared to supine position,[24] in awake animal models,[18,25-28] and in decerebrate animals.[14,29-31] The timing of each event and the degree of muscle activation may change according to bolus characteristics such as volume and viscosity,[32] but the pattern remains stable. From a motor control standpoint, the pharyngeal stage is considered "involuntary," or mediated by a central pattern generator.

Tongue Movement in the Pharyngeal Stage

Sensory information from the posterior movement of the bolus toward the base of the tongue sends information to the nucleus ambiguus, which initiates the pharyngeal swallow.[33] When the leading edge of the bolus passes the anterior faucial arches and the point where the tongue base crosses the lower rim of the mandible, the pharyngeal swallow should be triggered.[34] The genioglossus muscle contracts first in the pharyngeal stage to control the tongue as the bolus reaches the tongue base. Base of tongue approximation to the superior pharyngeal constrictor acting as part of the ventral wall of the pharynx is important during swallowing to create pressure for downward propulsion of the bolus. Other muscles that contract early in the pharyngeal stage include the mylohyoid and hyoglossus muscles that raise the hyoid bone.[20] The geniohyoid and mylohyoid act together to move the hyoid bone anteriorly.[20] The raising of the hyoid bone also elevates the larynx and tilts it anteriorly, placing it in a more protective posture and assists in the retroflexion of the epiglottis to help prevent foreign materials from entering the laryngeal vestibule.

Pharyngeal Muscle Movement

The palatopharyngeus closes off the nasopharynx and the levator veli palatini raises the soft palate to prevent nasal regurgitation and increase intrapharyngeal pressure that helps to propel the bolus inferiorly.[20] Two types of pharyngeal contractions propel the bolus in the pharyngeal stage. First the pharynx shortens along its axis decreasing its length. Second the shortening of the pharynx modifies the laryngeal shape to decrease pooling in the pharyngeal spaces of the valleculae and the pyriform sinuses.

When the bolus triggers a swallow response multiple muscle contractions occur in a rapid overlapping sequence and are mainly controlled by central pattern generators of the brain stem.[19] The pharyngeal stage incorporates: velopharyngeal closure to create pressure to propel the bolus, laryngeal closure to prevent aspiration, bolus propulsion toward the esophagus, and upper esophageal sphincter opening. The order of muscle movement in the pharyngeal stage remains constant while the temporal relationship among the muscles and the degree of muscle contraction may adapt to accommodate differences in bolus size and consistency.[20]

Esophageal Stage

The esophageal stage of swallowing occurs when the bolus passes from the pharynx through the upper esophageal sphincter (UES) and into the esophagus. Peristalsis moves the bolus from the proximal esophagus to the distal esophagus and into the stomach.[21] As the bolus passes through the UES motor control of the esophagus switches between somatic motoneurons located in the CNS to autonomic motoneurons in the periphery as muscle tissue changes from striated to smooth muscle.[20]

The UES is normally closed, which prevents air from going into the esophagus and prevents material in the esophagus from entering the pharynx. The muscle of the UES is the cricopharyngeus. It is a striated muscle innervated by motoneurons located in the nucleus ambiguus that sends information via the vagus nerve (X). The opening of the UES during swallowing is the result of three factors; 1) relaxation of UES by inhibition of tonic discharge to cricopharyngeus and inferior pharyngeal constrictor muscles, 2) elevation of hyoid by infrahyoid and suprahyoid muscles that creates passive opening of UES secondary to pulling it anteriorly, and 3) pressure from the bolus itself.[21]

The coordination of pharyngeal muscles involved in opening of the UES is controlled centrally by the brainstem involving the reticular formation with input to cranial motor nuclei.[20] Sensation from the upper esophagus is conveyed via the recurrent laryngeal nerve.[35]

Neural Controls of Swallowing

The neural control of swallowing is complicated. It involves motor control characteristics that range from central pattern generation to "voluntary" motor control. Most of what we know about the control of deglutition is from data examining the brainstem or cortex, which leaves us with a dearth of data on other important structures involved in motor control, such as the basal ganglia. Much of our understanding of the neural control of deglutition in the pharyngeal stage comes from the work of Jean and Bosma[25,36,37] in animal models and implicates brainstem structures as the primary controllers via central pattern generation. Additionally, chewing has been associated with a brainstem central pattern generator component.[17] More recently, through disease models and neuroimaging studies, cortical areas have been identified that are pertinent to the pharyngeal and oral stages of deglutition. Neuroimaging has also illuminated other subcortical structures that are active during all three stages of deglutition, such as the basal ganglia, cerebellum, and thalamus.[38] The pharyngeal stage is considered to be under more "involuntary control" while the oral stage has components of both "voluntary" and "involuntary" control (chewing).

Of all these central nervous system components, the brainstem has been most studied for its role in swallowing. Thus, the discussion about neural controls of deglutition will begin in the brainstem.

Pharyngeal Stage Swallow

Two main areas of the brainstem have been identified as the primary areas responsible for the pharyngeal swallow. These areas are in and near the reticular formation of the medulla bilaterally (rhombencephalic swallowing center), including the nucleus tractus solitarius in the dorsal medulla and the nucleus ambiguus in the ventrolateral medulla. Evidence for the nucleus tractus solitarius/nucleus ambiguus as the primary components of the pharyngeal swallow pathway came from experiments that demonstrated these structures are both necessary and sufficient for pharyngeal swallowing.[14,29-31] The first of these studies recorded from nucleus tractus solitarius and nucleus ambiguus during a bolus swallow in anesthetized rats. A simultaneous pattern of sequential bursting occurred in the nucleus tractus solitarius and the nucleus ambiguus associated with the external event of interest: the pharyngeal swallow (sufficient component).[12,15] Lesion studies showed that these structures were vital to the patterned motor response observed with the pharyngeal swallow. Ablation, severing connections, or blocking the action of these structures resulted in the inability to generate a pharyngeal swallow (necessary component).[12,14,16]

The nucleus tractus solitarius receives afferent input (touch, proprioception, pain/temperature) from the trigeminal (V), glossopharyngeal (IX), and vagus (X) nerves. Specifically, input from the superior laryngeal nerve of the vagus is paramount for eliciting a pharyngeal swallow via mechanoreceptors. It is responsible for triggering, shaping the degree and timing of efferent output, and the timing of the onset of the pharyngeal swallow.[25,29,33,39-41] The nucleus tractus solitarius projects bilaterally to the nucleus ambiguus that contains "switching neurons" that distribute drive to the motoneurons of the trigeminal (CN V), facial (CN VII), glossopharyngeal (IX), vagus (X), and hypoglossal (XII) cranial nerves for the patterned motor response of the pharyngeal swallow.[25,42] Stimulating the superior laryngeal nerve or nucleus tractus solitarius will generate a pharyngeal swallow. However, stimulating the nucleus ambiguus does not. Thus, the central pattern generator for a pharyngeal swallow resides in the interconnections between the nucleus tractus solitarius and the nucleus ambiguus.[25]

There has been considerable debate over whether the pharyngeal swallow is controlled by a central pattern generator. However, there is mounting evidence that supports the mechanisms underlying pharyngeal swallowing as a central pattern generator. Kandell defined a central pattern generator as a "neuronal network capable of generating a pattern of motor activity without phasic sensory input from a peripheral receptor."[43] Similarly, those who study the pharyngeal swallow central pattern generator define it as an "operational expression to designate an ensemble of neural elements whose properties and connectivity can give rise to characteristic patterns of rhythmic activity in the absence of external feedback."[18] Evidence of central pattern generator networks for the pharyngeal swallow is found in the neuronal cellular membranes. The neurons in the nucleus tractus solitarius have three distinct firing patterns that cause rhythmic bursting.[42] Furthermore, membrane conductance in nucleus tractus solitarius and nucleus ambiguus neurons can cause rhythmic waves of firing.[13,15,36,44]

The cellular properties of the brainstem neuronal network associated with the pharyngeal swallow were consistent with the defined properties of a central pattern generator. That is, neurotransmitters released at synapses in pathways associated with the pharyngeal swallow produced both excitation (serotonin, glutamate) and inhibition (dopamine, norepinephrine) in the post-synaptic cell.[25,45,46]

The "trigger" of a pharyngeal swallow was shown to occur when the primary sensory nerves from the pharynx or sensory pathways within the brainstem were stimulated with electrical or a pharyngeal bolus stimulus. The superior laryngeal nerve, the glossopharyngeal nerve (IX), or neural pathways from the pons to the nucleus tractus solitarius, elicited a pharyngeal swallow in anesthetized rats.[25] Stimulating the nucleus ambiguus or motor cranial nerve nuclei did not successfully trigger a pharyngeal swallow. Thus, it is demonstrated that the pharyngeal swallow does not require phasic sensory input, meeting the requirements of a central pattern generator.

Patterns of connectivity among neurons in the brainstem swallow center, such as local and projection interneurons, are both inhibited and excited, meaning that they are capable of generating patterns of activity.[25,36] For example, the nucleus tractus solitarius pharyngeal swallow network consists of cells that fire in a sequence of activity that commences with excitation of the proximal portions of the swallowing tract and inhibition to that of distal portions. As the bolus progresses through the aerodigestive pathway, the proximal portions are inhibited and the distal portions are excited. This occurrence implies the existence of excitatory and inhibitory connections between interneurons in the brainstem swallow network.[36,47,48]

In summary, the pharyngeal swallow exhibits a stable sequence of muscle activation that can not be modified or interrupted. This sequence is triggered by sensory stimulation through the superior laryngeal nerve or by stimulation of the primary sensory tract nucleus within the brainstem, the nucleus tractus solitarius. However, this does not require phasic sensory input. The sequence of efferent output from the nucleus ambiguus is a stable sequence that is present in deafferented and paralyzed animal,[17] animals with bilateral nerve resection.[17] Humans with positional and bolus delivery changes could theoretically cause the bolus to stimulate more distal areas of the pharynx before the proximal areas but still yield initial proximal muscle contraction.[24]

In addition to the brainstem contribution to the pharyngeal swallow, recent evidence demonstrates that other cortical structures are involved as well. The patterned motor response of the pharyngeal swallow can be elicited by stimulation of a "cortical swallowing region" located in the inferior portion of the prefrontal gyrus, near the insula.[49] Kern and Shaker demonstrated that the pharyngeal swallow is represented in the primary sensory/motor cortex, bilateral insula, cingulate, parietal/occipital regions.[49] This has also been demonstrated in primate models.[50] Thus it appears that the motor control of the pharyngeal swallow also involves cortical components.

Cortical and Subcortical Control of Deglutition

Cortical and subcortical structures have been shown to be involved in all three stages of deglutition. The afferent messages that trigger and adjust the swallowing program at the brainstem level are simultaneously conveyed to higher nervous system structures such as the thalamus and basal ganglia for integration of the voluntary and involuntary aspects of deglutition.[36] The oral stage of swallowing involves "voluntary" motor acts, such as conscious chewing and bolus manipulation, and "involuntary" chewing patterns that are controlled by a central pattern generator.[50] Volitionally, one can decide how much or how long to chew and hold a bolus before transporting it to the pharynx. Furthermore, one can inhibit a pharyngeal swallow (eg, resisting onset of a swallow during dental work in the mouth). The more voluntary aspects of the oral stage are attributed to primary motor and sensory areas of the cortex. Sensory information is relayed via the thalamus to the primary and secondary somatosensory cortical areas. These areas are involved in perception of temperature, touch, position, and stereognosis. Subcortical systems, such as the basal ganglia and cerebellum have been implicated as well but their role(s) are not understood.

Recent PET and fMRI studies implicate the inferior precentral gyrus and insula in both voluntary (to command) and vegetative swallowing.[38] Not surprisingly, the basal ganglia have been shown to respond to both types of swallowing.[38] Furthermore, lesions and diseases affecting only the cortex or basal ganglia can affect all three stages of deglutition. This evidence suggests that deglutition is a complex sensori-motor process requiring integration of the CNS and PNS to function properly. Because the basal ganglia are involved in other types of voluntary and involuntary motor control, it is not surprising that they would be active during both voluntary and involuntary aspects of swallowing.

Volitional swallowing is represented in multiple regions of the CNS, including the primary sensory/motor cortex, insular, prefrontal/cingulate gyrus, and cuneus and precuneus regions. Research demonstrates that deglutition actually involves a "large-scale distributed network" and "the nature of this network helps to explain how so many neurological conditions produce dysphagia,"[38] rather than those limited to the brainstem. A positron emission tomography study (PET) examined regional cerebral blood flow during voluntary swallowing, lateral tongue movements (to control for movement), and rest. They found that voluntary swallowing produced strong regional blood flow increase within the inferior precentral gyrus bilaterally, right insula, left cerebellum, and right temporal lobe.[38] Again, the putamen (basal ganglia) and the thalamus, which is part of the basal ganglia circuitry, were active during swallowing.[38] A functional magnetic resonance imaging (fMRI) study examined deglutition during automatic saliva swallowing, voluntary saliva swallowing, and water bolus swallowing. They found that automatic swallowing produced activation of the lateral pre- and post-central gyri, right insula, and superior temporal gyrus.[50] Additional areas that were not as strongly activated include the superior temporal gurus, the middle and inferior frontal gyri, and the frontal operculum. Voluntary saliva and voluntary water swallowing produced activation in the caudal anterior cingulate cortex. Again, the focus has been primarily on the role of the brainstem or cortex for deglutition. However, there are imaging data that support that the basal ganglia are clearly active during swallowing.[38] Because the basal ganglia are known to be involved in motor control, it is paramount that we better understand how they are involved in deglutition.

The only current evidence available about the basal ganglia and swallowing is that the putamen shows an increase in hemodynamic response during vegetative and voluntary swallowing.[50] However, it has not been demonstrated if the basal ganglia are activated in the planning stages before the oral stage commences, whether they remain active throughout all three stages of deglutition, if the nature of activation changes during the different stages of deglutition, or if the nature of the response changes with alterations of bolus volume or consistency. It is also unclear what specific structures of the highly complex basal ganglia system contribute to deglutition. These parameters are important to study in order to make predictions of how the basal ganglia are involved in deglutition. However, due to the timing and spatial resolution issues mentioned earlier, neuroimaging is not yet the most effective model for examining deglutition, especially for the pharyngeal swallow.

SWALLOWING CHANGES ASSOCIATED WITH PD

Disordered swallowing was identified by James Parkinson in his original essay on PD. He described difficulty with ingesting solid food and weight loss as being associated with PD.[51] The neuropathology of PD involves the progressive degeneration of neurons in subcortical and brain stem regions. The degeneration of the basal ganglia and brainstem including the medulla, may account for oral and pharyngeal phase swallowing changes.[52] People with PD also demonstrate an abnormal presence of Lewy bodies in the basal ganglia following neuronal loss and in the dorsal motor nucleus and the medullary reticular formation.[53] The dorsal motor nucleus of the vagus and the medullary reticular formation are known to be important in swallowing and damage to these areas may contribute to changes in the pharyngeal phase of swallowing.[5] Further, the involvement of the dorsal vagal nuclei may account for esophageal swallowing stage changes seen in PD.[52]

Dysphagia typically occurs in the mid to late stages of PD.[20] Dysphagia is implicated in dehydration, malnutrition, pulmonary disease, and death. The "gold standard" in dysphagia diagnosis, management, and research is videofluoroscopy (moving X-ray of deglutition using food and liquid mixed with a radio-opaque substance, "barium"), also called a "modified barium swallow study."[54] Other techniques such as ultrasound, endoscopy, and EMG are used to both study and diagnose dysphagia. Dysphagia associated with PD can occur in all three stages of deglutition, although most research focuses on the oral and pharyngeal stages. Dysphagia in PD is an impairment of motility in the both the oral and pharyngeal stages, meaning difficulty forming the bolus and effectively transferring the bolus to the pharynx and esophagus.

Although PD may occur in individuals at any age, the incidence of PD increases with age. The average age of diagnosis for PD is 60 years. The prevalence of PD in the United States is expected to triple over the next 50 years,[55] so it is critical that we understand the underlying mechanisms of swallowing disorders in PD and the appropriate treatment strategies. Since most people diagnosed with PD are over 60 years of age, swallowing disorders in PD likely result from a combination of these factors associated with normal aging and PD specifically.

Oral Stage Findings in PD

Swallowing changes associated with normal aging in the oral phase may include reduced labial closure with increased drooling, reduced lingual strength, and decreased lingual coordination for bolus formation and control that can result in delayed oral transit time, and changes in dentition that can make chewing and bolus control difficult.[60,61] The most common abnormalities in the oral stage of deglutition in individuals with PD are impaired mastication and lingual movements,[56] increased number of swallows per bolus (ie, piecemeal deglutition),[57,58] tongue pumping,[56-58] premature or uncontrolled loss of bolus from the oral cavity[58] increased oral transit duration,[19,58] decreased suction pressure,[59] and residue on the tongue and anterior and lateral sulci.[58] Robbins et al[5] described five lingual dysphagia characteristics in the oral phase of swallow associated with PD: lingual rocking of the bolus, lingual tremor, repetitive tongue pumping, prolonged ramp-like posture, and piecemeal deglutition. These authors noted that repetitive tongue pumping and piecemeal deglutition increased as bolus viscosity increased. Oral phase changes in PD that included tongue tremor, piecemeal bolus transit, decreased tongue mobility, and residue in the oral cavity were also described.[1,7]

Pharyngeal Stage Findings in PD

Changes in the pharyngeal phase associated with normal aging may include delayed initiation in pharyngeal swallow, longer oropharyngeal transit time,[65] decreased amplitude of pharyngeal contraction, and decreased duration of upper esophageal sphincter (UES) opening.[4] Logemann et al[54] compared swallow characteristics of younger and older men and found longer pharyngeal delay in men over 80 years of age as well as significantly reduced maximum vertical and anterior hyoid movement and decreased width of cricopharyngeal opening. Interestingly, in a study that examined swallow characteristics in women over 80 years of age it was found that laryngeal and hyoid elevation was better preserved than in men over 80 suggesting that women maintain muscular reserve for swallowing better than men.[54] Decreased muscular reserve could place an individual at greater risk for dysphagia, especially in the presence of a degenerative disease such as PD.

The most common abnormalities in the pharyngeal stage of deglutition are prolonged trigger of the pharyngeal swallow reflex,[19,57,58,62,63] prolonged laryngeal movement,[62] decreased pharyngeal contraction pressure,[4] vallecular and pyriform sinus residue,[56-58,63] inability to adapt hyoid bone movement with changes in bolus characteristics,[63] and aspiration.[58] Robbins et al[5] described a delayed pharyngeal response in all PD subjects studied as well as aspiration in two subjects, neither of whom demonstrated a cough response (silent aspiration). Aspiration occurred before the swallow secondary to premature spillage with penetration of the laryngeal vestibule and reduced laryngeal closure. Aspiration after the swallow was secondary to significant amounts of pharyngeal residue that was inhaled after respiration was resumed. The two subjects who aspirated in the Robbins et al study[5] were both in Stage V of the disease as rated by the Hoehn & Yahr disease severity scale.[66] Delayed triggering of the swallow reflex and prolongation of laryngeal movements during swallow was also noted in patients with PD and these deficits can increase the risk of aspiration.[19,62]

These signs of dysphagia in the oral and pharyngeal stages can be attributed to reduced movement (hypokinesia), slowness of movement (bradykinesia), and in the case of tongue pumping, hesitation of movement (akinesia). More explicitly, impaired mastication and lingual movements, multiple swallows, and decreased suction pressure are likely due to reduced muscle force of the jaw and tongue. Increased oral transit duration is related to reduced force and overall slowness of lingual muscle action. Prolonged trigger of the swallow reflex is a more complicated issue and is probably related to some sensory abnormality. Sensory deficits are associated with PD and likely contribute to decreased efferent output. Prolonged pharyngeal transit and laryngeal movement are related to bradykinesia and/or hypokinesia of the pharyngeal, laryngeal, and suprahyoidal musculature and also probably a result of reduced lingual force driving the bolus. Decreased pharyngeal contraction pressure and residue are again linked to reduced muscle force (hypokinesia). Aspiration is more complicated, but likely due to the hypokinesia and bradykinesia affecting the degree timing of laryngeal elevation and adduction for airway protection.

Given these signs and evidence that people with PD have a harder time adapting to bolus characteristic changes,[64] the basal ganglia are implicated in the initiation of the oral preparatory and oral transit phases of the oral stage, and for modification of the oral and pharyngeal stage motor plans to adjust to changes in bolus volume and viscosity. This role has been ascribed to the basal ganglia from evidence from neural disease that affects the basal ganglia, such as PD.[20] Although characteristics of dysphagia related to PD are well-described in the literature, the role of the basal ganglia and its specific structures in normal deglutition and in dysphagia is still largely unknown.

Esophageal Stage Findings

In the esophageal stage, weak peristalsis may result in food remaining in the esophagus or backflow into the pharynx in normal aging. In addition, anatomic and physiologic stores that provide the ability to adapt to stress are reduced with aging, putting older individuals at increased risk for dysphagia.[65,67] In a study comparing a group of 72 PD subjects with matched controls, Eadie and Tyrer[2] found a higher incidence of esophageal swallow changes in the PD subjects than in the age-matched controls. Changes included esophageal spasm, hiatal hernia, and gastroesophageal reflux. Leopold and Kagel[56] found that 40/71 subjects had gastroesophageal reflux and that 10 of those 40 had a hiatal hernia.

Considerations

Because PD is a chronic condition that results in gradual changes in functional status, nutritional status, and the ability to maintain pulmonary hygiene, dysphagia and aspiration are likely complications of PD as the disease progresses. The frequency of occurrence of swallowing disorders in PD has been reported to range from 50%[6] to as high as 95%.[68] The discrepancy in statistics about swallowing in PD may be partly accounted for by how researchers define dysphagia. For example, Hunter et al[1] described swallowing dysfunction in PD as symptomatic in 50% of patients but identified swallowing dysfunction in

	TABLE 12-1

List of Symptoms for Patients

The following is a list of symptoms that could indicate a swallowing problem. If you experience one or several of these symptoms you should consult your physician and/or ask for a consultation with a qualified speech-language pathologist.

- Increased coughing or choking at mealtimes
- A frequently wet or gurgly voice quality
- More difficulty than usual swallowing pills
- New difficulty eating foods that were not difficult before
- Eating a meal takes an unusually long time
- A sensation that you can not make the food go down or that food gets stuck in your throat
- Excessive drooling
- Weight loss
- Pneumonia/respiratory problems

90% of patients on videofluoroscopy. Although the severity of swallowing disorders in PD cannot be predicted by severity of the disease, people with end-stage PD at Stage V of the Hoehn & Yahr scale,[66] have the most significant swallowing disorders.[3-5,63]

Damage to the basal ganglia can result in changes in swallow function that are thought to be caused not only by reduced motor control but by impaired sensory feedback as well. The basal ganglia influence sensory components in the trigeminal system and may contribute to abnormalities in sensorimotor responses throughout the swallow.[5,69] Therefore, people with PD may have symptoms of dysphagia but be unaware of them.

Bushmann et al[7] studied 20 patients with PD. They asked the patients whether they had any swallowing complaints and analyzed swallow function using videofluoroscopy. They found that the patients' report of any swallowing difficulties had a poor correlation with findings on videofluoroscopy. Only 7 of 20 patients reported complaints of swallowing difficulties whereas videofluoroscopy identified swallowing abnormalities, including silent aspiration, in 15 out of 20 patients. Robbins et al[5] found that three out of six subjects studied denied difficulty swallowing although all six subjects had disordered swallowing and the subject with the most disordered swallow was one of the subjects who denied having swallowing difficulties. Potulska et al[62] studied swallowing in 18 patients with PD and identified swallowing disorders in all patients although only 13/18 patients presented with swallowing complaints. Table 12-1 lists symptoms that may reflect a swallowing disorder. This can be used as a reference for referring people for a swallow evaluation, keeping in mind that many patients may not indeed recognize these as a swallowing problem.

Treatment for Dysphagia Associated With PD

Traditional Swallow Treatment in PD

Appropriate treatment for swallowing disorders should address the underlying physiology that causes the disorder. Although people with PD share common symptoms of the disease there could still be a variety of causes for a swallowing disorder. People with PD may demonstrate some or all of the signs/symptoms described in the previous section on swallowing disorders of the various phases of swallowing and the specific causes for an individual determine the appropriate treatment regimen. Traditional behavioral treatment techniques carried out by speech-language pathologists have focused on environmental modifications, postures, compensatory maneuvers, and diet modifications to assist the person with PD in maximizing safe and pleasurable oral intake. Environmental considerations include eating smaller portions more frequently if excessive time is needed for oral mastication.[52] If anterior to posterior bolus transport is impaired then posterior placement of the food bolus can facilitate swallowing. An example of a postural change may include tucking the chin to the chest, which facilitates elevating the larynx and protecting the airway. An example of a compensatory strategy is a double swallow if there is residue in the oropharyngeal tract. Another example of a compensatory strategy is the Mendelsohn manuever if there is reduced laryngeal elevation with decreased ability to protect the airway. The Mendelsohn maneuver teaches the patient to feel the larynx lift and hold it upward during the swallow. This maneuver is based on biomechanics of increasing width and duration of cricopharyngeal opening with laryngeal elevation. If weakness of oropharyngeal musculature is identified as contributing to dysphagia then strengthening exercises may be appropriate. Diet modification includes altering the consistency of liquids and solids. For example, liquids can be thickened using commercially available thickener to increase the viscosity of thin liquids to varying levels of thickness, such as nectar, honey, and pudding-thick liquids. Solids can be made softer with a more uniform consistency, such as puree, ground, chopped, and mechanical soft. Sometimes it is necessary to consider alternatives to oral feeding such as a nasogastric tube or Dobhoff tube (considered a more temporary solution) or a surgical implantation of a perenteral gastrostomy tube (more permanent alternative to oral feeding). It should be noted that a combination of environmental changes, postural changes, compensatory strategies, strengthening exercises, and diet modification is often the most clinically salient therapeutic approach. These decisions are based on results from physiologic testing using videofluoroscopy or fiberoptic endoscopic evaluation of swallowing (FEES) and careful monitoring of pulmonary and nutritional status by the interdisciplinary team.

Pharmacological Treatments and Swallowing

The most common motor symptoms of PD are rigidity, weakness, bradykinesia, hypokinesia, and tremor. Pharmacological treatment of these symptoms includes the use of levodopa but it has had inconsistent effects on speech.[70,71] There have been inconsistent findings for the effects of medications on swallowing as well. Because it is possible for people with PD to have tremor in the oral structure without apparent limb tremor it has been suggested that basal ganglia mechanisms of tremor may have distinct effects on the corticobulbar and corticospinal pathways and that non-dopaminergic dysfunction underlies disordered speech and swallow in PD.[1,5,58] Some research studies have demonstrated beneficial effects of pharmacological treatment on swallow function[3,63,72] while others have not.[1,5,7] Thus, it remains unclear if pharmacological treatment indeed functionally changes swallowing.

Deep Brain Stimulation and Swallowing

Deep Brain Stimulation (DBS) is a surgical treatment for PD that places quadripolar electrodes in one of three locations: 1) the thalamus (currently less common), 2) the subthalamic nucleus (STN), or 3) the globus pallidus internal segment (GPi).[73] Electrodes are typically placed bilaterally. The electrode settings can be adjusted for voltage, current, pulse width, and stimulus frequency by a programmer unit used by the physician in the clinic. DBS is a newer technique that is often used in place of ablation surgeries because it causes less permanent damage to neural structures and can be modulated incrementally, thus providing optimal settings. When the stimulator is turned on, it provides high-frequency stimulation to the neural area that is adjacent to the placement of the electrodes and causes modulation of these structures. Stimulating the GPi or STN may modulate thalamocortical or brainstem neural areas and alleviate motor symptoms (tremor, freezing, decreased ability to ambulate). This leads to increased independence for activities of daily living.[74] Side effects of stimulation in these locations include: diplopia, dysarthria, increased drooling, and dysphagia. These side effects are not well understood, but are suspected to relate to current spread to descending corticobulbar fibers and visual pathways that are in close proximity to the electrodes. It appears that DBS generally improves the bradykinesia and hypokinesia associated with PD. However, it affects distinct types of movements (limb, voice, speech, oral force, and posture) differently.[75-77]

A study was performed examining the oral and pharyngeal stages of deglutition during the DBS ON and OFF conditions during a 12-hour medication "wash-out" study in participants with PD.[9] It was hypothesized that DBS in the ON condition would yield improvement in the following dependent variables: oral total composite score, pharyngeal total composite score, pharyngeal transit time, and maximal hyoid bone excursion. Statistically significant differences (improvement) were found for the pharyngeal composite score and pharyngeal transit time in the DBS ON condition.[9]

Findings of this study demonstrated that DBS in the ON condition helps to alleviate some of the bradykinesia and hypokinesia associated with PD on the pharyngeal stage of deglutition, as the participants demonstrated improvement on the pharyngeal total composite score (a composite of qualitative measures that was scored and transformed into a quantitative score) and pharyngeal transit time. Dysphagia is occasionally reported as a side-effect of DBS and it is likely due to current spread to corticobulbar fibers and not a result of the treatment effects. Although not statistically significant, it also appears that oral stage deglutition is to a degree improved in the DBS condition. The fact that oral stage parameters did not appear to improve in the DBS ON condition may be due to the high amount of variability among participants, or that the oral stage is mediated through differing basal ganglia connections.

The Trial and Bolus Effects that were found in this study are also important to note, as they may reflect a decline in motor response over time that is occurring, even in the small number of trials (nine for each condition).[9] This progressive decline in performance could be a critically important feature of PD and merits further investigation. These findings suggest that parkinsonian swallowing dysfunction is not solely related to nigrostriatal dopamine deficiency, which is purported to be the primary means of DBS alleviation of motor signs and may be due to an additional non-dopamine-related system of deglutition found in the brainstem, such as the pedunculopontine nucleus or related structures in the medulla.[1] Thus, it is paramount that we examine other structures and the connections of the basal ganglia and its circuitry to continue to shape our understanding of the role of the basal ganglia in deglutition.

Benefits from LSVT-LOUD and Swallowing

Preliminary data from a study by Sharkawi et al[10] demonstrated improvement in swallow function following LSVT-LOUD, a behavioral voice treatment developed for people with PD. It has been proposed that the reasons for the efficacy of LSVT-LOUD for improving voice and speech include: 1) A focus on increasing loudness provides a single motor organizing theme that maximizes generalization of effects to other speech systems such as respiration and articulation,[78-80] 2) The intensive mode of administration is consistent with theories of motor learning and appear essential to obtain optimum treatment results,[80,81] and 3) In addition to training the motor speech system, LSVT-LOUD trains sensory awareness so that the patient with PD understands the level of effort and loudness necessary to produce intelligible speech.[82] The positive effect of LSVT-LOUD on swallowing ability may reflect the spreading of effects of focusing on the phonatory system to swallow function.

SUMMARY

Swallowing disorders are a significant problem associated with PD. They can occur in all stages of the swallow and pose potential health risks that range from interfering with taking oral medications to contributing to aspiration pneumonia that leads to death. It has been suggested that non-dopaminergic dysfunction underlies disordered swallow in PD and the ability of pharmacological treatments such as synthetic dopamine to improve swallowing function in PD has not been clearly demonstrated. Furthermore, the effects of neurosurgery are still unclear. There are a number of behavioral interventions available for ameliorating swallowing disorders in people with PD, including postural changes, strengthening exercises, and compensatory strategies. Further, diet modifications, including alternatives to oral routes of nutrition and hydration, are often indicated, especially in advanced stages. The recent findings of Sharkawi et al[10] suggest that LSVT-LOUD may be another tool in the speech-language pathologist's repertoire for treating swallowing disorders in PD as well as for treating voice and speech disorders. The original intent of LSVT-LOUD was to improve functional communication for people with PD through intensive training of increased vocal loudness. The spreading of effects of treatment to swallowing was an unexpected finding. However, given the interaction of motor aspects of voice, speech, and swallow production, perhaps it is not so surprising. Interpretation of these data must be made cautiously until further research can be completed with additional subjects including a control group. Finally, diet modification based on instrumented assessment is paramount to complete the treatment picture.

As with any treatment of dysphagia, it is important to consider the complexity of each individual. This includes disease state and progression (keeping in mind that PD is neurodegenerative and is likely to change over time), environment of care (independent living vs. varying levels of assistance), nutrition/hydration status, personal preferences, and compliance with recommendations. It is strongly recommended that an interdisciplinary team approach is used, including the patient, caregivers, physicians, nurses, dieticians, speech-language pathologist, and other health care providers all being involved in the decision-making process.

REFERENCES

1. Hunter PC, Crameri J, Austin S, Woodward MC, Hughes AJ. Response of parkinsonian swallowing dysfunction to dopaminergic stimulation. *J Neurol Neurosurg Psychiatry*. 1997;63(5):579-583.
2. Eadie MJ, Tyrer JH. Alimentary disorder in Parkinsonism. *Australas Ann Med*. 1965;14:13-22.

3. Monte FS, Silva-Junior FP, Braga-Neto P, Nobre e Souza MA, Sales dB, V. Swallowing abnormalities and dyskinesia in Parkinson's disease. *Mov Disord.* 2005;20(4):457-462.

4. Ali GN, Wallace KL, Schwartz R, DeCarle DJ, Zagami AS, Cook IJ. Mechanisms of oral-pharyngeal dysphagia in patients with Parkinson's disease. *Gastroenterology.* 1996;110(2):383-392.

5. Robbins JA, Logemann JA, Kirshner HS. Swallowing and speech production in Parkinson's disease. *Ann Neurol.* 1986;19(3):283-287.

6. Lieberman AN, Horowitz L, Redmond P, Pachter L, Lieberman I, Leibowitz M. Dysphagia in Parkinson's disease. *Am J Gastroenterol.* 1980; 74(2):157-160.

7. Bushmann M, Dobmeyer SM, Leeker L, Perlmutter JS. Swallowing abnormalities and their response to treatment in Parkinson's disease. *Neurology.* 1989;39(10):1309-1314.

8. Calne DB, Shaw DG, Spiers AS, Stern GM. Swallowing in Parkinsonism. *Br J Radiol.* 1970;43(511):456-457.

9. Ciucci MR, Barkmeier-Kraemer JM, Sherman S. Subthalamic nucleus deep brain stimulation improves deglutition in Parkinson disease. *Mov Disord.* 2008 (in press).

10. Sharkawi AE, Ramig L, Logemann JA, Pauloski BR, Rademaker AW, Smith CH et al. Swallowing and voice effects of Lee Silverman Voice Treatment (LSVT): a pilot study. *J Neurol Neurosurg Psychiatry.* 2002; 72(1):31-36.

11. Jean A. Brainstem organization of the swallowing network. *Brain Behav Evol.* 1984;25(2-3):109-116.

12. Jean A. [Effect of localized lesions of the medulla oblongata on the esophageal stage of deglutition]. *J Physiol.* (Paris) 1972;64(5):507-516.

13. Jean A. [Localization and activity of medullary swallowing neurones]. *J Physiol.* (Paris) 1972;64(3):227-268.

14. Doty RW, Richmond WH, Storey AT. Effect of medullary lesions on coordination of deglutition. *Exp Neurol.* 1967;17(1):91-106.

15. Kessler JP, Jean A. Inhibition of the swallowing reflex by local application of serotonergic agents into the nucleus of the solitary tract. *Eur J Pharmacol.* 1985;118(1-2):77-85.

16. Weerasuriya A, Bieger D, Hockman CH. Interaction between primary afferent nerves in the elicitation of reflex swallowing. *Am J Physiol.* 1980; 239(5):R407-R414.

17. Jean A. Brainstem control of swallowing: localization and organization of the central pattern generator for swallowing. In: Taylor A, ed. *Neurophysiology of the Jaws and Teeth.* London: MacMillan Press; 1990.

18. Rossignol S, Dubuc R. Spinal pattern generation. *Curr Opin Neurobiol.* 1994;4(6):894-902.

19. Ertekin C, Tarlaci S, Aydogdu I, Kiylioglu N, Yuceyar N, Turman AB et al. Electrophysiological evaluation of pharyngeal phase of swallowing in patients with Parkinson's disease. *Mov Disord.* 2002;17(5):942-949.

20. Miller AJ. Oral and pharyngeal reflexes in the mammalian nervous system: their diverse range in complexity and the pivotal role of the tongue. *Crit Rev Oral Biol Med.* 2002;13(5):409-425.

21. Crary MA, Carnaby Mann GD, Groher ME. Biomechanical correlates of surface electromyography signals obtained during swallowing by healthy adults. *J Speech Lang Hear Res.* 2006;49(1):186-193.

22. Van Daele DJ, McCulloch TM, Palmer PM, Langmore SE. Timing of glottic closure during swallowing: a combined electromyographic and endoscopic analysis. *Ann Otol Rhinol Laryngol.* 2005;114(6):478-487.

23. Perlman AL, Palmer PM, McCulloch TM, Vandaele DJ. Electromyographic activity from human laryngeal, pharyngeal, and submental muscles during swallowing. *J Appl Physiol.* 1999;86(5):1663-1669.

24. Barkmeier JM, Bielamowicz S, Takeda N, Ludlow CL. Laryngeal activity during upright vs. supine swallowing. *J Appl Physiol.* 2002;93(2):740-745.

25. Jean A. Brain stem control of swallowing: neuronal network and cellular mechanisms. *Physiol Rev.* 2001;81(2):929-969.

26. Lund JP. Mastication and its control by the brain stem. *Crit Rev Oral Biol Med.* 1991;2(1):33-64.

27. Jean A. Control of the central swallowing program by inputs from peripheral receptors: A review. *J Autonomic Nervous Sys.* 1990;10:225-233.

28. Chandler SH, Tal M. The effects of brain stem transections on the neuronal networks responsible for rhythmical jaw muscle activity in the guinea pig. *J Neurosci.* 1986;6(6):1831-1842.

29. Doty RW, Bosma JF. An electromyographic analysis of reflex deglutition. *J Neurophysiol.* 1956;19(1):44-60.

30. Grill HJ, Norgren R. The taste reactivity test. I. Mimetic responses to gustatory stimuli in neurologically normal rats. *Brain Res.* 1978; 143(2):263-279.

31. Kornblith CL, Hall WG. Brain transections selectively alter ingestion and behavioral activation in neonatal rats. *J Comp Physiol Psychol.* 1979; 93(6):1109-1117.

32. Kendall KA, Leonard RJ. Pharyngeal constriction in elderly dysphagic patients compared with young and elderly nondysphagic controls. *Dysphagia.* 2001;16(4):272-278.

33. Miller AJ. Significance of sensory inflow to the swallowing reflex. *Brain Res.* 1972;43(1):147-159.

34. Robbins J, Hamilton JW, Lof GL, Kempster GB. Oropharyngeal swallowing in normal adults of different ages. *Gastroenterology.* 1992;103:823-829.

35. Hamdy S, Rothwell JC, Aziz Q, Thompson DG. Organization and reorganization of human swallowing motor cortex: implications for recovery after stroke. *Clin Sci* (Lond). 2000;99(2):151-157.

36. Gust J, Wright JJ, Pratt EB, Bosma MM. Development of synchronized activity of cranial motor neurons in the segmented embryonic mouse hindbrain. *J Physiol*. 2003;550(Pt 1):123-133.

37. Car A, Jean A, Roman C. [Deglutition: physiologic and neurophysiologic aspects]. *Rev Laryngol Otol Rhinol*. (Bord) 1998;119(4):219-225.

38. Zald DH, Pardo JV. The functional neuroanatomy of voluntary swallowing. *Ann Neurol*. 1999;46(3):281-286.

39. Roman C, Car A. [Deglutitions and oesophageal reflex contractions produced by stimulation of the vagal and superior laryngeal nerves]. *Exp Brain Res*. 1970;11(1):48-74.

40. Car A, Roman C. [Deglutitions and oesophageal reflex contractions induced by electrical stimulation of the medulla oblongata]. *Exp Brain Res*. 1970;11(1):75-92.

41. Miller AJ. Characteristics of the swallowing reflex induced by peripheral nerve and brain stem stimulation. *Exp Neurol*. 1972;34(2):210-222.

42. Tell F, Fagni L, Jean A. Neurons of the nucleus tractus solitarius, in vitro, generate bursting activities by solitary tract stimulation. *Exp Brain Res*. 1990;79(2):436-440.

43. Kandell ER, Schwartz JH, Jessell TM. *Principles of Neural Science*. New York: McGraw-Hill, 2000.

44. Sumi T. The activity of brain-stem respiratory neurons and spinal respiratory motoneurons during swallowing. *J Neurophysiol*. 1963;26:466-477.

45. Bieger D. Neuropharmacologic correlates of deglutition: lessons from fictive swallowing. *Dysphagia*. 1991;6(3):147-164.

46. Sessle BJ, Henry JL. Neural mechanisms of swallowing: neurophysiological and neurochemical studies on brain stem neurons in the solitary tract region. *Dysphagia*. 1989;4(2):61-75.

47. Amri M, Car A. Projections from the medullary swallowing center to the hypoglossal motor nucleus: a neuroanatomical and electrophysiological study in sheep. *Brain Res*. 1988;441(1-2):119-126.

48. Cunningham ET, Jr., Sawchenko PE. Central neural control of esophageal motility: a review. *Dysphagia*. 1990;5(1):35-51.

49. Kern MK, Shaker R. Cerebral cortical registration of subliminal visceral stimulation. *Gastroenterology*. 2002;122(2):290-298.

50. Martin RE, Kemppainen P, Masuda Y, Yao D, Murray GM, Sessle BJ. Features of cortically evoked swallowing in the awake primate (Macaca fascicularis). *J Neurophysiol*. 1999;(823):1529-1541.

51. Parkinson J. *An Essay on Shaking Palsy*. London: Whittingham and Rowland for Sherwood, Neely and Jones; 1817.

52. Groher ME. *Dysphagia: Diagnosis and Management*. 3rd ed. Newton, MA: Butterworth-Heinemann, 1997.

53. Dickson D.W. Neuropathology of parkinsonian disorders. In: Jankovic JJT, ed. *Parkinson's Disease and Movement Disorders*. Philadelphia: Lippincott Williams & Wilkins; 2002:256-269.

54. Logemann JA, Pauloski BR, Rademaker AW, Kahrilas PJ. Oropharyngeal swallow in younger and older women: videofluoroscopic analysis. *J Speech Lang Hear Res*. 2002;45(3):434-445.

55. Tanner CM, Goldman SM, Ross GW. Etilogy of Parkinson's disease. In: Jankovic JJ, Tolosa E, eds. *Parkinson's Disease and Movement Disorders*. Philadelphia: Lippincott Williams & Wilkins: 2002.

56. Leopold NA, Kagel MC. Pharyngo-esophageal dysphagia in Parkinson's disease. *Dysphagia*. 1997;12(1):11-18.

57. Bird MR, Woodward MC, Gibson EM, Phyland DJ, Fonda D. Asymptomatic swallowing disorders in elderly patients with Parkinson's disease: a description of findings on clinical examination and videofluoroscopy in sixteen patients. *Age Ageing*. 1994;23(3):251-254.

58. Nagaya M, Kachi T, Yamada T, Igata A. Videofluorographic study of swallowing in Parkinson's disease. *Dysphagia*. 1998;13(2):95-100.

59. Nilsson H, Ekberg O, Olsson R, Hindfelt B. Quantitative assessment of oral and pharyngeal function in Parkinson's disease. *Dysphagia*. 1996; 11(2):144-150.

60. Robbins J, Hamilton JW, Lof GL, Kempster GB. Oropharyngeal swallowing in normal adults of different ages. *Gastroenterology*. 1992; 103(3):823-829.

61. Hartelius L, Svensson P. Speech and swallowing symptoms associated with Parkinson's disease and multiple sclerosis: a survey. *Folia Phoniatr Logop*. 1994;46(1):9-17.

62. Potulska A, Friedman A, Krolicki L, Spychala A. Swallowing disorders in Parkinson's disease. *Parkinsonism Relat Disord*. 2003;9(6):349-353.

63. Fuh JL, Lee RC, Wang SJ, Lin CH, Wang PN, Chiang JH et al. Swallowing difficulty in Parkinson's disease. *Clin Neurol Neurosurg*. 1997; 99(2):106-112.

64. Wintzen AR, Badrising UA, Roos RA, Vielvoye J, Liauw L. Influence of bolus volume on hyoid movements in normal individuals and patients with Parkinson's disease. *Can J Neurol Sci*. 1994;21(1):57-59.

65. Robbins J, Levine R, Wood J, Roecker EB, Luschei E. Age effects on lingual pressure generation as a risk factor for dysphagia. *J Gerontol A Biol Sci Med Sci*. 1995;50(5):M257-M262.

66. Hoehn MM, Yahr MD. Parkinsonism: onset, progression and mortality. *Neurology*. 1967;17(5):427-442.

67. Logemann JA, Pauloski BR, Rademaker AW, Colangelo LA, Kahrilas PJ, Smith CH. Temporal and biome-chanical characteristics of oropharyngeal swallow in younger and older men. *J Speech Lang Hear Res.* 2000; 43(5):1264-1274.

68. Logemann JA, Blonsky ER, Boshes B. Editorial: Dysphagia in parkinsonism. *JAMA.* 1975;231(1):69-70.

69. Labuszewski T, Lidsky TI. Basal ganglia influences on brain stem trigeminal neurons. *Exp Neurol.* 1979;65(2):471-477.

70. Larson KK, Ramig LSRC. Acoustic and glottographic voice analysis during drug-related fluctuations in Parkinson's disease. *J Med Speech Lang Path.* 1994;2(3):227-230.

71. Schulz GM, Grant MK. Effects of speech therapy and pharmacologic and surgical treatments on voice and speech in Parkinson's disease: a review of the literature. *J Commun Disord.* 2000;33(1):59-88.

72. Fonda D, Schwarz J, Clinnick S. Parkinsonian medication one hour before meals improves symptomatic swallowing: a case study. *Dysphagia.* 1995; 10(3):165-166.

73. Dostrovsky JO, Hutchison WD, Lozano AM. The globus pallidus, deep brain stimulation, and Parkinson's disease. *Neuroscientist.* 2002;8(3):284-290.

74. Thobois S, Mertens P, Guenot M, Hermier M, Mollion H, Bouvard M et al. Subthalamic nucleus stimulation in Parkinson's disease: clinical evaluation of 18 patients. *J Neurol.* 2002;249(5):529-534.

75. Solomon NP, McKee AS, Larson KJ, Nawrocki MD, Tuite PJ, Eriksen S et al. Effects of pallidal stimulation in three men with severe Parkinson's disease. *Am J Speech Lan Path.* 2000;9:241-256.

76. Dromey C, Kumar R, Lang AE, Lozano AM. An investigation of the effects of subthalamic nucleus stimulation on acoustic measures of voice. *Mov Disord.* 2000;15(6):1132-1138.

77. Gentil M, Tournier CL, Pollak P, Benabid AL. Effect of bilateral subthalamic nucleus stimulation and dopa-therapy on oral control in Parkinson's disease. *Eur Neurol.* 1999;42(3):136-140.

78. Dromey C, Ramig LO. Intentional changes in sound pressure level and rate: their impact on measures of respiration, phonation, and articulation. *J Speech Lang Hear Res.* 1998;41(5):1003-1018.

79. Smith ME, Ramig LO, Dromey C, Perez KS, Samandari R. Intensive voice treatment in Parkinson disease: laryngostroboscopic findings. *J Voice.* 1995;9(4):453-459.

80. Fox C, Morrison C, Ramig L. Current perspectives on the Lee Silverman Voice Treatment (LSVT). *Am J Speech Lang Path.* 2002;11:111-123.

81. Schmidt RA, Lee TD. *Motor Control and Learning: A Behavioral Emphasis.* 3rd ed. Champaign, IL: Human Kinetics, 1999.

82. Ramig L, Pawlas ACS. Voice treatment for patients with Parkinson disease: development of an approach and preliminary efficacy data. *J Med Speech Lan Path.* 1995;2(3):191-209.

13

Speech Therapy Tips for Patients With Parkinson's Disease

Cynthia M. Fox, PhD, CCC-SLP; Lorraine Olson Ramig, PhD, CCC-SLP;
Angela Halpern, MS, CCC-SLP; Jill Cable, MS, CCC-SLP;
Leslie A. Mahler, PhD, CCC-SLP

Introduction

The purpose of this chapter is to provide speech-language pathologists with simple home practice exercises and strategies that are beneficial for patients with PD. Speech-language pathologists can reproduce the information in this chapter, based upon the LSVT®-LOUD (Lee Silverman Voice Treatment) (see Chapter 11), for use as a home speech exercise program or as an informative document to give to patients with PD (see shaded pages). This information is not meant to replace LSVT-LOUD training and certification for speech-language pathologists or LSVT-LOUD treatment for patients.

Speech Therapy

LSVT-LOUD focuses on improving vocal loudness by exercising the muscles of the voice box (larynx) and speech mechanism. One single goal—"speak LOUD"— improves respiratory, laryngeal, and articulatory function to maximize speech intelligibility[1] (Figure 13-1). Unlike traditional speech treatment, LSVT-LOUD is administered in 16 sessions in 1 month (four individual 60-minute sessions per week). In addition to stimulating the motor speech system, LSVT-LOUD incorporates sensory awareness training. Initially, when individuals with PD are trained to improve loudness, they often will say they feel as if they are shouting. LSVT-LOUD addresses this problem by helping patients recognize that their voice is too soft, convincing them that the louder voice is within normal limits, and making them comfortable with the new, louder voice[1,2] (Figures 13-2 and 13-3).

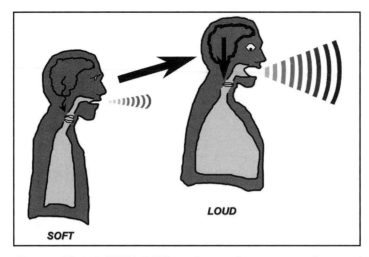

Figure 13-1. LSVT-LOUD is designed to improve the vocal source and scale up amplitude across the speech mechanism with the global variable "LOUD." Increases in loudness can trigger increases in respiratory volumes, vocal fold adduction, articulatory valving, and vocal tract opening. These factors may all contribute to improved speech intelligibility with the simple target of "LOUD." Reprinted with permission from GleeCo, LLC.

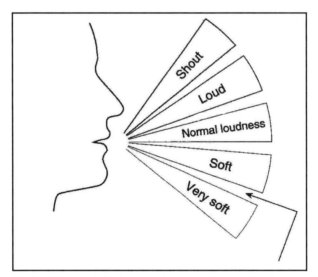

Figure 13-2. The middle box indicates Normal loudness. Notice the "amount of effort" necessary to move from Normal loudness to the higher boxes labeled Loud or Shout. For an individual with Parkinson's disease, his or her vocal loudness has dropped to one of the two lower boxes labeled Soft or Very soft. As a result, the individual with Parkinson's disease will need to use more vocal effort and loudness to be able to speak at the Normal loudness level. The amount of vocal effort he or she needs to use to reach a level of Normal loudness feels similar to the amount of vocal effort previously used to be Loud or to Shout. Reprinted with permission from GleeCo, LLC. (Adapted from Carolyn Mead Bonitati, 1987.).

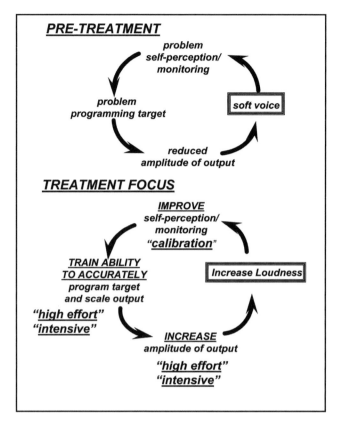

Figure 13-3. This figure graphically summarizes the hypothesized neural basis for the LSVT-LOUD approach to treating individuals with PD. Pretreatment (top circle) the "soft" voice of the patient may be a result of reduced amplitude of output to the speech mechanism. The "soft" voice is maintained because patients have reduced self-perception or self-monitoring and fail to realize that the voice is "too" soft. Therefore, when they program output for another utterance, they downscale the output and continue to produce a "soft voice." The LSVT-LOUD focus (bottom circle) addresses the "soft" voice at three levels. High effort, intensive treatment is designed to train increased amplitude of output to the respiratory phonatory system to generate increased loudness. Patients are then trained to improve self-perception or self-monitoring of effort so that they understand the relationship between increased effort and successful communication. In this way, when they generate an utterance on their own, they are able to "carry over" adequate effort and loudness for communication success outside the treatment room. Reprinted with permission from GleeCo, LLC.

Addressing speech and voice disorders early in the course of the disease is essential for individuals with PD if they are to maintain their ability to communicate.

Components of LSVT-LOUD

Patient Information Material

If you receive LSVT-LOUD, you will participate in all of the following exercises (this is the same everywhere in the world—there are no modifications). There is no such thing as "modified" LSVT-LOUD. Any changes to the standardized LSVT-LOUD protocol are NOT supported by research data and efficacy outcomes. All speech-language pathologists delivering LSVT-LOUD must be trained and certified to provide the treatment. The components of LSVT therapy include the following.[1,2]

- Treatment will consist of 4 days of therapy per week for 4 weeks
- Treatment session will last 50 to 60 minutes
- Treatment will be delivered individually
- The first half of the session will be spent on three daily tasks:

  *Sustain "AH" with increased loudness as long as you can (minimum 15 repetitions)

  *Sustain "AH" while going high/low in pitch—hold for 5 seconds (minimum 15 repetitions for high and 15 repetitions for low)

  *Repeat a list of 10 self-selected functional phrases 5 times each session (these phrases never change)

- The second half of the session will be spent on a speech hierarchy:

  *Week 1—words and phrases

  *Week 2—sentences

  *Week 3—reading

  *Week 4—conversation

The LSVT clinician will encourage you to bring in material for speech practice that is meaningful and interesting to you. This material will change every day of therapy. The entire second half of the session, you will be talking and practicing in your LOUD voice. If your speech therapist has done a good job, you will feel tired at the end of the session.

- Homework:

  You will have homework exercises to practice every day of the entire month of speech therapy. On days you have speech therapy (eg, Monday to Thursday), you will practice one other time a day for 5 to 10 minutes (completing daily tasks and hierarchy exercises). On days you do not have speech therapy (eg, Friday to Sunday), you will practice twice a day for 10 to 15 minutes (completing daily tasks and hierarchy exercises).

- Carryover exercises:

  Every day of the entire month of speech therapy (Monday to Sunday) you will have a carryover assignment. This is an assignment to use your LOUD voice with another person outside of the therapy room. The clinician will work with you to decide on a very specific task in which you will use your LOUD voice—as loud as you practice in the treatment room—in a real-life situation. These exercises help a person with PD realize that what feels and sounds too loud to them is actually within normal limits. The LSVT clinicians will make you accountable **every day** for doing your homework and carryover exercises. The daily homework and carryover exercises are an essential part of the treatment program, and must be completed daily.

How to Get Speech Therapy

Patient Information Material

Asking a Doctor for Referral and Prescription

If you are experiencing any changes in your speech or voice, be sure to tell your doctor. Ask for a referral for a speech evaluation. The sooner you get a speech evaluation and start speech therapy, the better! If you have not noticed changes in your speech, but a spouse, caretaker, or friend asks you to repeat, pay attention to their comments. One aspect of the speech disorder in PD is that the person with PD is often unaware of the changes in speech or voice. Individuals with PD feel as though they are speaking loudly enough, but others cannot hear or understand them. Communication is a **key** element in quality of life and can help individuals maintain confidence and a positive self-concept as they deal with the challenges of Parkinson's disease. We recommend beginning LSVT-LOUD early so that you can "keep your voice alive!"

Insurance Reimbursement

Speech therapy, including LSVT-LOUD, has been successfully reimbursed by many insurance providers and Medicare. There are certain provisions:
- Speech therapy must be included on your policy.
- If you have Medicare, you will need to receive speech therapy at a Medicare provider facility (typically hospitals, outpatient rehabs, etc). Currently, private practice speech therapists are unable to bill Medicare for services.
- You may need a prescription for speech evaluation/therapy from your primary care physician.

Locating a Speech-Language Pathologist

Speech-language pathologists work at a number of facilities including hospitals, outpatient rehabilitation centers, and private practice offices. It is best if the speech-language pathologist you are working with has experience treating people with PD. There are several referral sources for finding speech-language pathologists, including The American Speech-Language and Hearing Association (ASHA) (www.asha.org) and the LSVT Foundation (www.lsvt.org). the LSVT Foundation contains a list of professionals who are certified to provide LSVT-LOUD.

What If There Is Not Access to a Speech-Language Pathologist?

It is always recommended that you see a speech-language pathologist for a complete voice and speech evaluation prior to starting any exercise program for your voice. Home exercises and tips for improving communication are provided in the next section. These are not a replacement for a speech-language evaluation or therapy delivered by a speech-language pathologist. In addition, there is no research to support positive outcomes on speech of doing only home exercises instead of speech treatment. If you experience any pain or discomfort while using these exercises, stop and consult your speech-language pathologist or physician. If you experience persistent hoarseness, consult your physician. Although hoarseness is a symptom of PD, it can also be a symptom of other serious disorders, including gastric reflux disease or laryngeal abnormalities. Only an examination of the vocal folds conducted by an otolaryngologist (ear, nose, and throat doctor) can confirm the diagnosis. In addition, if you experience any difficulties with eating or swallowing, ask your physician for a referral for a swallowing examination.

Exercises for Voice and Speech

A Home Program for Patients With Parkinson's Disease

The speech exercises that follow are based on the LSVT-LOUD program and are designed for use by people with PD. They should only be used with approval of each person's speech-language pathologist and/or physician. These exercises are designed to be used in conjunction with or as a follow-up to LSVT-LOUD therapy. These exercises should not cause any pain in your voice. You may experience slight fatigue, similar to fatigue in your body after physical exercise (eg, walking, lifting weights). You should recover from this fatigue within 1 to 2 hours of completing your exercises. If you experience any pain or discomfort while using these exercises, STOP doing the exercises and consult your physician or speech-language pathologist.

Exercise 1: Maximum Duration Sustained Vowels

Instructions: Take a deep breath and say "AH" with increased loudness for as long as you can. Think about being LOUD and try to maintain the effort and loudness for the entire duration. **Do not shout**; you should just feel louder than you typically think you should be. It is more important to keep a good quality loud voice than to keep a longer duration. If your voice quality becomes poor because you are running out of air, stop, take a breath and then do your next AH. Do at least 6 repetitions of AH. Record your times.

Say "AH" loud for as long as you can. Check (✓) each line below as you complete the task or record your duration below:

_____   _____   _____   _____   _____

Exercise 2: Maximum Range of Sustained Vowels

Instructions: Take a deep breath and say "AH" with increased loudness going as high in pitch as you can and hold for 5 seconds. Think about being LOUD and try to maintain the same effort and loudness as in the sustained "AH" exercise. It is more important to keep a good quality loud voice than to go higher in pitch. Repeat the exercise going as low in pitch as you can. Once again, it is more important to keep a good quality loud voice than to go lower in pitch. Do both the high and low exercise for at least 6 repetitions.

Try to reach your highest pitch and sustain for 5 seconds. Check (✓) each line below as you complete the task:

_____   _____   _____   _____   _____

Try to reach your lowest pitch and sustain for 5 seconds. Check (✓) each line below as you complete the task:

_____   _____   _____   _____   _____

Exercise 3: Reading/Speaking Loud

Instructions: Spend 5 to 10 minutes each day reading aloud using the voice with increased loudness (**not a shout**) you warmed up with in the previous exercises. Be sure to maintain the same effort and loudness as in the sustained "AH" exercise. It is important to keep a good quality loud voice. Your voice will feel too loud to you, but to a listener (eg, spouse, co-worker, caretaker) it will sound within normal limits for loudness. If you are not sure about your loudness, ask someone to provide you feedback, or tape record yourself reading with a loud voice and play it back. When you first start these exercises try to read simple text and work towards more difficult text.

Why Work on Vocal Loudness?

The LSVT-LOUD approach centers on a very specific therapeutic target: increased vocal loudness. This key target acts as a "trigger" to increase effort and coordination across the speech production system. This focus provides a comprehensive motor organizing theme that impacts multiple levels of the motor output process in patients while limiting cognitive load, as individuals with neurological disorders often have difficulty with attention-demanding, complex tasks.[2] Our research has shown that a treatment with a simple focus (eg, "think loud" in speech production) may generalize to other systems (eg, articulation, speaking rate, swallowing, respiratory mechanics).[3]

Impact of Loudness on Respiration

When you work on vocal loudness, the majority of people automatically breathe more deeply. Therefore, we have observed that a direct focus on training respiration is not necessary and may even distract those patients with cognitive problems.[4] Because many patients have incomplete vocal fold closure, increasing vocal fold adduction and mouth opening are keys to improving vocal loudness.[5]

Impact of Loudness on Articulation

When you work on speaking loudly, most people automatically increase their mouth opening, increase lip movement, loosen their jaw, and drop their tongue. These automatic actions with the one goal of LOUD may have an impact on improving articulation.[6-8]

Strategies for Maximizing Communication With People With Parkinson's Disease

The following are tips for maximizing communication with people with PD. These tips can be employed by people with the disease who want to make themselves heard and understood. In addition, these tips can be used by family, friends, health care professionals, and others who want to communicate with people with PD. These tips are best used as an adjunct to participating in speech therapy.

Tips for Speakers With PD

THINK LOUD (Speak Loud)

- Speak with a **loud** voice. If you are asked to repeat, repeat in a "loud" voice.

- Focus on loudness only! Do not think about "slow down, speak clearly, and speak loud"—Loudness alone will facilitate slower, clearer, and louder speech.

- Speak in shorter sentences with a LOUD voice if someone is having difficulty understanding you or there is excessive background noise

- Seek out speech treatment—at least 89% of people with PD will have a voice or speech disorder. Do not wait—refer yourself immediately for a baseline assessment!

- Empower yourself to maintain effective communication by recognizing there is something you can do to improve your communication (beyond pharmacological and neurosurgical approaches). THINK LOUD!

Tips for Listening to People With PD

1. Suggest that the person with PD participate in speech treatment as soon as possible (eg, "You have important things to say, I want to understand you, let me help you find a speech clinician.")

2. Do not pretend that you understand what the client with PD is saying. Be honest and say, "I did not understand you. Could you say that again using a louder voice? I really want to understand what you said."

3. When the patient with PD speaks louder, express a positive reaction: "When you spoke louder, that really helped me hear and understand you."

BE AWARE OF MASKED EXPRESSION
- People with PD are feeling emotions that may not show through facial expression.
- Do not assume a person with PD is not understanding you—he or she is probably comprehending your message.
- Listen to the person's words; do not rely on an outward display of emotion.
- Avoid "talking down" to a person with PD or losing your own expressions and humor.

When the patient's speech disorder is severe, the following may be useful.

ELIMINATE BACKGROUND NOISE
- Shut the door to your office or treatment room.
- Turn off the radio, TV, or other noise-producing devices.
- Close car windows.

LISTEN CAREFULLY
- Look at the person with PD when he or she speaks.
- Use context to help decipher unintelligible speech.
- Focus on the task at hand and give the person with PD undivided attention.
- Be aware of masked face and listen for expression of emotions through words.

DECREASE BURDEN OF COMMUNICATION
- Ask questions that can be answered in short phrases.
- Provide choices for answers, eg, "Would you like tea or coffee with breakfast?"
- When possible, talk about topics that are familiar to the person with PD.

HAVE PATIENCE
- Allow the person with PD ample time to formulate answers and offer a response.
- Recognize that the person with PD may be embarrassed by tremors and/or dyskinesias, which make him or her nervous or self-conscious.
- Provide an open and accepting environment so the person with PD will feel comfortable communicating.

MAXIMIZING COGNITIVE PROCESSING[9]
- Reduce distractions.
- Use the strongest modality of input for a person with PD or a combination of modalities, eg, visual and auditory.
- Use simple, concrete, and frequently used words to communicate.
- Allow more time for cognitive processing—initiation and word-finding difficulties are common challenges to communication.

- Complete complex information processing tasks when medication is at its peak effectiveness.
- Eliminate time pressure.

What Devices Can Help Speech?

There are a number of devices and videos that have been designed to further assist communication for people with PD. These are supplements to what can be accomplished through behavioral speech treatment programs, such as LSVT-LOUD. The combination of interventions can be helpful for more advanced PD, or can motivate people who have completed LSVT-LOUD to keep practicing and using their loud voices. Sidebar 13-1 provides some information on these devices.

SUMMARY

Most patients with PD will eventually have a speech disorder that can progressively diminish quality of life. Speech treatment is an immediate, practical, and relatively inexpensive intervention for improving behavior. LSVT-LOUD empowers people with PD to participate in their treatment in fundamental ways and to gain control over one aspect of their PD—communication. The earlier a person with PD can receive a baseline speech evaluation and speech therapy, the more likely he or she will be able to improve speech and voice and maintain effective communication over the course of PD. Although direct speech therapy is the recommended course of action, there are home program voice exercises and other assistive communication devices that a person with PD can utilize. These exercises and devices have limited efficacy data and are most effective in combination with speech therapy. Further research into providing effective and efficient accessible speech treatment that can be delivered in home settings and potentially via Internet/ Web-based connections is ongoing. Communication is a key element in quality of life and can help people with PD maintain confidence and a positive self-concept as they deal with the challenges of the disease.

REFERENCES

1. Ramig L, Sapir S, Countryman S, Pawlas A, O'Brien C, Hoehn M, Thompson L. *Intensive voice treatment (LSVT) for individuals with Parkinson disease: a two-year follow-up. J Neurology, Neurosurgery, and Psychiatry.* 2001;71:493-498.
2. Fox CM, Morrison C, Sapir S. Current perspectives on the Lee Silverman Voice Treatment (LSVT) for people with idiopathic Parkinson's disease. *Am J Speech Lang Pathol.* 2002;22:111-123.
3. Ramig LO, Countryman S, Thompson LL, Horii Y. Comparison of two forms of intensive speech treatment for Parkinson disease. *J Speech Hear Res.* 1995;38(6):1232-1251.
4. Huber JE, Stathopoulos E, Ramig L, Lancaster S. Respiratory function and variability in individuals with Parkinson disease: pre and post Lee Silverman Voice Treatment (LSVT). *J Med Speech Lang Pathol.* 2003;11:185-201.
5. Smith ME, Ramig LO, Dromey C, Perez KS, Samandari R. Intensive voice treatment in Parkinson disease: laryngostroboscopic findings. *J Voice.* 1995;9(4):453-459.
6. Dromey C, Ramig LO. Intentional changes in sound pressure level and rate: their impact on measures of respiration, phonation and articulation. *J Speech Lang Hear Res.* 1998;41(5):1003-1018.
7. Dromey C, Ramig LO. The effect of lung volume on selected phonatory and articulatory variables. *J Speech Lang Hear Res.* 1998;41(3):491-502.
8. Sapir S, Spielman J, Ramig L, Story B, Fox C. Effects of intensive voice treatment (LSVT) on vowel articulation in dysarthritic individuals with idiopathic Parkinson's disease: acoustic and perceptual findings. *J Speech Lang Hear Res.* 2007;50:899-912.
9. Bayles KA, Tomoeda CK, Wood JA, Montgomery EB, Jr., Cruz RF, Azuma T et al. Change in cognitive function in idiopathic Parkinson disease. *Arch Neurol.* 1996;53(11):1140-1146.

SIDEBAR 13-1: DEVICES THAT CAN HELP SPEECH

- *Palatal lift.* This device is used for individuals who have severe speech intelligibility difficulties. This is most likely to occur in either advanced PD, or in some cases, post Deep Brain Stimulation surgery (DBS). When the opening between the oral (mouth) and nasal cavity can no longer close tightly during speech, too much air leaks out of the nose and greatly reduces speech intelligibility. The palatal lift is a dental apparatus that is similar to a retainer. It lifts the soft palate and stops air from escaping out of the nose during speech. These are products that are specially designed and fitted for each individual who requires one. A speech therapist can help a person decide if this device will be helpful.

- *Amplification.* A personal amplifier can be used to increase the volume of the voice. The amplifier also decreases voice fatigue. These devices work best in combination with behavioral speech therapy. Devices used alone may only work to amplify poor speech quality.

- *Loudness Indicator Lights Monitor (LIL).* This device was designed specifically for people with PD. The loudness level on this device can be set and a person with PD can monitor if he or she is speaking at an appropriate loudness level.

- *Augmentative Communication Devices.* Augmentative communication devices can help people with PD communicate when oral speech becomes too difficult. The technology can range from a board with pictures representing a person's daily needs to sophisticated electronic speech synthesizers. Computers with voice synthesizers and dedicated communication devices are available.

- *LSVT-LOUD Companion (LSVT-LOUDC).* This is a computer program for delivering LSVT-LOUD to people with PD either via a personal digital assistant (PDA) or computer. The LSVT-LOUDC was designed to meet the challenges of treatment accessibility and frequency that people with PD often encounter. The LSVT-LOUDC is specially programmed to collect data and provide feedback as it guides people through the LSVT-LOUD exercises, enabling them to participate in therapy sessions at home.

- *Speech Exercise Videos*: The LSVT Homework Helper is a 28-minute video that features voice and speech exercises based on LSVT-LOUD. A speech therapist guides the viewer through a series of exercises designed to maintain improvements in speech following delivery of LSVT-LOUD.

Assistive and Adaptive Technology to Enhance Functional Performance in Patients with Parkinson's Disease

Mary Frances Baxter, PhD, LOT

Introduction

Although medication often alleviates the symptoms of Parkinson's disease (PD), it does not fully remediate bradykinesia, tremors, decreased balance, and fine and gross motor deficits that can interfere with a person's ability to engage in daily activities.[1] Therapists should consider assistive and adaptive technology for those struggling with functional tasks. Assistive and adaptive technology can help patients maintain maximum function in their day-to-day routines and enable them to live meaningful lives.

The Technical Assistance to the States Act in 1987 defines assistive technology as "any item, piece of equipment, or product system—whether acquired commercially off the shelf, modified, or customized—that is used to increase, maintain or improve functional capabilities of individuals with disabilities" (Public Law 100-407).[2] In considering this definition there are two important concepts. First, the definition offers a wide range of technological applications, from simple "low-tech" tools to complicated multi-use systems utilizing advanced technology. Secondly, the definition focuses on "increasing, maintaining, or improving functional capabilities." The goal and end result of assistive technology should be increased function and improved participation in daily tasks.

When considering assistive or adaptive technology, it is important to keep in mind several factors that may make the difference between successful integration of the technology in the daily routine or abandonment of the device or system for other options. An important consideration is whether the person is willing to accept or try new devices, gadgets, or technology. This can be referred to as the person's "gadget tolerance." There is no empirical or subjective measure for a person's eventual acceptance of assistive technology, but there are some indications that could be used as guiding principles:

1. Does the person use some of the latest commercially available technology?

2. Does the person seem excited about the technology available to them to make life a bit easier?

If the answer to these questions is "Yes," the person is more likely to be willing to learn to use assistive or adaptive technology to enhance his or her life. If the answer to these questions is "No," the person is likely to abandon any technological device recommended and low-tech options should be considered.[3-6]

Frame of Reference for Service Delivery

There are several models for the delivery of assistive technology service delivery. Most models consider the person, the activity or task that needs to be done, and the assistive technology that can be used as a tool to enhance performance for specified activities. The human activity assistive technology (HAAT)[7] model (Figure 14-1) takes these concepts further and broadens the service delivery model to consider the context within which the person is participating in the activities that require technology.

Let's consider each of these components of the model.

- *Context* covers several situations in which the assistive technology is used. Context begins with the setting, which includes the physical location and environment as well as the tasks and conventions that rule the tasks and behaviors in the setting. For instance, a house can be identified by the physical location, but the home includes the other people and or animals in the house, and the rules that govern comfortable living, such as cleaning up the kitchen, answering the phone, and responding to the needs and requests of the others in the home. Setting includes home, place of employment, school, community. Social and cultural circumstances are also contextual considerations as part of AT service delivery. Social context is important because one of the functional outcomes of AT is to aid performance in communication, mobility, and manipulation, components of human performance that require or result in social interactions. Additionally, Krefting and Krefting[8] identify a "cultural screen" through which we view and interact with the world. This screen is a product of our family relationships, cultural heritage, experiences, and many other factors. Lastly, the conditions in the environment where the task is performed or the AT is used is referred to as the physical context. The temperature of the environment, the sound, and lighting are important considerations for successful use of AT. For example, some displays on communication boards are difficult to see in bright light.

- *Human* is the "operator" of the assistive technology system. According to Christiansen and Baum,[9] the intrinsic enablers including the sensory system, central processing, and motor output are basic functions of the human operator that need to be considered in the evaluation and intervention process.

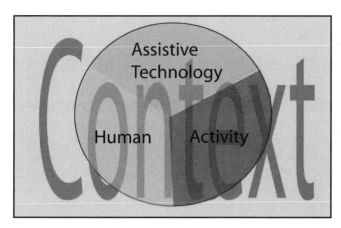

Figure 14-1. The human activity assistive technology (HAAT) model shows context of performance as an overarching consideration for the use of assistive technology. (Modified from Cook AM, Hussey SM. *Assistive Technologies: Principles and Practical Applications.* 2nd ed. St. Louis, MO: Mosby, Inc. 2002.)

- *Activity* is the basic component of the HAAT model. The need for assistive technology arises because a patient is unable or is having difficulty participating in or completing a functional task. Improved functional performance is the overall goal of assistive technology. Activities are categorized into three basic performance areas as defined by the American Occupational Therapy Association (1994): activities of daily living, work/productive activities, and play/leisure activities. There are a variety of AT devices or systems that can help a person complete the tasks in these performance areas. Additionally, activities consist of smaller tasks known as the components of the activity. For example, cooking can include cutting food, measuring ingredients, stirring ingredients together, and turning on and monitoring an oven or stove. Assistive technology, the third piece of the HAAT model, requires human interaction and can provide a variety of output. The end result of the technology should be improved human performance. Aids for mobility and communication as well as options for input and output are all considerations in the AT service delivery process. In an ideal situation, the abilities of the human are matched with the capabilities of the assistive technology for improved function.[7,10-12] The remainder of the chapter will be used to describe the potential assistive technology solutions for persons having difficulty in a variety of activities.

MOBILITY AND MOBILITY AIDS

Persons with disabilities often rate their quality of life based upon their degree of mobility. We require mobility in order to participate in many performance areas and daily roles—self-care, work, and leisure.[10,13-15] When a person with PD develops difficulties in balance or walking and has had a history of falling, it may be time to consider an aid for mobility. Often a cane is the first consideration to augment the person's gait and increase safety. When a cane is no longer enhancing mobility, specifically safety, a walker is the next recommendation. Walkers come with distinct features for safety and function, but the choice of one can also be based upon the user's personal preference. Features that the user might consider are adjustable height, folding frame, large wheels, hand brakes, and seats. When a person is unable to walk long distances or remain standing for longer periods, a wheelchair or scooter is an option. Wheeled mobility can be used for accessing the community, whether it is shopping, entertainment, or socializing. It is best to consult with an occupational therapist or physical therapist with skills in wheelchair assessment when considering wheeled mobility.[16,17]

ACCESS

When we use appliances, devices, and equipment in our daily lives, we require input or access to make them work. Human/technology interface is defined as interaction between a human and the technology.[7] The therapist must identify the access method or the input during the evaluation process for effective and efficient interface. Factors that affect a patient's ability to access appliances and devices in his or her environment include orthopedic and neuromuscular impairments, as well as cognitive and perceptual difficulties. Specifically, a patient with PD may experience access difficulties because of any individual or combination of symptoms. Tremors, bradykinesia, rigidity, and impaired fine motor skills may impede access to appliances and devices.[1,18] In addition to the patient's impairments, the limitations and access challenges that he or she faces are also based on predisposing characteristics.[19-22] Computer skills, fine motor coordination, learning style, motivation, and willingness to try new methods all contribute to successful access and use of AT. Because of individual differences and disease manifestations, it is important to identify the patient's abilities through a thorough assistive technology and/or occupational therapy or physical therapy evaluation.

Outcomes of Access

The ability to use knobs, switches, handles, and/or other mechanisms to control appliances and other pieces of equipment is important to support independence. Such appliances or devices include faucet handles, telephone buttons, light switches of various shapes and sizes, oven knobs, door handles, remote control devices, computer keyboard and mouse, and many others.

One of the first factors to consider when determining optimal access is to identify movement that is reliable, consistent, efficient, effective, and non-fatiguing. Ideally, the hands and fingers are the best access mode. When the hands are reliable access points, but may not be effective because of fine motor impairment, movement limitations, tremors or other factors, simple modifications of the knobs, switches, or buttons may be effective solutions. Enlarging handles, knobs, and touch controlled switches allow inexpensive, effective access for patients who have difficulty with small knobs and switches.[23,24]

When the hands and fingers are not capable, effective, or efficient for access, the therapist should consider other movements, body parts, or methods. When patients use other body parts, they usually accomplish access through the use of a switch.[7,25] Figure 14-2 shows a variety of switches available.

Additionally, Behrman and DeRuyter & Olson[25,26] suggest the following considerations for optimal access:

1. Can the patient perform the motion(s) required to complete the task with in a functional time?

2. Can the patient cognitively understand the access method?

3. Can the patient use visual, auditory, or tactile outputs? Does the access method provide the feedback?

4. Can the patient stabilizer the device to access it?

5. Can the patient access the device in all desired locations and positions?

We can divide methods of access into two categories: direct and indirect selection.[7,25] Indirect selection is further divided into scanning and encoding.

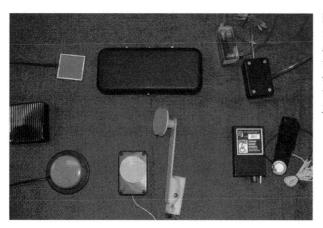

Figure 14-2. Special switches used for alternative access to electronic aids and assistive devices. From the top left: touch membrane switch, rocker switch, sip and puff switch, p-switch (responds to movements), light touch switch, and jelly bean switch.

We define direct selection as the user being able to directly interface with the device, whether by fingers, hands, typing stick, mouth stick, voice recognition, or alternative mouse devices.

When direct selection is not feasible, we consider indirect selection. Indirect selection refers to any method, often scanning or encoding, that excludes direct access operating the apparatus. Patients require evaluation and training when scanning and encoding are the desired access methods. A large selection of different switches is available, with many that can be accessed by body segments or methods other than the hand. The head, cheek, shoulder, wrist, elbow, foot, knee, or breath (plus others) can all be employed to access switches. As mentioned previously, the therapist must determine movement that is reliable, consistent, efficient, effective, and non-fatiguing for switch access.[27]

Computer Access

We usually access computers through two devices, the keyboard and the mouse. The keyboard is designed to be used by ten fingers, but many people are effective in using the keyboard with one or two finger typing. Users typically hold with the whole hand and slide it across a flat surface to move the cursor around the computer screen. The index finger is used on the "click" buttons to select the items viewed on the screen. Although this sounds fairly straightforward, computer use can be very complicated, requiring complex visual perceptual skills, variable motor tasks, and higher levels of cognitive functioning. The computer needs an integration of both input and output to make it functional and useful. We define input as the method(s) used to put information into the computer, including operation of a keyboard and mouse.[7,25] Output is information that is returned to the user. Types include the visual output on the computer screen, audio or voice output through the speakers, and hard copy output through the printer or fax. A person with PD may develop difficulties in accessing the computer because of deficits in visual perception and specific motor problems associated with the disease. There are solutions that may be helpful.[11,28]

Alternative Keyboards

Ergonomic—ergonomic keyboards are readily available at office and computer supply stores. They are designed to place the hands into a more comfortable position for keyboard use. Some ergonomic keyboards have built-in wrist rests that may help diminish involuntary movements.

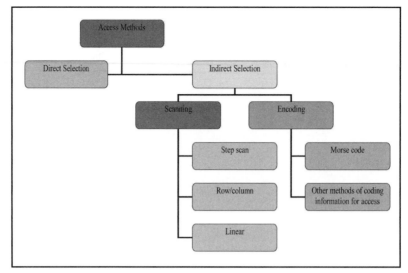

Figure 14-3. Diagram of the hierarchy and classes of various access methods.

Mini—a mini-keyboard is one that is much smaller than typical size; these are usually obtained through specially adapted computer resources. They require less movement of the elbow and shoulder and are useful for patients with motor control problems.

Enlarged—larger keyboards require more shoulder and elbow movements. They may be useful for persons with low vision and dyskinesia.

On-screen—on-screen keyboards are computer programs that display a keyboard on the computer monitor. They are accessed via the mouse or mouse emulation systems.

Chordic—Chordic keyboards have very few keys and are designed to respond to patterns of keystrokes. Just as a pattern of "fingering" produces a chord on a musical instrument, chordic keyboards produce letters and numbers by chords of keys (Figure 14-4).

Alternative Mouse Input

Ergonomic—there are a variety of ergonomic mouse options commercially available. Computer and office supply stores usually have several on display, and it is advisable to try the different options before purchase. Some patients find different ergonomic options uncomfortable or painful, depending upon their musculoskeletal predisposition.

Trackballs—when involuntary movements make access with a mouse difficult, trackballs are an option. Large trackballs are especially helpful for patients with limited fine motor control. If a person can generate fine motor coordination with the upper limb supported, then a small trackball may be an effective solution for mouse access.

Keystrokes for mouse—there are several programs available that allow keystrokes on the keyboard to reproduce mouse movements. Even without special programs, the arrow keys can move the mouse over most of the screen. Additionally, many operations that are done via pull-down menus and tool bars can be accomplished with keystrokes, common ones include "ctrl" + S = save, "ctrl" + C = copy, and "ctrl" + V = paste (Figure 14-5).

Other Input Methods

Other input methods that require consideration include voice recognition and switch use with an on-screen keyboard. Voice recognition software is available commercially

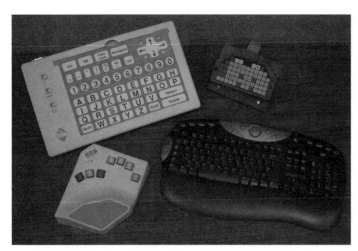

Figure 14-4. Examples of alternative keyboards. Circular from top right: a large sized keyboard, a miniature keyboard with alternative key arrangement, an ergonomic keyboard that users infrared (no chord), and a chordic keyboard that can be used with one hand.

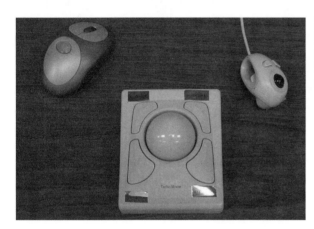

Figure 14-5. Alternative mouse options. From left to right, an ergonomic mouse that operates on infrared (no cord), a larger track ball, a small track ball that can be operated with the thumb.

and has improved considerably in recent years. It requires user training, as well as patience and persistence in creating a user profile. For a person with fine motor difficulties, voice recognition is a viable option for computer access. Unfortunately, persons with PD with speech impairments such as reduced volume or imprecise articulation may not be candidates for this type of software.[29,30]

Output Options

Persons with PD often have vision or visual perceptual deficits.[1,31] For Microsoft Office® users, there are built-in options that should be considered. Using the Control Panel and finding the Accessibility Options provides the patient with simple modifications such as high contrast visual display, correction of repetitive key strokes, and auditory signals for important key strokes and functions. Screen magnifiers clarify the images on the computer monitor. Patients benefit from consultation with a low-vision specialist to obtain the most appropriate equipment.

Another option for persons with low or impaired vision is voice output for text documents. Software is available that will "read" the letters, words, or sentences as the person types. Accuracy and typing can improve with voice output, and it is also available for "reading" anything that is displayed on the computer monitor. Screen reader software is designed to provide auditory feedback about mouse movements as the cursor moves over screen features. Screen readers are especially useful for persons with impaired vision who use multiple computer applications, including the tool and task bars and the Internet.[32]

Alternative and Augmentative Communication (AAC)

About 50% of persons with PD exhibit speech problems.[29,30,33] Augmentative and alternative communication (AAC) systems or strategies provide speech options for persons with a wide range of disabilities and some are suitable for PD patients.[33-38] AAC systems are an integrated group of components, symbols, aids, strategies, and techniques used to enhance communication.[34] AAC is appropriate for persons who have intent, need, and desire to communicate but cannot do so through standard means. The goal of AAC is to provide the most effective communication possible and facilitate potential for personal achievement.[40]

The evaluation process for determining optimal communication for a person should be completed by a team, including the client and his or her family, a speech language pathologist, and an occupational therapist or physical therapist, as there are multiple issues to consider. It is important to first evaluate positioning because of the effect posture has on functional and fine motor abilities.[17,41,42]

Specific positioning questions to ask related to AAC are:

1. In what positions will the system be used?

   - Sitting?

   - Reclining?

   - Wheelchair?

   - Standing?

2. What positions are effective for the patient?

3. How do the person's abilities change as a result of different positions?

   - Physical abilities

   - Visual perceptual abilities

As previously noted, how a person provides input or accesses an AAC device or system is a critical part of the successful use of the device or system. During the AAC evaluation, the therapist should address issues such as the position of the device or system in relation to the patient, and the patient's ability to effectively manipulate the upper extremity or another body part for access and switch use.

In addition to the motor, sensory, cognitive, and perceptual issues involved in accessing a communication system, it is also important to consider the features of the device. Features include the type of input or access the device requires, the visual display, the type of output, including the feedback provided, and the type of symbol system.[2,11,22,43] Let's look at each of these.

The fingers are the ideal input method for any AAC device or system. As noted previously, when the fingers are not reliable for access, the therapist should consider other methods such as the switch. Switch access for an AAC device requires that the apparatus has the capability for scanning—direct, indirect, or both.

The visual display is the "face" of the communication device. In the simplest form, the visual display on a low tech communication board is the letters, words, or graphics that the person points to. This type of visual display requires that the communication partner is in close proximity and comprehends the message the user is trying to relay. Additionally, the visual display can be electronic such as an LCD or a computer type display. In these high tech forms, the visual display can be simple or confusing, have a high or low contrast, or be static or dynamic in the way it presents the information. Each of these features can have an impact on the successful use of the AAC device or system. The therapist needs to evaluate the patient's visual, perceptual, and cognitive abilities to determine which of the visual display features are likely to be successful.[1,22,27]

The primary types of output that a device provides include auditory (speech) output, or visual, written output. AAC devices have become sophisticated in that there are a variety of voices that can be programmed as output, and the speech rate and pronunciation can be modified to match the user's and communication partner's needs. Additionally, the auditory output can include feedback such as verbal, clicking, or beeping sounds as keys are hit. This auditory feedback assists in device use, but can also interfere with effective communication.[43-46] It is important for the therapists, patients, and families to consider the patients' abilities and learning style when deciding on these features.

Symbols that are used on the display of the AAC device range from concrete to abstract. Literate adults will be able to use AAC devices that include the alphabet as part of the display. An alphabet allows the person to generate words, sentences, statements, and so on that may be personal, and the user is not limited to the phrases and words programmed into the device by the manufacturer or the therapist. Beyond the alphabet, symbols can include photographs, colored or black and white line drawings, and more abstract symbol sets such as Blissymbols, Pic-Syms, or Minspeak.[29,44,47-48]

Electronic communication devices rely on storage of messages that the user can retrieve when needed through a series of key strokes. Typing individual letters to spell words, phrases, or sentences for conversation can be time consuming and often frustrating. Message storage and retrieval techniques can increase the speed or rate of access and improve the system's efficiency. Strategies for message storage and retrieval include:

- The use of multiple levels of storage, so that all the information is not on the opening screen, but is accessed through various levels of screens. This is similar to storing documents in levels of folders on the computer.

- Encoding of the information so that commonly used phrases can be accessed through 2 to 4 "hits" on the keyboard. For example, "Good morning" might be accessed through two symbols on the keyboard or the letters "GM."

- Prediction of the next letter or word can help speed the access and increase the rate of interaction. The device provides the user with choices rather than contacting all the letters or words in a phrase.

- Use of symbols that have multiple meanings or can relay an idea in the form of a sentence.[7,40]

In addition to the above considerations, a functional communication device needs other features that are compatible with the person's lifestyle (Figure 14-6). The flexibility of the device is important to accommodate changes in environments and positions of use. Furthermore, if the therapist anticipates changes in the patient's physical abilities, cognitive status, or communication needs, the features on the apparatus need to be adaptable so the patient can continue to use it.

The therapist should appraise the portability of the device, especially if the patient is going to need it during ambulation. Weight and size of the device are also concerns when a person has to carry a communication device for any length of time. If the AAC user also requires a mobility aid, such as a wheelchair, scooter, or walker, there are mounting systems to attach the communication device. These mounting systems allow access and provide easy on and off mounting for use in other positions or situations.

Figure 14-6. Examples of AAC devices: Center bottom: a simple device with 16 programmable phrases, Top left: a mid-range device with lights used for cueing symbol sequences and Top right; a high-end device with dynamic display that is highly customizable and programmable.

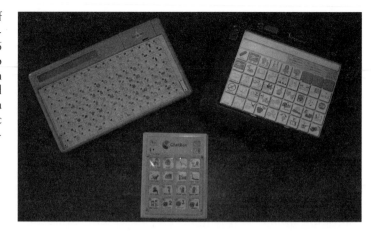

Any electronic device that is used frequently should be durable, and inclement weather, dropping, and/or rough handling should be always be anticipated. It is critical that the communication device be able to survive life's happenings.

When a person has multiple needs that are accommodated by electronics, the integration and compatibility with other assistive devices may be a factor in the overall AT assessment. Many AAC devices are capable and may be required to integrate with computers, home appliances, and electronic aids to daily living or wheelchair controls.

Other issues include the cost, warranty, and manufacturer support. High cost and poor manufacturer support can make some AAC devices prohibitive.

The American Speech and Hearing Association (ASHA) has outlined an evaluation process for augmentative and alternative communication.[40] ASHA suggests that at the end of the evaluation, the following questions should be answered:

1. What communication approaches (speech, standard augmentative, special augmentative) have been recommended and/or used in the past?

2. Which approaches will be used for:
   - Quick phrases and interjections?
   - Short messages?
   - Expressing feelings?
   - Giving and getting information?
   - Conversation with family? Friends? Teachers?
   - Employers? Strangers?
   - Written communication (to self and others)?
   - Communication at a distance?

3. If part of the system uses aided communication, how will choices on the board or device be indicated?

4. Will special equipment or switches need to be bought or made?

5. Will the equipment or switches work for other devices, such as televisions or computers?

6. What symbols (eg, letters, pictures, graphics, words, and phrases) will be used on boards or devices?

7. Is there enough flexibility in the recommended communication system so that communication is possible in a variety of settings (home, work, school, at play, in bed, on the floor, sitting down, standing up)?

8. What techniques can be used to get someone' s attention to start a conversation? To interrupt? To keep from being interrupted?

9. What body positions can be used to increase communication and function, including suggestions for mobility, hand movement, head control, eye contact, stability, and fatigue?

10. Can the recommended system be modified as capabilities and needs change?

11. What will the equipment and follow-up services cost, including information relating to maintenance and repairs?

12. Why were the recommended techniques chosen?

13. Which professionals will be carrying out the recommended communication plan and how often must they be seen?

Prior to purchasing an AAC system, the patient should talk with a current user to obtain feedback about the quality and function of the device. It is a complicated yet very personal process, and it is imperative that the user have as much input in the selection as possible.[4,43,48]

As part of the evaluation and prescription process, the therapist should think about the functional goals of intervention with augmentative or alternative communication devices or systems. Cook and Hussey[7] suggest some examples of communication goals including:

Improve conversational skills:
- In one on one communication
- By increasing the ability to catch another's attention
- By increasing interaction with peers as well as unfamiliar partners
- By increasing rate of communication output
- By increasing the size and complexity of the user's vocabulary
- Through use of the telephone
- By speaking to groups of people, or in classroom or meeting situations

Additionally, AAC can complement, supplement, or replace graphic communication skills. Goals to improve graphic communication might include:

1. By aiding, augmenting, or replacing handwriting

2. By aiding, augmenting, or replacing computer keyboard access

3. By aiding, augmenting, or replacing tasks such as note-taking, messages, editing, or correcting

4. By aiding or augmenting written math, drawing, plotting, or graphing.[7]

Successful communication that is assisted by augmentative or alternative communication devices or systems may be viewed along a continuum and includes the levels of context dependent, emerging communicator, and independent communicator (Table 14-1).

TABLE 14-1

Levels of Communication[3,30,42-45]

	Context Dependent	Emerging	Independent
Form of communication	Uses some symbolic display and strategies, but continues to be dependent on familiar communication partners.	Use of symbolic modes of communication is inconsistent.	Interacts on multiple topics with familiar and unfamiliar communication partners.
Personal factors	-Unfamiliar and occasionally familiar partners may not understand the AAC. -Vocabulary in AAC is insufficient or inappropriate to generate novel messages.	-Communicator could be very young or older with developmental delays or severe communication impairments. -AAC strategies and technologies that are appropriate may not be available or accessible.	-Can be independent while using AAC equipment. -Can be independent without age appropriate cognitive or language skills. -May rely on familiar communication partners for support.

ELECTRONIC AIDS TO DAILY LIVING

The daily tasks in which we all participate frequently require use of electronic devices and appliances. Lamps, televisions, radios, room fans, and others as well as minor appliances such as blenders or food processors make our lives easier. When a person with PD has difficulty accessing or managing these electronic gadgets, there are a range of options to foster their use. The electronic adaptations, devices, and systems that help patients access their environment and perform daily tasks are collectively known as electronic aides to daily living (EADLs).

For EADL to operate, there has to be a mechanism for the EADL control device to send a signal to the appliance and a mechanism for the appliance to understand and respond to the signal. EADL mechanisms operate through four primary signals: house electrical wiring, radio waves, infrared, or ultrasound transmissions. When the house alternating current (AC) wiring is used, the EADL consists of a control unit that sends a transmission and individual appliance modules, often referred to as X-10 units (Figure 14-7). The therapist or patient can easily obtain these systems through electronic or hardware stores such as Radio Shack or Home Depot. Each appliance is plugged into an individual module that is then plugged into a standard wall socket. Each module interprets the signal sent out by the control unit and translates the signal to generate the action requested (eg, turn the light on, turn the radio off). These systems are relatively inexpensive and easy to install, but can only perform simple functions such as on/off.

Additionally, it is important to understand the wiring when using the house circuitry. Houses often have multiple circuits for the different room outlets, switches, and appli-

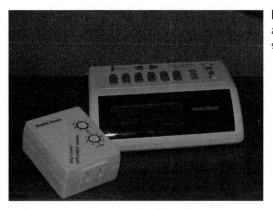

Figure 14-7. From left to right, an example of an X-10 unit and a control unit used for operating simple appliances such as lamps.

ances, and several control units may be needed. Some of the newer houses contain this type of control capability.[52,53]

Radio waves provide another way to make the link between the control unit and the appliance. Garage door openers are a common example of the use of radio wave technology. Radio waves have an advantage in that they are not blocked by walls and doors, so devices can be controlled in other rooms or from a distance away.

Anyone who has used remote control for the television should understand infrared transmission (IR). IR is used to control the multiple functions of TVs, VCRs and DVD players, radios, CD players, and others. Appliances that can be operated by IR require a receiver that can respond to the IR signal. Furthermore, IR requires that the controller and the receiver are in direct line of sight, although you may be able to effectively "bounce" signals off of reflective surfaces to reach the receiver. Another disadvantage is that because IR signals are light sensitive, devices that receive them may not work well in bright, sunny rooms. However, many of the high-end communication devices have the capability to send IR signals and can be used as EADL to control TVs, CD and DVD players, and other IR devices.[7]

Ultrasound transmission functions in a similar way as infrared, except that ultrasound transmission uses sound waves too high to be detected by the human ear. Additionally, ultrasound transmission systems require both a transmission unit and a receiving unit, similar to the house-wiring set-up. Whereas a house-wiring system can only do on–off, ultrasound systems can do a variety of functions on appliances such as TVs and VCRs (eg, channel change, volume change, stop, rewind, and play). As with infrared transmissions, ultrasounds are line of sight and cannot transmit through obstacles.

As our world becomes more electronically savvy and technology becomes more readily available, EADLs are also becoming more available and accepted by the general public. Therapists who are aware of EADL options to improve the functional abilities of persons with PD will provide better access to and training in their use.[53-55]

DRIVING

According to The National Highway Safety Administration (NHTSA), there are an estimated 383,000 registered vehicles that have been modified with adaptive equipment (based on 1995 data).[56] As noted in Chapters 5 and 9, driving becomes a difficult task for persons with PD. Difficulties with reaction time, visual perceptual tasks, turning one's head, and "freezing" lead to impaired driving.[57,58] When driving becomes problematic, it is best to consult with a nationally certified Driving Rehabilitation Specialist. The Association for Driver Rehabilitation Specialists (ADED) maintains standards for those who provide evaluation and training for persons with disabilities.[59] A Driver Rehabilitation Specialist evaluates the person's ability and potential to drive. An occupational therapist often performs the initial assessment, which includes:

- Visual, perceptual, and cognitive screening
- Physical skills evaluation
- Reaction time testing in an electronic car simulator

Evaluation and training in a driving simulator is a critical part of the adaptive driving program. The simulator creates a safe environment to assess skills and determine deficits while driving in a variety of computer-generated conditions and situations.

Some of the motor vehicle modifications that might be beneficial include:

- A wide array of mirrors, both rear-view and side mirrors that reduce the need to turn the head to see around the vehicle
- Adapted steering wheel aids including a variety of steering knobs
- A hand brake for use if the legs are unable to activate the foot brake in an effective and timely manner
- Hand controls for accessing the accelerator and brake when the lower extremities are unable to activate the accelerator and brake in an effective and timely manner

CONCLUSION

Although this chapter presented a great deal of information, it only scratches the surface when considering the assistive and adaptive technologies that are currently available and will be available in the future. When the symptoms of PD affect functional skills and the ability to perform daily tasks, from simple tasks such as turning on a lamp to more complex tasks such as using the computer, assistive and adaptive technologies are available to complement and supplement a person's abilities. Local hardware stores and electronic stores are valuable resources for finding easy to use technologies such as modified light switches, alarm systems, and X-10 units. The Internet is also a valuable resource for finding qualified professionals and needed equipment. Of course, a consult and thorough evaluation by the rehabilitation team can help PD patients find the best technologies to meet their needs.

Case Study

Raymond is a 52-year-old gentleman who was diagnosed with Parkinson's disease 5 years previously. He has the classic symptoms of PD including bradykinesia, tremors, decreased balance, and difficulty with fine motor dexterity. He is currently an office manager and does a large amount of work on a computer. He also attends meetings where he likes to take notes. His goal is to continue to work. His employer enlisted an ergonomic specialist to evaluate his work station and ensure that he is positioned appropriately in front of the computer following good ergonomic principles. He worked with the specialist to determine the best keyboard and mouse options. He currently uses a keyboard that is "split" in the middle and therefore positionable for comfort and access. The keyboard is also a bit smaller than normal requiring less movement and excursion of the forearm and hands. He chose to use a track ball instead of a mouse for moving the cursor about the screen. These devices required practice before Raymond adjusted to them. Additionally, Raymond has voice recognition software on the computer. It requires a microphone sensitive enough to pick up his voice, especially when it is not at its strongest. He is still learning how to use the software effectively and efficiently. Raymond now uses a tape recorder to take notes during meetings, which his secretary transcribes when needed. Raymond also negotiated with his company to work flexible hours to accommodate fluctuations in his condition.

At home, Raymond has an EADL control unit on his bedside table with X-10 units placed with lamps around the house. This enables him to get to bed with lights on and increases his safety. The control unit allows him to turn lights on and off while in bed. Additionally, this control unit can be programmed to operate the lights automatically, a feature he uses when he is away from home for several days.

Raymond also has motion sensing options attached to the overhead lights in the kitchen, den, and garage. As a person enters the room, the lights come on. After a few minutes of no movement, such as when a person leaves the room, the lights go out. This also increases the safety of the house by improving the lighting.

Raymond uses a universal remote control unit that has large-sized buttons, which make it easier for him to access. The universal remote is programmed to operate several different devices such as the TV, DVD player, and radio. In his car, Raymond has installed a wider rearview mirror, thus reducing his need to turn his head. He chooses to increase his driving safety by avoiding rush-hour traffic and following a planned route to familiar locations.

Raymond is not ready for a communication device, but he knows they are available when he needs one. He has looked at the options and believes that a device with a static display simple symbol system and an alphabet included will potentially meet his needs. He suspects that he may need to have a device with the potential for switch access and would really like the device to control his TV, DVD, CD, radio, and other appliances. When he is ready and needs the device, he will make an informed decision with the help of a speech language pathologist and/or occupational therapist.

REFERENCES

1. Samil A, Nutt J, Ransom B. Parkinson's disease. *Lancet.* 2004;363:1783-1793.
2. *Access to information technology by users with disabilities, initial guidelines.* Washington, DC: U.S. Department of Education, 1987.
3. Cornman JC, Freedman VA, Agree EM. Measurement of assistive device use: implications for estimates of device use and disability in late life. *Geront.* 2005; 45:347-358.
4. McCall F, Markova I, Murphy J, Moodie E, Collins S. Perspectives on AAC systems by the users and by their communication partners. *Eur J Disord Commun.* 1997;32:235-256.
5. Scherer MJ. Outcomes of assistive technology use on quality of life. *Disabil Rehabil.* 1996;18:439-448.
6. Scherer MJ, Sax C, Vanbiervliet A, Cushman LA, Scherer JV. Predictors of assistive technology use: the importance of personal and psychosocial factors. *Disabil Rehabil.* 2005;27:1321-31.
7. Cook AM, Hussey SM. *Assistive Technology: Principles and Practice.* St. Louis, MO: Mosby, Inc.; 2002.
8. Krefting L, Krefting D. Cultural influence on performance. In: Christiansen C, Baum C, eds. *Occupational Therapy.* Thorofare, NJ: SLACK Incorporated; 1991.
9. Christiansen C, Baum C. Person-environment occupational performance: a conceptual model for practice. In: Christiansen C, Baum C, eds. *Occupational Therapy: Enabling Function and Well Being.* Thorofare, NJ: SLACK Incorporated; 1997.
10. Amsterdam P. Choices in wheeled mobility. The importance of seeing the person behind the case. *Case Manager.* 1999;10:28-31.

11. Turpin G, Armstrong J, Frost P, Fine B, Ward C, Pinnington L. Evaluation of alternative computer input devices used by people with disabilities. *J Med Eng Technol.* 2005;29:119-129.

12. Verza R, Carvalho ML, Battaglia MA, Uccelli MM. An interdisciplinary approach to evaluating the need for assistive technology reduces equipment abandonment. *Mult Scler.* 2006;12:88-93.

13. Batavia AI, Hammer GS. Toward the development of consumer-based criteria for the evaluation of assistive devices. *J Rehabil Res Dev.* 1990;27:425-436.

14. Cooper RA. Improvements in mobility for people with disabilities. *Med Eng Phys.* 2001;23:v.

15. York J. Mobility methods selected for use in home and community environments. *Phys Ther.* 1989;69:736-747.

16. Meyers AR, Anderson JJ, Miller DR, Shipp K, Hoenig H. Barriers, facilitators, and access for wheelchair users: substantive and methodologic lessons from a pilot study of environmental effects. *Soc Sci Med.* 2002;55:1435-1446.

17. Trefler E, Taylor SJ. Prescription and positioning: evaluating the physically disabled individual for wheelchair seating. *Prosthet Orthot Int.* 1991;15:217-224.

18. Center UoMM. Signs and Symptoms of Parkinson's Disease: http:wwwumm.edu/cgi-bin/printpage.cgi, 10-9-2005.

19. Casali SP, Williges RC. Data bases of accommodative aids for computer users with disabilities. *Hum Factors.* 1990;32:407-422.

20. DeVries RC, Deitz J, Anson D. A comparison of two computer access systems for functional text entry. *Am J Occup Ther.* 1998;52:656-665.

21. Kruse D, Krueger A, Drastal S. Computer use, computer training, and employment. Outcomes among people with spinal cord injuries. *Spine.* 1996; 21:891-896.

22. Merrow SL, Corbett CD. Adaptive computing for people with disabilities. *Comput Nurs.* 1994;12:201-209.

23. MacNeil V. Electronic aids to daily living. *Team Rehabilitation Report.* 1998; 9:53-56.

24. Ostensjo S, Carlberg EB, Vollestad NK. The use and impact of assistive devices and other environmental modifications on everyday activities and care in young children with cerebral palsy. *Disabil Rehabil.* 2005;27:849-861.

25. DeRuyter F, Olson DA. *Clinician's Guide to Assistive Technology.* St. Louis, MO: Mosby, Inc.; 2002.

26. Behrman AL. Factors in functional assessment. *J Rehabil Res Dev Clin Suppl.* 1990:17-30.

27. Angelo J. Factors affecting the use of a single switch with assistive technology devices. *J Rehabil Res Dev.* 2000;37:591-598.

28. Lesher GW, Moulton BJ, Higginbotham DJ. Optimal character arrangements for ambiguous keyboards. *IEEE Trans Rehabil Eng.* 1998;6:415-423.

29. Armstrong L, Jans D, MacDonald A. Parkinson's disease and aided AAC: some evidence from practice. *Int J Lang Commun Disord.* 2000;35:377-389.

30. Johnson JA, Pring TR. Speech therapy and Parkinson's disease; a review and further data. *Euro J Disorders of Commun.* 1990;25:183-194.

31. Mosimann UP, Mather G, Wesnes KA, O'Brien JT, Burn DJ, McKeith IG. Visual perception in Parkinson disease dementia and dementia with Lewy bodies. *Neurology.* 2004;63:2091-2096.

32. Chiang MF, Cole RG, Gupta S, Kaiser GE, Starren JB. Computer and World Wide Web accessibility by visually disabled patients: problems and solutions. *Surv Ophthalmol.* 2005;50:394-405.

33. Zeitlin DJ, Abrams GM, Shah BK. Use of augmentative/alternative communication in patients with amyotrophic lateral sclerosis. *J Neurologic Rehabil.* 1995;9:217-220.

34. Jacobs B, Drew R, Ogletree BT, Pierce K. Augmentative and Alternative Communication (AAC) for adults with severe aphasia: where we stand and how we can go further. *Disabil Rehabil.* 2004; 26:1231-40.

35. Beukelman DR, Ball LJ. Improving AAC use for persons with acquired neurogenic disorders: understanding human and engineering factors. *Assist Technol.* 2002;14:33-44.

36. Soderholm S, Meinander M, Alaranta H. Augmentative and alternative communication methods in locked-in syndrome. *J Rehabil Med.* 2001;33:235-239.

37. Light JC, Roberts B, Dimarco R, Greiner N. Augmentative and alternative communication to support receptive and expressive communication for people with autism. *J Commun Disord.* 1998;31:153-178; quiz 179-180.

38. Schepis MM, Reid DH, Behrman MM. Acquisition and functional use of voice output communication by persons with profound multiple disabilities. *Behav Modif.* 1996;20:451-468.

39. American S-L-HA. Competencies for speech-language pathologists providing services in augmentative communication. *ASHA.* 1989;31:107-110.

40. Association ASaH. *Augmentative and Alternative Communication.* Vol. 2006: ASHA, 2005.

41. Hulme JB, Gallacher K, Walsh J, Niesen S, Waldron D. Behavioral and postural changes observed with use of adaptive seating by clients with multiple handicaps. *Phys Ther.* 1987;67:1060-1067.

42. O'Leary S, Mann C, Perkash I. Access to computers for older adults: problems and solutions. *Am J Occup Ther.* 1991;45:636-642.

43. Murphy J, Markova I, Collins S, Moodie E. AAC systems: obstacles to effective use. *Eur J Disord Commun.* 1996;31:31-44.

44. Blackstone SW, Williams MB, Joyce M. Future AAC technology needs: consumer perspectives. *Assist Technol.* 2002;14:3-16.

45. Demasco P. Human factors considerations in the design of language interfaces in AAC. *Assist Technol.* 1994;6:10-25.

46. Schepis MM, Reid DH. Effects of a voice output communication aid on interactions between support personnel and an individual with multiple disabilities. *J Appl Behav Anal.* 1995;28:73-77.

47. Diener BL, Bischof-Rosarioz JA. Determining decision-making capacity in individuals with severe communication impairments after stroke: the role of augmentative-alternative communication (AAC). *Top Stroke Rehabil.* 2004;11:84-88.

48. Dickerson SS, Stone VI, Panchura C, Usiak DJ. The meaning of communication: experiences with augmentative communication devices. *Rehabil Nurs.* 2002; 27:215-220.

49. Alm N, Parnes P. Augmentative and alternative communication: past, present and future. *Folia Phoniatr Logop.* 1995;47:165-192.

50. Dowden PA, Marriner NA. Augmentative and alternative communication: treatment principles and strategies. *Semin Speech Lang.* 1995;16:140-157; quiz 157-158.

51. Light JC, Binger C, Agate TL, Ramsay KN. Teaching partner-focused questions to individuals who use augmentative and alternative communication to enhance their communicative competence. *J Speech Lang Hear Res.* 1999;42:241-255.

52. Lansley P, McCreadie C, Tinker A. Can adapting the homes of older people and providing assistive technology pay its way? *Age Ageing.* 2004;33:571-576.

53. LaPlante M, Hendershot G, Moss A. The prevalance of need for assistive technology devices and home accessibility features. *Technology and Disability.* 1997;6:17-28.

54. Fisher P, Toczek M, Seeger BR. Technology for people with disabilities: a survey of needs. *Assist Technol.* 1993;5:106-118.

55. Kanny EM, Anson DK. Current trends in assistive technology education in entry-level occupational therapy curricula. *Am J Occup Ther.* 1998;52:586-591.

56. US Department of Transportation. *Estimating the Number of Vehicles Adapted for Use by Persons with Disabilities.* Washington, DC: National Center for Statistics & Analysis—Research & Development; 1997:3.

57. Heikkila VM, Turkka J, Korpelainen J, Kallanranta T, Summala H. Decreased driving ability in people with Parkinson's disease. *J Neurol Neurosurg Psychiatry.* 1998;64:325-330.

58. Borromei A, Caramelli R, Chieregatti G et al. Ability and fitness to drive of Parkinson's disease patients. *Funct Neurol.* 1999;14:227-234.

59. Specialists TAfDR. ADED Training Program—Fundamentals of Driver Rehabilitation. http://www.driver-ed.org/i4a/pages/index.cfm?pageid=1, 2006.

APPENDICES

THE UNIFIED PARKINSON'S DISEASE RATING SCALE (UPDRS)

Fahn S, Elton RL, and members of the UPDRS Development Committee, "Unified Parkinson's Disease Rating Scale." In Fahn S, Marsden CD, Goldstein M, et al. eds. Recent developments in Parkinson's Disease II. New York: Macmillan; 1987:153-163.

Description: Scale most commonly used by movement disorder specialists to assess patients with Parkinson's disease.

Application: Assessment of parkinsonism in routine clinical, research setting.

Duration: Approximately 40 minutes.[28]

Score range: 0 to 154 points (> score = > disability) Scores are determined for each extremity separately, in both "on" (under optimal medication effect) and "off" (absent or sub-optimal medication effect) states.

I. Mentation, Behavior, and Mood

  1. Intellectual impairments

    0. None

    1. Mild, consistent forgetfulness with partial recollection of events and no other difficulties.

    2. Moderate memory loss, with disorientation and moderate difficulty handling complex problems; mild but definite impairment of function at home with need of occasional prompting.

    3. Severe memory loss with disorientation for time and often to place; severe impairment in handling problems.

    4. Severe memory loss with orientation preserved to person only; unable to make judgments or solve problems; requires much help with personal care; cannot be left alone at all.

  2. Thought disorder (due to dementia or drug intoxication)

    0. None

    1. Vivid dreaming.

    2. "Benign" hallucinations with insight retained.

    3. Occasional to frequent hallucinations or delusions; without insight; could interfere with daily activities.

    4. Persistent hallucinations, delusions, or florid psychosis; not able to care for self.

  3. Depression

    0. Not present.

    1. Periods of sadness or guilt greater than normal, never sustained for days or weeks.

    2. Sustained depression (one week or more).

    3. Sustained depression with vegetative symptoms (insomnia, anorexia, weight loss, loss of interest).

    4. Sustained depression with vegetative symptoms and suicidal thoughts or intent.

4. Motivation/initiative
- 0. Normal.
- 1. Less assertive than usual; more passive.
- 2. Loss of initiative or disinterest in elective (non-routine) activities.
- 3. Loss of initiative or disinterest in day to day (routine) activities.
- 4. Withdrawn, complete loss of motivation.

II. Activities of Daily Living

5. Speech
- 0. Normal
- 1. Mildly affected; no difficulty being understood.
- 2. Moderately affected; sometimes asked to repeat statements.
- 3. Severely affected; frequently asked to repeat statements.
- 4. Unintelligible most of the time.

6. Salivation
- 0. Normal
- 1. Slight but definite excess of saliva in mouth; may have nighttime drooling.
- 2. Moderately excessive saliva; may have minimal drooling.
- 3. Marked excess of saliva with some drooling.
- 4. Marked drooling; requires constant tissue or handkerchief.

7. Swallowing
- 0. Normal
- 1. Rare choking.
- 2. Occasional choking.
- 3. Requires soft diet.
- 4. Requires NG tube or gastrostomy feeding.

8. Hand writing
- 0. Normal
- 1. Slightly slow or small.
- 2. Moderately slow or small; all words are legible.
- 3. Severely effected; not all words are legible.
- 4. The majority of the words are not legible.

9. Cutting food and handling utensils
- 0. Normal
- 1. Somewhat slow and clumsy, but no help needed.
- 2. Can cut most foods, although clumsy and slow; some help needed.
- 3. Food must be cut by someone, but can still feed slowly.
- 4. Needs to be fed.

10. Dressing
- 0. Normal
- 1. Somewhat slow, but no help needed.

2. Occasional assistance with buttoning, or with getting arms in sleeves.

3. Considerable help required, but can do some things alone.

4. Helpless

11. Hygiene

0. Normal

1. Somewhat slow, but no help needed.

2. Needs help to shower or bathe; or very slow in hygienic care.

3. Requires assistance for washing, brushing teeth, combing hair, going to bath room.

4. Foley catheter or other mechanical aids.

12. Turning in bed and adjusting bed clothes

0. Normal

1. Somewhat slow and clumsy, but no help needed.

2. Can turn alone or adjust sheets, but with great difficulty.

3. Can initiate, but not turn or adjust sheets alone.

4. Helpless

13. Falling (unrelated to freezing)

1. None

2. Rare falling.

3. Occasional falls, less than once per day.

4. Falls on average of once a day.

5. Falls more than once per day.

14. Freezing when walking

0. None

1. Rare freezing when walking; may have start hesitation.

2. Occasional freezing when walking.

3. Frequent freezing; occasional falls from freezing.

4. Frequent falls from freezing.

15. Walking

0. Normal

1. Mild difficulty; may not swing arms or may tend to drag leg.

2. Moderate difficulty, but requires little or no assistance.

3. Severe disturbance of walking, requiring assistance.

4. Cannot walk at all, even with assistance.

16. Tremor

0. Absent

1. Slight and infrequently present.

2. Moderate; bothersome to patient.

3. Severe; interferes with many activities.

4. Marked; interferes with most activities.

17. Sensory complaints related to parkinsonism
- 0. None
- 1. Occasionally has numbness, tingling, or mild aching.
- 2. Frequently has numbness, tingling, or aching; not distressing.
- 3. Frequent painful sensations.
- 4. Excruciating pain.

III. Motor Examination

18. Speech
- 0. Normal
- 1. Slight loss of expression, dictation, and/or volume.
- 2. Monotone, slurred but understandable; moderately impaired.
- 3. Marked impairment, difficult to understand.
- 4. Unintelligible

19. Facial expression
- 0. Normal
- 1. Minimal hypomimia, could be normal "poker face."
- 2. Slight but definitely abnormal diminution of facial expression.
- 3. Moderate hypomimia; lips parted some of the time.
- 4. Masked or fixed facies; lips parted ¼ inch or more.

20. Tremor at rest
- 0. Absent
- 1. Slight and infrequently present.
- 2. Mild in amplitude and persistent; or moderate in amplitude, but only intermittently present.
- 3. Moderate in amplitude and present most of the time.
- 4. Marked in amplitude and present most of the time.

21. Action or postural tremor of hands
- 0. Absent
- 1. Slight; present with action.
- 2. Moderate in amplitude, present with action.
- 3. Moderate in amplitude with posture holding as well as action.
- 4. Marked in amplitude; interferes with feeding.

22. Rigidity
- 0. Absent.
- 1. Slight; present with action.
- 2. Mild to moderate.
- 3. Marked, but full range of motion easily achieved.
- 4. Severe, range of motion achieved with difficulty.

23. Finger taps
- 0. Normal
- 1. Mild slowing and/ or reduction in amplitude.

2. Moderately impaired; definite and early fatiguing; may have occasional arrests in movement.

3. Severely impaired; frequent hesitation in initiating movements or arrests in ongoing movements.

4. Can barely perform the task.

24. Hand movements

0. Normal

1. Mild slowing and/or reduction in amplitude.

2. Moderately impaired; definite and early fatiguing; may have occasional arrests in movement.

3. Severely impaired; frequent hesitation in initiating movements or arrests in ongoing movements.

4. Can barely perform the task.

25. Rapid alternating movements of hands

0. Normal

1. Mild slowing and/or reduction in amplitude.

2. Moderately impaired; definite and early fatiguing; may have occasional arrests in movement.

3. Severely impaired; frequent hesitation in initiating movements or arrests in ongoing movements.

4. Can barely perform the task.

26. Leg agility

0. Normal

1. Mild slowing and/ or reduction in amplitude.

2. Moderately impaired; definite and early fatiguing; may have occasional arrests in movement.

3. Severely impaired; frequent hesitation in initiating movements or arrests in ongoing movements.

4. Can barely perform the task.

27. Arising from chair

0. Normal

1. Slow; or may need more than one attempt.

2. Pushes self up from arms of seat.

3. Tends to fall back and may have to try more than one time, but can get up without help.

4. Unable to arise without help.

28. Posture

0. Normal erect.

1. Not quite erect; slightly stooped posture; could be normal for older person.

2. Moderately stooped posture, definitely abnormal; can be slightly leaning to one side.

3. Severely stooped posture with kyphosis; can be moderately leaning to one side.

4. Marked flexion with extreme abnormality of posture.

29. Gait

    0.   Normal

    1.   Walks slowly, may shuffle with short steps, but no festination or propulsion.

    2.   Walks with difficulty, but requires little or no assistance; may have some festination, short steps, or propulsion.

    3.   Severe disturbance of gait, requiring assistance.

    4.   Can not walk at all, even with assistance.

30. Postural stability

    0.   Normal

    1.   Retropulsion, but recovers unaided.

    2.   Absence of postural response; would fall if not caught by examiner.

    3.   Very unstable, tends to lose balance spontaneously.

    4.   Unable to stand without assistance.

31. Body bradykinesia and hypokinesia

    0.   None

    1.   Minimal slowness, giving movement a deliberate character; could be normal for some persons; possibly reduced amplitudes.

    2.   Mild degree of slowness and poverty of movement that is definitely abnormal; alternatively, some reduction in amplitude.

    3.   Moderate slowness, poverty, or small amplitude of movement.

    4.   Marked slowness, poverty, or small amplitude of movement.

V1. Complications of Therapy (in the past week)

  A. Dyskinesias

32. Duration: What proportion of the waking day are dyskinesias present?

    0.   None

    1.   1 to 25% of day

    2.   26 to 50% of day

    3.   51 to 75% of day

    4.   76 to 100% of day.

33. Disability: How disabling are the dyskinesias?

    0.   Not disabling

    1.   Mildly disabling

    2.   Moderately disabling

    3.   Severely disabling

    4.   Completely disabled

34. Painful dyskinesias: How painful are the dyskinesias?

    0.   No painful dyskinesias

    1.   Slight

    2.   Moderate

    3.   Severe

    4.   Marked

35. Presence of early morning dystonia
    0. No
    1. Yes

B. Clinical Fluctuations

36. Are any "off" periods predicable as to timing after a dose of medication?
    0. No
    1. Yes

37. Are any "off" periods unpredictable as to timing after a dose of medication?
    0. No
    1. Yes

38. Do any of the "off" periods come on suddenly, eg over a few seconds
    0. No
    1. Yes

39. What proportion of the waking day, is the patient "off" on average?
    0. None
    1. 1 to 25% of day
    2. 26 to 50% of day
    3. 51 to 75% of day
    4. 76 to 100% of day

C. Other complications

40. Does the patient have anorexia, nausea, or vomiting?
    0. No
    1. Yes

41. Does the patient have any sleep disturbances, for example, insomnia or hyper-somnolence?
    0. No
    1. Yes

42. Does the patient have symptomatic orthostasis?
    0. No
    1. Yes

Record the patient's blood pressure, pulse, and weight on scoring form.

HOEHN AND YAHR STAGING SCALE

Hoehn MM, Hahr MD. Parkinsonism: onset, progression and mortality. *Neurology*. 1967;17:427-442.

Masur H, Papke K, Althoff S. *Scales and Scores in Neurology: Quantification of Neurological Deficits in Research and Practice*. Stuttgart: Thieme; 2004.

Goetz CG, Poewe W, Rascol O, Sampaio C, Stebbins GT, Counsell C, Giladi N, et al. Movement Disorder Society Task Force Report on the Hoehn and Yahr Staging Scale: Status and recommendations. *Mov Disord*. 2004;19(9):1020-1028.

Description: This scale classifies the disease state into different stages, based on disease severity and distribution and postural stability.

Application: Assessment of severity of PD symptoms.

Duration: A few minutes

Score range: Stage I to V (> stage = > disability)

Stage: **Description**:
1   Unilateral involvement only; usually minimal or no functional disability.
2   Bilateral or midline involvement without balance impairment.
3   First sign of impaired righting reflexes. This is evident by unsteadiness as the patient turns or is demonstrated when he is pulled from standing equilibrium with feet apart and eyes open. Functionally, the patient is somewhat restricted in his activities but may have some work potential depending upon the type of employment. Patients are physically capable of leading independent lives, and their disability is mild to moderate.
4   Fully developed, severely disabling disease; the patient is still able to walk and stand unassisted but is markedly incapacitated.
5   Confinement to bed or wheelchair unless aided.

MODIFIED HOEHN AND YAHR STAGING SCALE (FROM GOETZ ET AL)[18]

Stage 1.0   Unilateral involvement only
Stage 1.5   Unilateral and axial involvement
Stage 2.0   Bilateral involvement without impairment of balance
Stage 2.5   Mild bilateral disease with recovery on pull test
Stage 3.0   Mild to moderate bilateral disease; some postural instability; physically independent
Stage 4.0   Severe disability; still able to walk or stand unassisted
Stage 5.0   Wheelchair bound or bedridden unless aided

SCHWAB AND ENGLAND ACTIVITIES OF DAILY LIVING SCALE

Schwab R, England A. Projection technique for evaluating surgery in Parkinson's disease. In: Gillingham FJ, Donaldson IML, eds. *Third Symposium on Parkinson's Disease E&S*. Edinburgh: Livingstone; 1969.

Description: Rates the PD patient's ability to perform activities of daily living.

Application: The Schwab and England allows the clinician to categorize a patient's functional ability in terms of daily living activities.

Duration: A few minutes

Score range: 0 to 100% (< % = > disability)

Scale:

100%   Completely independent. Able to do all chores without slowness, difficulty or impairment. Essentially normal. Unaware of any difficulty.

90%   Completely independent. Able to do all chores with some degree of slowness, difficulty and impairment. Might take twice as long. Beginning to be aware of difficulty.

80%   Completely independent in most chores. Taking twice as long. Conscious of difficulty and slowness.

70%   Completely independent. Most difficulty with some chores. Three to four times as long as some. Must spend a large part of day with chores.

60%   Some dependency. Can do most chores but exceedingly slowly and with much effort. Errors; some impossible.

50%   More dependent. Difficulty with everything.

40%   Very dependent. Can assist with all chores but few alone.

30%   With effort now and then does a few things alone or begins alone. Much help needed. Part invalid.

20%   Nothing alone. Can be slight help with some chores. Severe invalid.

10%   Totally dependent, helpless. Complete invalid.

PARKINSON'S DISEASE QUESTIONNAIRE—PDQ39

Peto V, Jenkinson C, Fitzpatrick R, Greenhall R. The development and validation of a short measure of functioning and well being for individuals with Parkinson's Disease. *Qual Life Res.* 1995;4:241-248. ©University of Oxford.

Description: An instrument used to gauge quality of life issues in patients with Parkinson's disease.

Score range: 0 to 156 (> score = < Health-related QoL)

Duration: Highly variable among patients depending on cooperation and cognition.

DUE TO HAVING PARKINSON'S DISEASE, how often have you experienced the following, during the last month?

Due to having Parkinson's disease, how often during the past 30 days have you ….

	Never	Rarely	Sometimes	Often	Always
1. Had difficulty looking after your home, for example, housework, cooking, or yardwork?					
2. Had difficulty doing the leisure activities you would like to do?					
3. Had difficulty carrying shopping bags?					
4. Had problems walking half a mile?					
5. Had problems walking 100 yards (approximately 1 block)?					
6. Had problems getting around the house as easily as you would like?					
7. Had difficulty getting around in public places?					
8. Needed someone else to accompany you when you went out?					
9. Felt frightened or worried about falling in public?					
10. Being confined to the house more than you would like?					

11. Had difficulty showering or bathing?					
12. Had difficulty dressing?					
13. Had difficulty with buttons or shoelaces?					
14. Had problems writing clearly?					
15. Had difficulty cutting up your food?					
16. Had difficulty holding a drink without spilling it?					
18. Felt isolated and lonely?					
17. Felt depressed?					
19. Felt weepy or tearful?					
20. Felt angry or bitter?					
21. Felt anxious?					
22. Felt worried about the future?					
23. Felt you had to hide your Parkinson's from people?					
24. Avoided situations which involved eating or drinking in public?					
25. Felt embarrassed in public?					
26. Felt worried about other people's reaction to you?					
27. Had problems with your close personal relationships?					
28. Received the support you needed from your spouse or partner?					
If you do not have a spouse or partner, please mark here					
29. Received the support you needed from your family or close friends?					

30. Unexpectedly fallen asleep during the day?					
31. Had problems with your concentration, for example, when reading or watching TV.					
32. Felt your memory was failing?					
33. Had distressing dreams or hallucinations?					
34. Had difficulty speaking?					
35. Felt unable to communicate effectively?					
36. Felt ignored by people?					
37. Had painful muscle cramps or spasms?					
38. Had aches or pains in the joints?					
39. Felt uncomfortably hot or cold?					

SELF-REPORTED DISABILITY SCALE IN PATIENTS WITH PARKINSONISM

Brown RG, MacCarthy B, Gotham AM, Der GJ, Marsden CD. Accuracy of self-reported disability in patients with parkinsonism. Arch Neurol. 1989;46(9):955-959.

Masur H, Papke K, Althoff S, Oberwittler, C. Scales and Scores in Neurology: Quantification of Neurological Deficits in Research and Practice. Thieme: Stuttgart; 2004.

Biemans M, Dekker J, van der Woude LH. The internal consistence and validity of the Self-assessment Parkinson's Disease Disability Scale. Clinical Rehabilitation. 2001;15:221-228.

Description: A self-assessment measure for patient's to rate their ability to perform activities of daily living and instrumental activities of daily living.

Application:

Duration: 15 to 30 min

Score range: 25 to 125 (> score = > disability)

Scale:
Please read the instructions below. For each item circle the number which describes best how easy or difficult it is for you to perform that activity. If you are more able at some times than others, indicate how you are in general at the times of the day you would normally perform these activities. If you use a frame or walking stick or any special aids to help you, please answer according to how well you would manage without the aid.

1. Able to do alone without difficulty.
2. Able to do alone with a little effort.
3. Able to do alone with a lot of effort or a little help.
4. Able to do only with a lot of help
5. Unable to do at all.

1. Get out of bed

0	1	2	3	4	5

2. Get up from armchair

0	1	2	3	4	5

3. Walk around the house/flat

0	1	2	3	4	5

4. Walk outside, for example, to the local shops

0	1	2	3	4	5

5. Travel by public transport

0	1	2	3	4	5

6. Walk up stairs

0	1	2	3	4	5

7. Walk down stairs

0	1	2	3	4	5

8. Wash face and hands

0	1	2	3	4	5

9. Get into a bath

0	1	2	3	4	5

10. Get of a bath

0	1	2	3	4	5

11. Get dressed

0	1	2	3	4	5

12. Get undressed

0	1	2	3	4	5

13. Brush your teeth

0	1	2	3	4	5

14. Open tins/cans (not using an electric opener)

0	1	2	3	4	5

15. Pour milk from a bottle or carton

0	1	2	3	4	5

16. Make a cup of tea or coffee

0	1	2	3	4	5

17. Hold a cup and saucer

0	1	2	3	4	5

18. Wash and dry dishes

0	1	2	3	4	5

19. Cut food with a knife and fork

0	1	2	3	4	5

20. Pick up an object from the floor

0	1	2	3	4	5

21. Insert and remove an electric plug

0	1	2	3	4	5

22. Dial a telephone

0	1	2	3	4	5

23. Hold and read a newspaper

0	1	2	3	4	5

24. Write a letter

0	1	2	3	4	5

25. Turn over in bed

0	1	2	3	4	5

RESOURCES FOR ASSISTIVE AND ADAPTIVE TECHNOLOGY

Organizations and Conferences

RESNA: http://www.resna.org/

CSUN: http://www.csun.edu/cod/

Closing the Gap: http://www.closingthegap.com/

Products (General)

Kentucky Assistive Technology Service (KATS) Network Fact Sheet # 3 - Choosing Appropriate Assistive Technology:
http://www.katsnet.org/fact3.html

Able Data: http://www.abledata.com/

Rehab Tool: http://www.rehabtool.com/

Ablenet: http://www.ablenetinc.com/

Ability Hub: http://www.abilityhub.com/

Products (by Category)

Adaptive Computer Products: http://www.makoa.org/computers.htm

Communication Devices: http://wata.org/resource/communication/Tour/index.htm

EADL's: http://snow.utoronto.ca/technology/products/daily-living-aids.html

Adaptive Driving: http://www.adaptivedriving.com/

PATIENT RESOURCE INFORMATION

State & National Associations Supporting PD Education and Research

American Academy of Neurology
- This is a professional organization for neurologists. Neurology Now, is a new patient- and family-focused magazine, with feature stories and regular sections providing information and support to individuals living with neurological diseases. http://www.aan.com/

American Parkinson Disease Association (APDA) (800) 345-223-2732
- This organization focuses its energies on research, patient support, education and raising public awareness of the disease. http://www.apda.org

Dystonia Medical Research Foundation (504) 254-2455.
- Helps fund research to find a cure, provides patient service and awareness activities, and educational programs.

  http://www.dystonia-foundation.org/

Huntington's Disease Society of America (800) 345-HDSA
- Helps to promote research to find a cure, helps people and families affected by this disease, and educates the public and healthcare professionals about HD. http://www.hdsa.org

International Essential Tremor Foundation (888) 387-3667 http://www.essentialtremor.org/

Michael J. Fox Foundation for Parkinson's Research (800) 708-7644
- This organization is committed to the pursuit of all ethical avenues of research promising improved therapies and ultimately a cure for people living with Parkinson's disease. http://www.michaeljfox.org/

Movement Disorder Society (MDS)
- An international professional society of clinicians, scientists, and other healthcare professionals, who are interested in PD and related neurodegenerative and neuro-developmental disorders.

  http://www.movementdisorders.org/links.shtml

National Institutes of Health
- Includes a special section—National Institute of Neurological Disorders and Strokes—that contains information about PD.

  http://health.nih.gov/result.asp/502

National Organization for Rare Disorders (NORD) (800) 999-6673
- Federation of health organizations that helps people with rare diseases.
  http://www.rarediseases.org

National Parkinson Foundation (NPF) (800) 327-4545
- This is the largest PD organization that supports an international network of research, treatment, education and support centers. Contact them for free booklets about medication, speech, memory problems, exercise, activities of daily living, nutrition, and coping.
  http://www.parkinson.org

Normal Pressure Hydrocephalus (NPH)
- Includes education about NPH & a listing of publications, organizations, & support groups.
  http://www.ninds.nih.gov/disorders/normal_pressure_hydrocephalus/normal_pressure_hydrocephalus_pr.htm

Parkinson's Action Network (PAN) (800) 437 MOV2
- Scientific research and legislative issues addressed.
  http://www.parkinsonaction.org

Parkinson's Disease Consortium
- The Consortium is designed to network nationally dispersed VA clinicians with expertise and/or interest in the fields of Parkinson's disease and related movement disorders. It serves as a channel for collaboration and development in the areas of clinical care, scientific research and educational outreach.
  http://www.va.gov/padrecc/

Parkinson's Disease Foundation (PDF) (800) 457-6676.
- The Parkinson's Disease Foundation (PDF) is a national organization devoted to research, education, and advocating for persons with PD.
  http://wwwpdf.org

Parkinson's Disease Research, Education and Clinical Centers (PADRECCs)
- These are six nationwide sites established for veterans living with PD. Medical evaluation, research, education and support are provided at these centers located in Houston, Northwest (Portland and Seattle), Philadelphia, San Francisco, Southeast (Richmond, VA), and West Los Angeles (Southwest).
   www.va.gov/padrecc_houston/

People Living with Parkinson's (PLWP)
- Provides resources and web sites from government funding, medical centers to caregiver support.
  http://www.plwp.org

Shy-Drager Syndrome (Multiple System Atrophy) (866) SDS-4999.
- • Information about support groups and educational programs.
  http://www.shy-drager.com

Society for Progressive Supranuclear Palsy (PSP) (800) 457-4777.
- • This society is dedicated to increasing awareness of PSP, to advancing a cure, providing hope, support, education.
  http://www.psp.org

The Parkinson Alliance (PA) (800) 579-8440
- • This group lists PD research, events, & provides links to other sites.
  www.parkinsonalliance.net/home.html

The Parkinson's Web
- • Provides links to private groups, government aid, & health centers
  http://www.pdweb.mgh.harvard.edu

We Move 204 West 84th Street, New York, NY 10024.
- • Provides worldwide education and information about all movement disorders.
  http://www.wemove.org

Other National Agencies/Organizations

American Healthcare Association (202) 479-1200.
- • Federation of state organizations that represents long term care communities to the nation.
  http://www/ahca.com

American Massage Therapy Association (AMTA) (888) 843-2682.
  http://www.amtamassage.org/

American Occupational Therapy Association (AOTA) (301) 652-2682.
  http://www.aota.org/

American Physical Therapy Association (APTA) (800) 999-2782
  http://www.apta.org//AM/Template.cfm?Section=Home

Elder Care Locator Service (800) 677-1116
- • (Part of Administration on Aging).
  http://www.eldercare.gov/

National Council on Aging (202) 479-1200
- Promotes vital aging in America.
  http://www.ncoa.org/index.cfm?bType=ie4

National Council on Disability (202) 272-2004.
- Promotes an improved quality of life for all Americans.
  http://www.ncd.gov/

Emergency Alerts, Medications, Products, Videos, Voice

Catalogs of products
- AdaptAbility Catalog (800) 243-9232 http://www.ssww.com/store/browse/grp=HCR
- Partnership For Care Athena Rx Home Pharmacy (800) 528-4362.
- Clothing Solutions (800) 336-2660). http://www.clothingsolutions.com
- Sammons Preston Rolyon (800) 323-5547 http://www.sammonsprestonrolyan.com
- Sears Health and Wellness. (800) 326-1750 http://searshealthandwellness.com/products.asp?CATEGORY_ID=5

Canes, walkers, lifts, wheelchairs, mobility vehicles
- HurryCane Products, Inc./Stepover Wand (818) 789-9612. http://www.stepover.com
- In-Step Mobility Products, Inc. (800) 558-7837) U-Step Walking Stabilizer http://www.1800wheelchair.com/asp/view product.asp?product_id=960
- Hoveround (800) 542-7236. HoverLift www.hoveround.com
- The Scooter Store (866) 603-7369 www.thescooterstore.com

Emergency alerts
- Med Alert (800) 985-4357. Medical Alert systems, alarms. http://www.1800medalert.com
- Lifeline Systems, Inc. (800) 543-3546 Security alert button in home. http://www.lifelinesys.com
- Medications Electronic medication reminders. The products have been featured on TV & in the press. http://epill.com/nsearch.html

Videos/DVDs
- Gentle Fitness (800) 566-7780 www.gentlefitness.com
- Sit and Be Fit (509) 448-9438 www.sitandbefit.com
- Videos on PD (Australian) www.enable.net.au
- Managing Parkinson's www.waparkinsons.org

Voice Amplification Systems (call for catalogs)

- Park Surgical Co. (800) 633-7878 http://www.parksurgical.com
- Luminaud (800) 255-3408 http://www.luminaud.com/amplifier.htm\
- One-to-One Communications (913) 764-4072
- Radio Shack http://www.radioshack.com

Other Health-Related Web sites

- www.parkinsonshealth.com Serving the Parkinson's disease community.
- www2.aahsa.org American Association of Homes & Services for the Aged.
- www.caregiver.com Caregiver's Guide.
- www.medicare.gov/Publications/Pubs/pdf/nhguide A Guide for Choosing A Nursing Home.
- www.healthatoz.com The Search Engine for Health & Medicine.
- www.medhelp.org MedHelp Internatl.
- www.geohealthweb.com Geo Health
- www.caregiver911.com Caregiver Survival Resources
- www.nfcacares.org National Family Caregivers Association.
- www.herbalgram.org American Botanical Council.
- www.amazon.com Optimal Health.
- www.lifeextension.com Health Products.
- www.healthfind.com Health Information.
- www.NCBI.NLM.NIH.GOV/PUBMED NIH Literature Reference Website
- www.webMD.com Consumer-focused health care information.
- www.alz.org National Alzheimer's Association.
- www.aarp.org AARP

Index